# Aids to Clinical
# Pharmacology and Therapeutics

# Aids to Clinical Pharmacology and Therapeutics

## Howard Rogers

MA MB BChir PhD MRCP

Professor of Clinical Pharmacology,
Guy's Hospital Medical School,
United Medical Schools, London

## Roy Spector

MD PhD FRCP FRCPath

Professor of Applied Pharmacology,
Guy's Hospital Medical School,
United Medical Schools, London

CHURCHILL LIVINGSTONE
EDINBURGH LONDON MELBOURNE AND NEW YORK 1984

CHURCHILL LIVINGSTONE
Medical Division of Longman Group Limited

Distributed in the United States of America by
Churchill Livingstone Inc., 1560 Broadway, New
York, N.Y. 10036, and by associated companies,
branches and representatives throughout the
world.

First published 1984
Reprinted 1985

ISBN  0-443-02680-7

British Library Cataloguing in Publication Data
Rogers, Howard
    Aids to clinical pharmacology and therapeutics.
    1. Chemotherapy
    I. Title       II. Spector, Roy
    615.5'8        RM262

Library of Congress Cataloging in Publication Data
Rogers, H. J. (Howard John)
    Aids to clinical pharmacology and therapeutics.

    1. Pharmacology — Handbooks, manuals, etc. 2.
Drugs — Handbooks, manuals, etc. 3.
Chemotherapy — Handbooks, manuals, etc. I.
Spector, R. G. (Roy Geoffrey) II. Title. [DNLM: 1.
Pharmacology, Clinical — Handbooks. 2. Drugs
therapy — Handbooks. QV 38 R726a]
RM300.R668    1984       615'1       83–7798

Produced by Longman Singapore Publishers (Pte) Ltd.
Printed in Singapore

# Preface

We all differ in our approach to learning in the medical course. In general, 'Aids' and 'Notes' have greater popularity with students than with their teachers. One possible explanation of this phenomenon is that such short-cut texts are academically poor and do not represent the real world because a practised doctor does not sieve through lists when confronted with a clinical problem. Students, on the other hand, gain confidence in seeing the imposition of some sort of order on the chaos of facts which confront them. Of course, in a subject such as clinical pharmacology, which is imperfectly understood in terms of mechanism and whose subject matter is in a constant state of flux, order may be spurious and illusory. Despite this, we have made an attempt to tame the facts and the material presented contains the nucleus of our courses at Guy's Hospital Medical School. Around this core is other material which may be of use for students taught elsewhere. Practice is geographically variable and a drug used widely in our hospital may be substituted by another in another institution. Therefore this book is in some respects over-comprehensive. Our advice is to use it in conjunction with a pen to emphasise the drugs and practices which are of importance in your hospital and medical course.

We believe this subject cannot be learnt in abstraction from a book but that the student should learn therapeutics at the bedside. The drug chart and the patient's response to each item on it should be sought with that eager attention with which you strain to hear an opening snap or pleural rub on your patients. In addition you should consult larger textbooks for discussion in depth of those aspects of particular relevance to the treatment of a difficult clinical problem. Of all the subjects in the medical curriculum, clinical pharmacology is the one which will be most widely applicable in your future career: the surgeon, psychiatrist or general practitioner requires just as sound a background in therapeutics as the cardiologist or gastroenterologist. All are users of drugs but all may also be abusers of drugs to the detriment of their patients. We hope that this little book may also assist qualified doctors reading for higher examinations or perhaps just reading. Students in other faculties such as pharmacy may also find some of the lists and tables a useful summary of the information required in their examinations.

Our secretaries, Carmel Kennedy and Christine Wier, performed, as usual, a minor miracle in sorting out our handwritten manuscript to produce immaculate typescript with never a cross word. Nicola Schmidt-Renfree drew the diagrams with care. Professor John Trounce and Dr Helen Kinsella have helped us by their encouragement and comments on various parts of the text. We are indebted to them all for their assistance.

London,                                                      H.J.R.
1984                                                         R.G.S.

# Contents

# Contents

# Drug absorption, distribution, metabolism and excretion

## DRUG ABSORPTION

### Transmembrane movement of drugs
Drugs must pass several membranes to reach site of action.
1. *Passive diffusion* — commonest and most important
   — no energy required
   — not saturable or inhibited by metabolic inhibitions
   — non-selective
   — obeys Fick's law (so concentration gradient important)
   — non-ionised drug is lipid soluble and diffuses easily (so oil/water partition coefficient, pH and p$K_a$ important).
2. *Active* — relatively unusual
   — specific, e.g. iodide, amino acids
   — competition for transport can occur
   — drugs resembling natural substrate can be transported, e.g. methyldopa, levodopa, 5-fluorouracil, methotrexate uptake in gut; renal tubular secretion of weak acids and bases
   — requires energy
   — can occur against concentration gradient.
3. *Facilitated* — carrier-mediated but no energy required e.g. $B_{12}$-intrinsic factor complex but not important for drugs.
4. *Pinocytosis* — physical engulfment by cell
   — little importance for drugs; vitamins A, D, E, K absorbed this way.

## BIOAVAILABILITY

Relative amount of administered drug dose reaching systemic circulation and rate at which this occurs,
   Formulation can contain same amount of drug but availability to body may be vastly different.

*Bioequivalence* — two or more pharmaceutical formulations produce comparable bioavailability characteristics in an individual when administered in equivalent dosage regimes.
*Bioinequivalence* — statistically significant difference in bioavailability between preparations.
*Therapeutic inequivalence* — clinically important difference in bioavailability.
*Absolute bioavailability* — availability of a drug product relative to i.v. administration.
*Relative bioavailability* — availability as compared to recognised standard preparation.

**Factors influencing bioavailability**
1. Drug characteristics
    (i)  instability
    (ii)  incomplete absorption
    (iii)  first pass elimination.
2. Formulation characteristics
    (i)  Excipients and other ingredients
    (ii)  Compression and physical factors affecting formulation dissolution and solubility
    (iii)  State of drug, e.g. surface area, particle size.
3. Interactions with other substances in gut — food, drugs.
4. Patient characteristics — disease (e.g. malabsorption, hepatic dysfunction)
    — gastro-intestinal factors (motility, pH, blood flow)
    — genetic factors, e.g. acetylator status.

**Bioavailability assessment**
1. *Plasma data — single dose*
    (i)  time of peak plasma concentration
    (ii)  peak plasma concentration
    (iii)  area under plasma concentration, time curve (AUC).
    Usually oral and i.v. doses (D) given in random order to panel of subjects.

Since $(AUC)_{p.o.} = \dfrac{FD}{kV}$ & $(AUC)_{i.v.} = \dfrac{D}{kV}$

where F is bioavailability fraction if k and V remain constant between doses (k = elimination rate constant V = distribution volume)

$$F = \frac{(AUC)_{p.o.}}{(AUC)_{i.v.}}$$

— *multiple dose*: as (i), (ii), (iii) above during a single dosage interval.

2. *Urine data*
   (i)  total fraction of dose excreted
   (ii)  rate of drug excretion
   (iii)  time of maximum excretion.
3. *Clinical observation and pharmacological effects*, e.g. salivary secretion, heart rate.

## Potential for bioinequivalence of dosage forms

| *Low* | *Intermediate* | *High* |
|---|---|---|
| Elixirs | Capsules | Compressed tablets |
| Syrups | Suspensions | Enteric-coated tablets |
| Solutions | Chewable tablets | Sustained release formulations |
| | | Suppositories |

Examples of drugs for which bioinequivalence demonstrated among marketed oral formulations:

| Aspirin | Digoxin | Phenytoin |
|---|---|---|
| Chloramphenicol | Nitrofurantoin | Prednisolone |
| Chlordiazepoxide | Oxytetracycline | Warfarin |

Therapeutic inequivalence shown in most of the above. Bioinequivalence often results in therapeutic inequivalence if therapeutic index low.

## Sustained release preparations
Aim to prolong action of drugs with short $T_{\frac{1}{2}}$ by pharmaceutical means, e.g. resin coated pellets in capsules, drug enclosed in wax or plastic matrix.

*Potential advantages*
1. Prolonged effects
2. Improved compliance
3. Comparable or improved efficacy
4. Improved tolerability
May be valuable if
   (i)  Short $T_{\frac{1}{2}}$ (1 – ?8h)
   (ii)  Prolonged treatment necessary (improves compliance)
   (iii)  Constant plasma levels needed for efficacy.

*Potential disadvantages*
1. Cost — more expensive than conventional tablets
2. Delayed absorption — delayed onset of action
   — increased first-pass effects
   — ? increased effect on gut flora
3. Prolonged toxicity
4. Risk of overdose — dosage form failure
   — intentional
5. Increased risk of gut toxicity

**Enteric coated tablets or granules**
Film coat (polymer like cellulose acetate phthalate) which resists
dissolution by stomach acid but disrupts or dissolves in alkaline
intestinal juice. Occasionally used to reduce gastric irritation, e.g.
aspirin, prednisolone.

## FACTORS AFFECTING GASTRO-INTESTINAL DRUG ABSORPTION

1. **Drug**
   a. Molecular weight
   b. Lipophilicity (e.g. oil/water partition coefficient)
   c. pKa
   d. Metabolism by gut enzymes (e.g. monoamine oxidase,
      sulphatase, non-specific esterase)
   e. Metabolism by gut bacteria
   f. Stability in gut contents, e.g. low pH of stomach.

2. **Formulation**
   a. Disintegration time
   b. Dissolution rate
   c. Excipients and adjuvents.

3. **Patient**
   a. pH of gut
   b. Rate of gastric emptying
   c. Intestinal motility (transit time)
   d. Surface area available for absorption
   e. Gastro-intestinal disease
   f. Presence of food in gut
   g. Interactions with drugs in gut.

## EFFECT OF FOOD ON DRUG ABSORPTION

| *Decreased absorption* | *Increased absorption* |
|---|---|
| Penicillin V | Nitrofurantoin |
| Cephalexin | Propranolol |
| Tetracycline (milk, cottage cheese) | Metoprolol |
| Aspirin | Dicoumarol |
| Erythromycin | Diazepam |
| Methotrexate (milk) | Hydrochlorothiazide |
| Isoniazid | Hydralazine |

## ROUTES OF DRUG ADMINISTRATION

### Sublingual/buccal absorption
1. Rapid absorption
2. Avoids first-pass gastro-intestinal/hepatic elimination.

Examples: glyceryl trinitrate, oxytocin, methyltestosterone, testosterone propionate.

### Rectal administration
1. Only partially avoids first-pass metabolism.
2. Small surface area (passive absorption only) and drug may be expelled so absorption rate and bioavailability erratic.
3. Unsuitable for irritant drugs.
4. Drugs given as solution (retention enema) more rapid and efficient than given as solid formulation with wax base (suppository).
5. Useful if patient vomiting.
6. Used for systemic (e.g. theophylline, prochlorperazine, aspirin, indomethacin) or local (e.g. corticosteroids for inflammatory bowel disease) effects.

### Intramuscular injection
1. Gastro-intestinal and hepatic first-pass elimination avoided.
2. Absorption influenced by
   (i) local blood flow, massage and movement (e.g. exercise increases absorption; morphine absorption decreased after myocardial infarct; insulin absorption increased by sauna).
   (ii) site, e.g. lignocaine absorption absorbed faster from deltoid than vastus lateralis or gluteus maximus.
   (iii) physical properties of drug — poorly water soluble drugs, e.g. diazepam, phenytoin precipitate in muscle and are poorly and erratically absorbed.
   (iv) sex of patient — females may absorb less from gluteal injection.
   Thus absorption less reliable than i.v. but solubility of drug not necessary.
3. Compliance ensured.
4. Onset of action more rapid than oral route.
5. Prolonged absorption can be produced by modification of injection
   — high viscosity vehicles like glycerin
   — fatty acid esters which slowly hydrolyse, e.g. fluphenazine decanoate for maintenance therapy in schizophrenia
   — water insoluble suspensions, e.g. procaine penicillin.

6. Complications
    (i) Pain, e.g. benzypenicillin (maximum volume by i.m. is 4–5 ml)
    (ii) Muscle and skin necrosis, e.g. digoxin, sterile or septic abscesses, pigmentation, e.g. iron
    (iii) Sciatic nerve damage following gluteal injection
    (iv) Elevated CPK may confuse diagnosis of myocardial infarction
    (v) Inadvertant intravascular injection.

**Intravenous injection**
1. Only route (apart from intra-arterial) when bioavailability considerations immaterial. Useful if:
    (i) drug not absorbed p.o., e.g. gentamicin
    (ii) high first-pass elimination, e.g. lignocaine
    (iii) too irritant for i.m. or p.o. route, e.g. nitrogen mustard.
2. Almost instantaneous response but bolus of highly concentrated drug may cause cardiac, respiratory etc complications so i.v. injections should usually be slow over 1–2 minutes (circulation time).
3. Rate of administration flexible, e.g. nitroprusside, lignocaine, and plasma levels can be accurately maintained.
4. Drug administered may not be recalled c.f. p.o. when absorption can be reduced.
5. Only water-soluble or aqueous miscible systems can be given.
6. Tonicity of solution and lack of irritant properties important, some preparations cause thrombophlebitis, e.g. diazepam.
7. Risks
    (i) anaphylaxis — greater with this route than others
    (ii) infection especially in immunosuppressed and seriously ill
    (iii) tissue damage if irritant drug extravasates, e.g. doxorubicin, actinomycin D, thiopentone.

**Subcutaneous injection**
1. Absorption influenced by same factors as i.m. injection but absorption slower and more erratic. Can sometimes increase bioavailability with hyaluronidase, local heat, massage, exercise.
2. Sustained release effect obtained from pellets of solid drug, e.g. testosterone replacement. Duration of insulin action controlled by crystalline size, e.g. semilente, lente, ultralente insulins
3. Some injections painful, may cause necrosis or abscesses.

**Percutaneous absorption**
1. Drug absorption increased
    (i) polythene occlusion increases skin hydration (N.B. danger of systemic steroid overdosage)
    (ii) lipid solubility, e.g. poisoning by absorption of nicotine, organic phosphates through skin

(iii) loss of stratum corneum
(iv) site — plantar < scalp < posterior auricular (depends on thickness of stratum corneum and number of hairs and sweat glands)
(v) age — steroids absorbed more readily in children than adults
(vi) vehicle.
2. Topical application minimises systemic absorption — but can occur, e.g. steroids.
3. Route can be utilised to avoid first-pass elimination and prolong systemic action, e.g. glyceryl trinitrate.

**Pulmonary absorption**
1. Almost instantaneous absorption (large surface area).
2. Difficult to deliver drug into lung and to dose accurately — particles > 10 $\mu$m impact in pharynx and nose and are swallowed. Optimum size is 1–2 $\mu$m which may reach alveoli and terminal bronchiole. Tidal volume and bronchial anatomy also important.
3. Mainly for local therapy, e.g. disodium cromoglycate, dexamethasone, isoprenaline but can use for systemic effects, e.g. ergotamine.

**DRUG DISTRIBUTION**

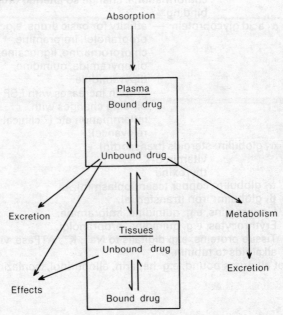

**Protein binding of drugs**
Drugs can bind to tissue proteins but plasma protein binding best understood.

*1. Characteristics of binding*
Electrostatic interaction between drugs and charged groups ($-NH_3$ of lysine and N-terminal amino acids; $-S^-$ of cysteine; $-COO^-$ of aspartate, glutamate; $-NH^+$ of histidine) plus van der Waals and hydrogen bonding.
   Usually but not always reversible.
   Competition for binding may occur between drugs or drugs and endogenous compounds.

*2. Proteins responsible for binding.*
   (i)   Albumin — affinity for acidic drugs.
               — 2 sites: I (warfarin site) also binds frusemide, phenytoin, valproate, phenylbutazone, indomethacin, glibenclamide, bilirubin.
                  II (diazepam site) also binds probenecid, ethacrynic acid, cloxacillin, salicylate, glibenclamide, tryptophan.
               — fatty acids bind at separate site but can cause conformational change so altering drug binding.
   (ii)  $\alpha_1$ acid glycoprotein — affinity for basic drugs, e.g. propranolol, imipramine, chlorpromazine, lignocaine, disopyramide, quinidine, dipyramidole.
                              — protein increases with ESR so binding changes with inflammation etc (? clinical relevance).
   (iii)  $\alpha_1$ globulin: steroids (transcortin)
                      vitamin $B_{12}$
                      thyroxine
   (iv)  $\alpha_2$ globulin: copper (caeruloplasmin).
   (v)  $\beta_1$ globulin: iron (transferrin).
   (vi)  Lipoproteins, e.g. quinidine, imipramine.
   (vii)  Erythrocytes, e.g. quinidine, propranolol.
   (viii)  Tissue proteins, e.g. digitalis to $Na^+$, $K^+$, ATPase, vinca alkaloids to tubulin.
N.B.  Not all drugs bound, e.g. heparin, allopurinol, isoniazid.

3. *Consequences of binding*
   (i)  drug transport within body.
   (ii)  drug reservoir if binding high.
   (iii)  only unbound ('free') drug may be available for action or metabolism so reduced binding may increase toxicity and clearance.
   *Renal excretion* : only unbound drug filtered at glomerulus so increased binding prolongs $T_{\frac{1}{2}}$ if drug not secreted or metabolised. If drug secreted binding usually unimportant — may increase excretion by retaining drug in blood for delivery to tubules.
   *Hepatic excretion* : depends if drug has flow-dependent hepatic metabolism (e.g. propranolol) when increased binding delivers more drug or flow-independent (e.g. warfarin) where only unbound drug is eliminated.
   (iv)  bound drug cannot diffuse into tissues so binding determines volume of distribution and penetration into tissues, e.g. CSF, and secretions, e.g. saliva.
   (v)  displacement from binding clinically important if:
      a.  drug highly bound (e.g. change from 99% to 98% binding increases free drug by 100%)
      b.  small volume of distribution (follows from a).
      c.  low therapeutic index with steep dose-response curve.
*BUT* new steady-state reached and free drug concentration reaches previous level so drug effects only increase transiently.
   (vi)  saturation of binding produces non-linear pharmacokinetics, e.g. phenylbutazone, prednisolone, disopyramide.
N.B. for highly bound drugs with large $V_d$ displacement interactions have no significant pharmacological effects.
Examples of displacement interactions:

| Displaced drug or substance | Displacing agent |
| --- | --- |
| Bilirubin | Sulphonamides, Salicylates |
| Methotrexate | Sulphonamides, Salicylates |
| Tolbutamide | Phenylbutazone, Salicylates |
| Warfarin | Salicylates, Clofibrate, Phenytoin, Sulphinpyrazone, Phenylbutazone |

N.B. some interactions may result from more than one action e.g. phenylbutazone inhibits metabolism of most active (S−) isomer of warfarin.

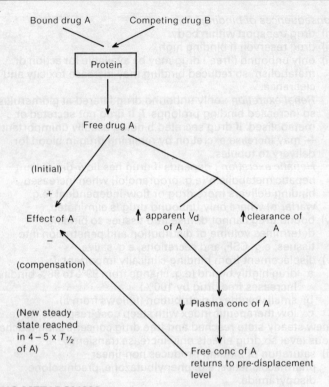

## DRUG METABOLISM

Drug metabolism chemically modifies drugs and may:

a. Abolish the activity (e.g. oxidation of barbiturates, phenytoin, alcohol; hydrolysis of suxamethonium, acetylcholine; conjugation of isoprenaline, salicylate).

or

b. Promote or increase activity (e.g. conversion of chloral to trichlorethanol; conversion of phenacetin to paracetamol; activation of cyclophosphamide to alkylating metabolites).

or

c. Produce no change in activity (e.g. dealkylation of tricyclic anti-depressants, benzodiazepines).

   Metabolism usually produces a more polar molecule which increases drug elimination since it is less susceptible to tubular reabsorption or active uptake in renal tubules or biliary system. Two phases of metabolism:

Phase I — Metabolic modification (e.g. oxidation, reduction, hydrolysis)

Phase II — Synthesis — i.e. conjugation (e.g. with glucuronic acid, glycine, glutamine, sulphate, acetate)

|  | *Phase I*<br>oxidising etc |  | *Phase II*<br>conjugating |  |
|---|---|---|---|---|
| Drug | $\longrightarrow$<br>enzymes | metabolites | $\longrightarrow$<br>enzymes | conjugated<br>metabolites |

## PHASE I METABOLISM

Occurs in 3 areas of cell:
  (i) smooth endoplasmic reticulum, e.g. barbiturates, pethidine
 (ii) cytosol, e.g. ethanol, chloral
(iii) mitochondria, e.g. oxidation of tyramine by MAO.
  May also occur in plasma, e.g. succinylcholine hydrolysis by plasma pseudocholinesterase.
  Not all drugs broken down by enzymes, e.g. melphalan undergoes spontaneous hydroxylation to inactive metabolites.

## PHASE II METABOLISM

Conjugation with
     (i) glucuronic acid, e.g. salicylate, chloramphenicol, morphine.
    (ii) glycine, e.g. salicylate, nicotinic acid.
   (iii) glutamine, e.g. p-aminosalicylic acid.
   (iv) acetate, e.g. isoniazid, hydralazine, dapsone.
    (v) methyl, e.g. thiouracil.
   (vi) sulphate, e.g. chloramphenicol, oestrogen, ,isoprenaline.
  (vii) mercapturate, e.g. some sulphonamides.
 (viii) ribosides, e.g. 6-mercaptopurine.

## ENZYME INDUCTION

Enhancement of enzyme activity due to increase in the amount of enzyme protein present in the cell. Induction of enzymes concerned with drug metabolism usually accelerates destruction of drugs and reduces their action. The process is usually studied in the liver parenchyma, but it also occurs in other cells, e.g. fibroblasts, lymphocytes.
  Not only enzyme content of liver increased but organ size and blood flow also enhanced.
  Non-microsomal metabolism is not inducible.

**Three groups of inducing agents**
a. Substances which stimulate metabolism in many pathways, e.g. barbiturates.
b. Polycyclic hydrocarbons (e.g. 3-methyl cholanthrene; 3–4 benzo (a) pyrine) produce limited metabolic stimulation.

c. Steroids: mainly microsomal enzyme stimulation.
   Most inducing agents produce maximal effects within 2
   weeks.
   Induction is dependent on dose of inducer.
   Wide inter-individual variation in inducibility at least partially
   under genetic control.

**Effects of some enzyme inducers on metabolism of endogenous
and exogenous chemicals**

| Enzyme inducing agent | Substances whose metabolism is enhanced |
| --- | --- |
| Barbiturates | Barbiturates, coumarins, phenytoin, griseofulvin, digitoxin, chlorpromazine, phenylbutazone, cortisol, testosterone, bilirubin, vitamin $D_3$, tricyclic antidepressants, contraceptive pill |
| Glutethimide | Glutethimide, warfarin, vitamin $D_3$ |
| Phenylbutazone | Digitoxin, cortisol, aminopyrine |
| Phenytoin | Digitoxin, dexamethasone, cortisol, thyroxine, dieldrin, DDT, tricyclic antidepressants, contraceptive pill, (the synthesis of cholesterol is also stimulated), vitamin $D_3$ |
| Ethanol | Ethanol, warfarin, phenytoin, barbiturates, meprobamate, tolbutamide, bilirubin |
| DDT, gamma benzene hexachloride (Lindane) | Cortisol, phenylbutazone, bilirubin, phenytoin, phenazone |
| Phenothiazines | Phenothiazines |
| Griseofulvin | Warfarin |
| Rifampicin | Steroids, including contraceptive steroids, digitoxin, tolbutamide, quinidine |

Smoking accelerates the metabolism of:
    nicotine
    paracetamol
    amitriptyline
    imipramine
    pentazocine
    dextropropoxyphene
    chlorpromazine
    phenobarbitone
    glutethimide
    ascorbic acid
    caffeine
    theophylline

Smoking does not affect the metabolism of:
    phenytoin (and other highly protein bound drugs)
    pethidine
    ethanol
    nortriptyline
    chlordiazepoxide
    diazepam

## Inhibition of drug metabolism

| Drug | Substance whose metabolism is inhibited |
|---|---|
| Isoniazid | Phenytoin |
| Chloramphenicol | Phenytoin, tolbutamide |
| Sulthiame | Phenytoin |
| Phenylbutazone | Tolbutamide |
| Ethanol (single large dose) | Chloral, tolbutamide, phenytoin, warfarin |
| Coumarins | Tolbutamide |
| Disulfiram | |
| Sulphonylureas | |
| Metronidazole | Acetaldehyde (from ethanol) |
| Citrated calcium carbimide | |
| Procarbazine | |
| Oral contraceptives | Diazepam, caffeine, antipyrine |
| Cimetidine | Diazepam, chlordiazepoxide, warfarin, caffeine, theophylline, propranolol, phenytoin. |

## Environmental inhibitors of microsomal enzymes
    organophosphorus insecticides
    pesticide synergists (methylene dioxyphenyl derivatives)
    carbon tetrachloride
    ozone
    carbon monoxide

## Pulmonary drug metabolism
Importance recently realised.
1. Several pulmonary cell types contain drug metabolising enzymes (pulmonary macrophages, types I and II pneumocytes, Clara cells, endothelial cells).
2. Total blood volume passes through lungs several times each minute.
3 Compounds given i.v. or inhaled must pass through lungs before entering systemic circulation (pulmonary first-pass metabolism).

## Compounds metabolised by lungs — examples
1. Endogenous — 5-hydroxytryptamine
   Angiotensin I
   Noradrenaline
   Bradykinin
   Testosterone
   Prostaglandins (E & F)
2. Exogenous — chemicals (? relation to carcinogenesis)
   Benzo (a) pyrine
   Benzanthracene
   Benzene
   Aniline
   — pesticides (? *agricultural hazard*)
   Parathion
   Carbaryl
   — drugs (not usually the major site of metabolism but may contribute significantly; as yet mostly animal evidence)
   Isoprenaline (especially when inhaled)
   Ifosfamide
   Ethylmorphine
   Imipramine

## Metabolism by gut flora
Flora is a mixture of aerobic and anaerobic organisms mainly in colon with large inter- and intra-individual variations in numbers and types of organisms. Gut transit time affects exposure of drug to their enzymes.
 (i) Microbial breakdown of hepatic conjugates frequently essential part of enterohepatic circulation.
(ii) Drug metabolism in lumen as yet not well recognised in man, e.g. sulindac, sulphinpyrazone, sulphasalazine.

## Metabolism by gut mucosa
Mainly conjugations rather than Phase I metabolism in mucosal cells.

Probably important for morphine, pentazocine, isoprenaline, tyramine, levodopa, oestrogens, progestogens, pivampicillin, flurazepam.

Enzymes may be induced, e.g. foodstuffs and inhibited, e.g. MAOIs.

## DRUG ELIMINATION

1. Metabolism (see above)
2. Storage — highly lipid soluble drugs in fat (e.g. DDT), heavy metals in bone, colloids in reticulo-endothelial system.
3. Excretion
   (i) milk, sweat, tears, saliva. Usually quantitatively minor routes but may be of importance for toxicity, e.g. for baby in milk (dapsone, phenobarbitone, lithium).
   or
   can be used for therapeutic advantage, e.g. rifampicin for nasal carriage of meningococci.
   (ii) bile — secretion depends on structure, polarity, MW (? needs to be < 325 in man)
      — carrier mediated active transport
      — competition within each compound class but not between classes
        e.g. organic anions: penicillin, bile acids, bromsulphthalein
        organic cations: tubocurarine, procainamide
        unionised molecules: cardiac glycosides.
      — some drugs excreted unchanged in bile, e.g. rifampicin, adriamycin, erythromycin, others as conjugates, e.g. indomethacin, oestradiol, morphine, carbenoxolone.
   (iii) renal — often most important route of elimination of parent drug and/or metabolites if water-soluble and low MW < 500.

Three mechanisms
a. Glomerular filtration — small molecules (< 500 MW) so tightly protein bound not filtered.
b. Active tubular secretion — active carrier-mediated (requires energy, shows competition and saturation effects). 2 systems:
   1. Weak acids, e.g. acetazolamide, nitrofurantoin, penicillins, probenecid, phenobarbitone, salicylic acid, sulphathiazole.
   2. Weak bases, e.g. amphetamine, chloroquine, imipramine, quinine.

c. Tubular reabsorption — may be active or passive
— reabsorption governed by pH of tubular fluid and $pK_a$ of drug
— acids best eliminated in alkaline urine; bases best in acid urine.

For weak acids:

$$\frac{\text{Conc in urine}}{\text{Conc in plasma}} = \frac{1 + 10^{(pH_{urine} - pKa)}}{1 + 10^{(pH_{plasma} - pK_a)}}$$

For weak bases:

$$\frac{\text{Conc in urine}}{\text{Conc in plasma}} = \frac{1 + 10^{(pK_a - pH_{urine})}}{1 + 10^{(pK_a - pH_{plasma})}}$$

*Renal clearance* ($CL_R$)

$$CL_R = \frac{dAe/dt}{C}$$

where dAe/dt is rate of excretion of drug in urine and C is plasma drug concentration. In practice it is found from UV/P where U = concentration of drug excreted over a short period (say 1 hour); V = volume of urine produced in that period; P = plasma conc at mid-point of time period.

If $CL_R$ > GFR tubular secretion must occur.
If $CL_R$ < GFR tubular reabsorption must occur.

*But* both processes may occur and obscure this simple pattern.

## ENTEROHEPATIC CIRCULATION

Examples: thyroxine, oestrogens, stilboestrol, rifampicin, digitoxin, sulindac, spironolactone.

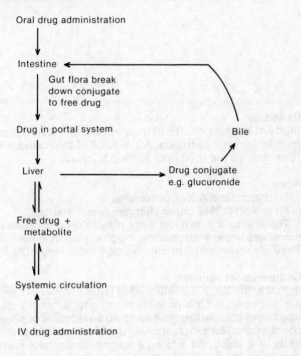

# Pharmacokinetics

**Definition**
Study of the time course of drug absorption, distribution, metabolism and excretion (ADME) and of the mathematical relationships required in modelling this data.

**Aims**
To understand ADME processes.
To predict ADME under changed circumstances.
These aims are possible since plasma drug concentration often correlates better with pharmacological response than does dose. They are achieved by mathematically modelling ADME processes.

**Compartment concept**
In reality the body is composed of large number of compartments, e.g. each cell, but it is possible to lump together organs and tissues into larger compartments having no anatomical or physiological counterpart. The simplest pharmacokinetic model considers the body as a 'black box' or single homogeneous (well stirred) compartment the volume of which determines the plasma concentration resulting from total amount of drug in the body. This *apparent volume of distribution* V is defined as

$$V = \frac{A}{C}$$

where A = amount of drug in body,
    C = plasma drug concentration
i.e.   A = VC                                    (1)
so that V is a proportionality factor relating dose to concentration.

V — has no physiological or anatomical meaning
   — seldom corresponds to anatomical body spaces
   — may exceed total body volume if drug concentrates in some region, e.g. fat.
C varies with time as drug undergoes ADME.

Many drugs eliminated by *first-order kinetics*. This implies: rate of process $\propto$ amount of drug present (c.f. rate of emptying of a bath which depends on amount of water in it). Sometimes called *linear kinetics*.

so
$$-\frac{dA}{dt} \propto A$$

(minus because amount of drug decreases with time)

so
$$\frac{dA}{dt} = -kA$$

and
$$\frac{dC}{dt} = -kC \text{ (since C = A/V)} \qquad (2)$$

k is the first order elimination rate constant (units $[\text{time}]^{-1}$ e.g. $h^{-1}$, $\min^{-1}$). Integrating from t = 0 when a dose of A(0) is given produces

$$A = A(0)e^{-kt}$$

and
$$C = C(0)e^{-kt} \qquad (3)$$

These exponential equations are similar to those familiar from elementary physics, e.g. decay of radio-isotopes, discharge of a condenser.

Thus after a rapid (bolus) i.v. injection the plasma concentration, time curve is exponential for first order elimination.

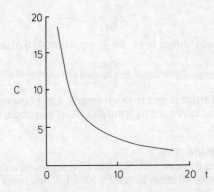

This may be converted to a straight-line plot (easier to handle mathematically) by plotting

$$\log C = \log C(0) - \frac{kt}{2.303}$$

i.e. ordinate intercept at t = 0 is C (0)

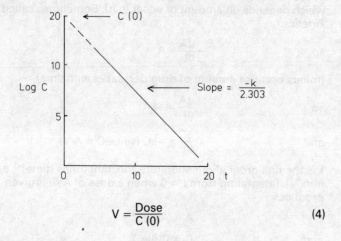

$$V = \frac{Dose}{C(0)} \tag{4}$$

but this is of limited practical use for finding V since an i.v. drug injection is required.

More useful is to integrate equation (3) from t = 0 to ∞ which gives the area under the plasma concentration, time curve (AUC)

$$AUC = \int_0^\infty C(0)\, e^{-kt}$$

$$= \frac{C(0)}{k}$$

which can be substituted for C (0) in equation 4 to give

$$V = \frac{Dose}{k(AUC)} \tag{5}$$

AUC is found from direct measurement, e.g. planimeter, weighing cut-out curve, or by mathematical methods, e.g. trapezoidal rule.

**Elimination half-life (T½)**
Commonly used indicator of rapidity of drug elimination is time for any drug concentration to fall by half, i.e. has units of time (e.g. h, min).

As log C versus t plot is linear, $T_{\frac{1}{2}}$ is same over entire time period

$$T_{\frac{1}{2}} = \frac{\log_e 2}{k} = \frac{0.693}{k} \tag{6}$$

## Elimination clearance

As descriptors of drug elimination rate $T_{\frac{1}{2}}$ and k are unsuitable because they also depend upon V. Clearance does not have this deficit.

*Definition*

Volume of biological fluid cleared of drug in unit time

$$CL = \frac{\text{Rate of elimination}}{\text{Concentration}}$$

Concentration of drug in plasma, blood or the concentration of unbound (free) drug in plasma define, respectively, plasma, blood or unbound drug clearance.

Rewriting equation (2) in terms of mass/unit time by multiplying by V (using equation 1) gives

$$-\frac{dC}{dt} \cdot V = kCV \quad (7)$$

$$= \text{rate of drug elimination}$$

$$= CL.C \quad (8)$$

Comparison of equations (6) and (7) reveals that

$$CL = kV$$

$$= \frac{0.693V}{T_{\frac{1}{2}}}$$

Substituting for kV in equation (5) gives

$$CL = \frac{\text{Dose}}{\text{(AUC)}}$$

It is a physiologically meaningful parameter with units of flow (e.g. ml/min).

Total body clearance = sum of clearances by each eliminating organ (e.g. liver, kidneys).

N.B.  $T_{\frac{1}{2}} = \frac{0.693V}{CL}$

so drug $T_{\frac{1}{2}}$ can be long either because CL is low or V is large.

## Extraction ratio (E)

= proportion of drug removed by a single transit of blood through an organ

$$E = \frac{C_{in} - C_{out}}{C_{in}}$$

where $C_{in}$, $C_{out}$ are drug concentrations in afferent and efferent blood.

Clearance across an organ = organ blood flow × E

e.g. for the liver $CL_H = Q_H E_H$
where $Q_H$ is hepatic blood flow, $E_H$ is hepatic extraction ratio

i.e. $CL_H = \dfrac{Q_H (C_{in} - C_{out})}{C_{in}}$

As the ability of the liver to extract drug from the blood increases $C_{out} \rightarrow 0$ and $E_H \rightarrow 1$. For such drugs $CL_H$ approaches and becomes limited by $Q_H$ so that clearance reflects hepatic blood flow rather than changes in the ability of the liver to extract such drugs (e.g. enzyme induction). This intrinsic eliminating capacity is defined in terms of the intrinsic clearances $CL_{int}$ relating the rate of hepatic drug elimination to the unbound drug concentration in the liver $(C_{H,u})$

$$CL_{int} = \frac{\text{Rate of elimination}}{C_{H,u}}$$

## First pass effects

Drugs with high hepatic extraction ratios tend to have high first-pass (or pre-systemic) elimination after oral absorption, i.e. large proportion of drug is eliminated by the liver before it reaches general circulation.

Hepatic first-pass metabolism explains why despite complete absorption from the gut a drug may be much less effective than after i.v. dosing.

First-pass effects also occur due to intestinal mucosal metabolism (after oral administration), e.g. isoprenaline, chlorpromazine, and pulmonary metabolism (after aerosol inhalation), e.g. isoprenaline, nicotine.

Extent of first-pass elimination is predictable since

$$E = \frac{CL_H}{Q_H}$$

and the fraction of an orally administered drug reaching the systemic circulation

$$f_o = 1 - E$$

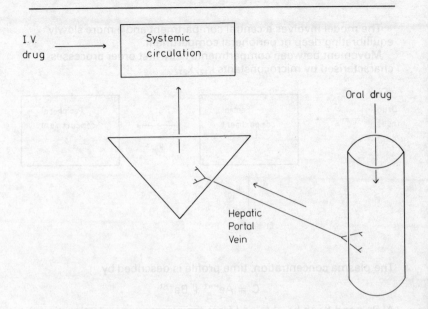

Drugs with high hepatic first-pass elimination include:
  Several β-blockers, e.g. propranolol, labetalol.
  Organic nitrates, e.g. glyceryl trinitrate.
  Tricyclic antidepressants, e.g. imipramine, nortriptyline.
  Some opiates, e.g. morphine, dextropropoxyphene, pethidine.
  Some hormones, e.g. cortisone, aldosterone.
  Some amines, e.g. 5-hydroxytryptamine, dopamine.

**Two-compartment** models may be needed to explain the biphasic
fall in log plasma concentration seen after i.v. drug injection:

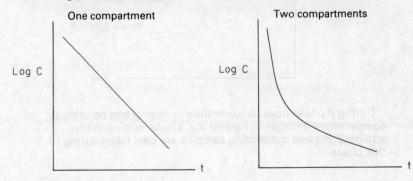

The model involves a central compartment and a more slowly equilibrating deep or peripheral compartment.

Movement between compartments is by first order processes characterised by microconstants $k_{12}$, $k_{21}$.

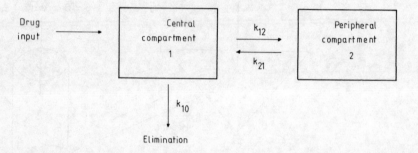

The plasma concentration, time profile is described by

$$C = Ae^{-\alpha t} + Be^{-\beta t}$$

A, B, $\alpha$ and $\beta$ can be obtained from the plasma concentration, time curve

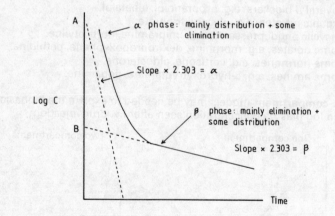

During $\beta$-phase drug concentration in central and peripheral compartment declines in parallel (i.e. kinetic homogeneity attained). Plasma monitoring samples are best taken during this phase.

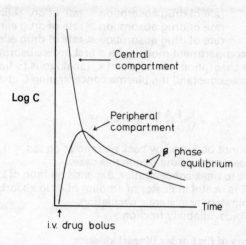

$$\text{Distribution half life} = T_{\frac{1}{2}\alpha} = \frac{0.693}{\alpha}$$

$$\text{Disposition half life} = T_{\frac{1}{2}\beta} = \frac{0.693}{\beta}$$

If unspecified, $T_{\frac{1}{2}\beta}$ is 'half-life' for 2-compartment drug.

**Oral and i.m. injections**
Produce plasma concentration, time profiles which rise to peak then fall again.

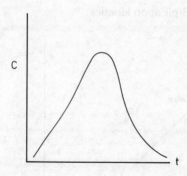

At peak     : rate of drug absorption = rate of drug elimination
Before peak  : rate of drug absorption > rate of drug elimination
After peak   : rate of drug absorption < rate of drug elimination

For a one compartment model with a first order absorption process with absorption rate constant $k_a$ (analogous to first order elimination rate constant) the plasma concentration C at any time t is given by

$$C = \frac{k_a\, F\, A\,(0)}{V\,(k_a - k)}\, (e^{-kt} - e^{-k_a t})$$

N.B. 1. V cannot be found by back extrapolation to t = 0 on a log concentration, time plot in this case.
      2. Time to peak concentration depends on ratio of $k_a/k$.
      3. AUC is useful indicator of amount of drug absorbed and eliminated by systemic circulation.
      4. F is bioavailability fraction

## Consequences of first order (linear) kinetics
1. $T_{\frac{1}{2}}$ is constant
2. AUC $\propto$ dose
3. Composition of drug products excreted independent of dose
4. Amount of drug excreted unchanged in urine $\propto$ dose
5. $C_{ss} \propto$ dose.

## Saturation or zero order kinetics
In some cases the rate of ADME processes may not be proportional to drug amount or concentration. Many ADME processes occur via enzymes or carrier mediated systems which for some drugs become saturated in the therapeutic dose or concentration range. This results in
(i) non-linear elimination kinetics:

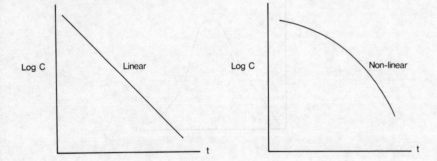

(ii) $T_{\frac{1}{2}}$ increases with dose.

(iii) AUC is not proportional to amount of available drug — as corollary steady state plasma concentration not directly proportional to dose.

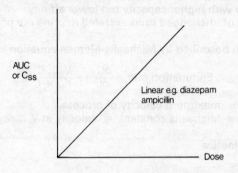

AUC or $C_{SS}$

Linear e.g. diazepam ampicillin

Dose

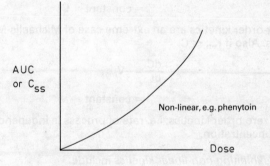

AUC or $C_{SS}$

Non-linear, e.g. phenytoin

Dose

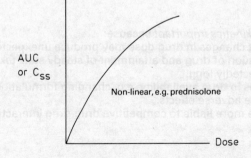

AUC or $C_{SS}$

Non-linear, e.g. prednisolone

Dose

(iv) Saturation of capacity limited processes may be affected by other drugs requiring same process, i.e. drug interactions common.
 (v) Composition of drug metabolites may vary with dose as one pathway becomes saturated and drug 'spills-over' into another pathway with higher capacity but lower affinity.
(vi) Amount of unchanged drug excreted in urine not proportional to dose.
   Elimination described by Michaelis-Menten equation

$$\text{Elimination rate} = \frac{dC}{dt} = -\frac{V_{max}\,C}{K_m + C}$$

where $V_{max}$ = maximum velocity of process,
      $K_m$  = Michaelis constant = velocity at $V_{max}/2$

**Non-linear kinetics**
If $K_m \gg C$

$$\frac{dC}{dt} = \frac{-V_{max}\,C}{K_m}$$

$$= \text{constant} \times C$$

i.e. first-order kinetics are an extreme case of Michaelis-Menten kinetics. Also if $K_m \ll C$

$$\frac{dC}{dt} = -V_{max}$$

$$= \text{constant}$$

This is zero order kinetics, i.e. rate of process is independent of drug concentration.

*Drugs exhibiting non-linear kinetics* include:
ethanol; phenytoin; aspirin and salicylates; prednisolone; dicoumarol; theophylline (?); chloroquine (?); overdoses with barbiturates and tricyclic antidepressants (?); 5-fluorouracil; vincristine.

*Non-linear kinetics important* because:
 (i) modest changes in drug dose may produce unexpected toxicity
 (ii) elimination of drug and attainment of steady state takes unexpectedly long.
(iii) changes in drug availability, e.g. changing formulation can produce adverse effects.
(iv) may be more liable to competitive drug-drug interactions.

**Intravenous infusions**
Drug accumulates until a steady state is attained when
Rate drug infused = Rate drug eliminated.
If $R_0$ = rate of constant infusion

$$\frac{dA}{dt} = R_0 - kA$$

and at steady state $R_0 = kA$
Divide through by V to get concentration at steady state.

$$\frac{A}{V} = C_{ss} = \frac{R_0}{kV} = \frac{\text{Infusion rate}}{\text{Clearance}} \qquad (9)$$

so knowing desired $C_{ss}$, k and V, infusion rate can be calculated
C at any time t during infusion is given by

$$C = \frac{R_0}{VK}(1 - e^{-kt}) \qquad (10)$$

Rate at which steady state is achieved is *independent* of rate of drug infusion since substitution from (9) into (10) gives

$$C = C_{ss}(1 - e^{-kt})$$

and          $\dfrac{C}{C_{ss}}$ = fraction of steady state attained

$$= 1 - e^{-kt}$$

Substituting for $T_{\frac{1}{2}}$ from (6) gives

$$\frac{C}{C_{ss}} = 1 - e^{-(0.693/T_{\frac{1}{2}})t}$$

| Thus     *Fraction of steady state attained* | *Number of half lives* |
|:---:|:---:|
| 0.5 | 1 |
| 0.75 | 2 |
| 0.875 | 3 |
| 0.94 | 4 |
| 0.97 | 5 |
| 0.98 | 6 |

Thus for drugs *obeying linear kinetics* 97% of steady state is reached after $5 \times T_{\frac{1}{2}}$.
No simple analogous rule exists for drugs obeying non-linear kinetics.

**Multiple dosing**

When drug is given in multiple doses if dose interval ($\tau$) is small relative to $T_{\frac{1}{2}}$ drug accumulates in the body until a steady state is achieved when amount of drug given in dose interval = amount of drug eliminated in dose interval.

$$\bar{C} = \text{mean steady state concentration} = \frac{\text{AUC in one dose interval}}{\tau}$$

$$\bar{C} = \frac{\text{dose}}{\tau} \times \frac{1}{\text{clearance}}$$

since dose/$\tau$ is analogous to infusion rate

$$= \frac{\text{dose}}{kV}$$

as $k = 0.693/T_{\frac{1}{2}}$ and $1/0.693 = 1.44$

$$\bar{C} = \frac{1.44 \times \text{dose} \times T_{\frac{1}{2}}}{V_{\tau}}$$

If $F < 1$ (bioavailability $< 1$)

$$\bar{C} = \frac{1.44F \times \text{dose} \times T_{\frac{1}{2}}}{V_{\tau}}$$

Assuming $F = 1$ and constant $V$ during multiple dosing, a drug will accumulate in the body if it is given at intervals less than 1.4 times its half-life. The ratio of accumulation is defined as

$$R = \frac{1.4T_{\frac{1}{2}}}{\tau}$$

$$= \frac{\bar{C}}{\text{dose}}$$

i.e. R defines by what multiple $\bar{C}$ exceeds the amount given in a single dose. For a given dose it is possible to calculate the value of $\tau$ necessary to achieve a desired $\bar{C}$ from $\tau = \text{AUC}/\bar{C}$. Fluctuations in blood levels when plateau is reached:

Maximum level – Minimum level = Dose

$$\frac{C_{max}}{C_{min}} = 2^{(\tau/T_{\frac{1}{2}})}$$

e.g. if doses are given every 2 half-lives

$$\frac{C_{max}}{C_{min}} = 2^2 = 4$$

i.e. maximum blood level is 4 times minimum level (just before next dose).

As for i.v. infusion time to reach steady state *solely* depends on $T_{\frac{1}{2}}$, e.g. for digoxin $T_{\frac{1}{2}} = 36$ h so time to reach steady state on repeated maintenance dose is about $5 \times 36 = 180$ h. A loading dose L can be given to achieve steady state more rapidly

$$L = \frac{\text{Maintenance dose}}{1 - e^{-k\tau}} \text{ (for rationale see diagram)}$$

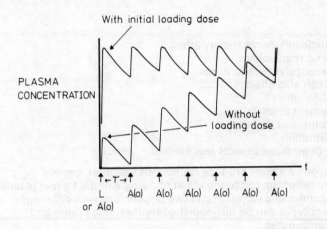

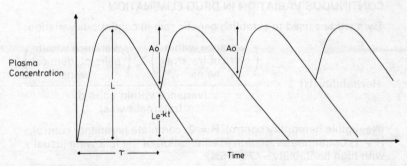

L = Loading dose
$A_0$ = Maintenance dose

# Pharmacogenetics

Genetic influences mainly affect:
   drug metabolism
   responsiveness to drugs
but can also affect:
   absorption
   protein binding
   volume of distribution
   excretion
although these aspects less studied.

*Polygenic effects* produce continuous variation; *genetic polymorphism* (often the result of a single mutant gene) results in discontinuous variation and two populations with differing phenotypes can be distinguished representing homo- and heterozygotes.

## CONTINUOUS VARIATION IN DRUG ELIMINATION

Twin studies used to establish genetic role in continuous variation:

$$\text{Heritability (H)} = \frac{\left(\begin{array}{c}\text{variance within} \\ \text{pairs of fraternal} \\ \text{twins}\end{array}\right) - \left(\begin{array}{c}\text{variance within} \\ \text{pairs of identical} \\ \text{twins}\end{array}\right)}{\left(\begin{array}{c}\text{variance within pairs of} \\ \text{fraternal twins}\end{array}\right)}$$

(Negligible hereditary control, H = 0; complete hereditary control, H = 1) Continuous variation in elimination of the following (usually with high heritability — 75–95%):

| | | |
|---|---|---|
| alcohol | bishydroxycoumarin | warfarin |
| antipyrine | phenylbutazone | phenytoin |
| aspirin | halothane | nortriptyline |
| amylobarbitone | chlorpromazine | imipramine |

## CONTINUOUS VARIATION IN PROTEIN BINDING

e.g. Warfarin

| | Heritability Index |
|---|---|
| Warfarin-albumin association constant | 0.89 |
| Number of drug binding sites/albumin molecule | 0.85 |

## DISCONTINUOUS VARIATION IN DRUG METABOLISM

### Acetylation polymorphism

Due mainly to difference in activity and amount of hepatic N-acetyltransferase; several primary amine drugs show bimodal acetylation in man. Classically populations termed fast and slow acetylators because $T_{\frac{1}{2}}$ isoniazid is 50–100 minutes in former and 100–250 minutes in latter. Some drugs, e.g. dapsone, have same $T_{\frac{1}{2}}$ in both phenotypes but ratio of acetylated metabolite to parent compound greater in fast acetylators.

*Inheritance* Rapid acetylation is autosomal dominant.

*Prevalence*

| Ethnic group | % Rapid acetylators |
|---|---|
| Canadian eskimos | 100 |
| Japanese | 88 |
| American Indians | 80 |
| Black Americans | 52 |
| Swedes | 49 |
| Britons | 38 |
| Egyptians | 18 |

*Clinical relevance*

| Drug | Phenotype | Clinical effect |
|---|---|---|
| Isoniazid | Slow | Develop SLE more frequently. Peripheral neuropathy commoner. More prone to phenytoin toxicity if given isoniazid. |
| | Fast | ?More prone to isoniazid hepatitis. ?Less rapid control of TB on once weekly isoniazid regimes. |
| Procainamide | Slow | Develop antinuclear antibodies and SLE more frequently. |
| Hydralazine | Slow | Develop antinuclear antibodies and SLE more frequently (but HLA-Dw4 more highly correlated). |
| | Fast | ?Require higher doses to control hypertension. |

| Sulphapyridine (and sulphasalazine which generates sulphapyridine) | Slow | More prone to side effects (haematological). |
| Dapsone | Slow | ?More prone to side effects (haematological). |
| Phenelzine | Slow | ?More prone to side effects (headache) |
| | Fast | ?Less improvement of depression on standard doses. |

Other drugs showing acetylation polymorphism are sulphadimidine (most sulphas do not), aminoglutethimide and amino metabolites of nitrazepam and clonazepam.

Some evidence that slow acetylators more likely to develop 'spontaneous' SLE and diabetic peripheral neuropathy.

**Polymorphism of oxidation phenotype**
Few isolated pedigrees (p-oxidation of phenytoin; O-de-ethylation of phenacetin) reported. Recent intensive investigation of two systems:

*a. Oxidation of debrisoquine.* Based on 0–8 h urine following 10 mg dose p.o.:

$$\text{Metabolic ratio} \quad = \quad \frac{\text{\% dose as debrisoquine}}{\text{\% dose as 4-hydroxydebrisoquine}}$$

Poor hydroxylators have ratio > 20.
Extensive hydroxylators have ratio < 12.5.

*Inheritance* Poor hydroxylation is autosomal recessive.

*Prevalence* Poor hydroxylators:U.K.   9%
Arabs   1%
Hong Kong Chinese   30%
*Drugs with metabolism associated with debrisoquine 4-hydroxylation*
Metoprolol; Timolol; Propranolol
Guanoxan
Carbocysteine
4-methoxyamphetamine; Nortriptyline (E-10 hydroxylation)
Phenformin
Phenytoin
Phenacetin O-dealkylation
Perhexiline
Encainide

*Clinical relevance*
1. Oxidation status determines efficacy of debrisoquine and guanoxan as hypotensives.
2. Efficacy of metoprolol, timolol, propranolol as beta-blockers.
3. Phenformin lactic acidosis occurs in poor metabolisers.
5. Vertigo and confusion after nortriptyline commoner in poor metabolisers.
6. Possibly phenacetin-induced methaemoglobinaemia commoner in poor metabolisers.
7. Possibly captopril-induced agranulocytosis commoner in poor metabolisers.

*b. N-oxidation of sparteine* (uterine stimulant used in Germany) Based on 0–12 h urine sample after 100 mg sparteine sulphate.

$$\text{Metabolic ratio} \quad = \quad \frac{\%\ \text{dose excreted as sparteine}}{\%\ \text{dose as sparteine metabolites}}$$

Non-inheritors have log (metabolic ratio) $\approx 3\ 2$.
*Inheritance*  Non-metabolism is autosomal recessive.
*Prevalence*  Non-metabolism:  Canadian Chinese 30%
Germany 5%
Canada 9%
*Relationship to debrisoquine polymorphism*  Both determined by relative amount of form of hepatic cytochrome P450. May be closely related but not identical cytochromes since in a few people there is discordance between debrisoquine and sparteine phenotypes.

Unlikely that this cytochrome P450 contributes to oxidation of antipyrine, amylobarbitone or acetanilide (metabolism not correlated with debrisoquine or sparteine metabolism).

**Suxamethonium sensitivity**
Suxamethonium-induced muscular paralysis usually lasts 5–10 mins due to rapid hydrolysis of drug by plasma pseudo-cholinesterase. Several variants of enzyme described, some of which cause prolonged paralysis requiring mechanical ventilation for some hours. Most common variant is $E_1^a E_1^a$ inherited as autosomal recessive (1 in 2500 in UK but absent in Japanese and Eskimos, rare in Africans).

## DISCONTINUOUS VARIATION IN DRUG RESPONSE

### Glucose 6-phosphate dehydrogenase (G6PD) deficiency

*Inheritance*
Sex-linked (X chromosome) defect of intermediate dominance determining activity of G6PD. Affects about 100 million people in world: African negros; some Mediterranean races; Kurdish and Iraqi Jews; some Philipinos; Chinese and S.E. Asians.

Heterozygous females have 2 red cell populations (+ and − enzyme), proportion varies from 1−99% sensitive-cells: approximately ⅓ heterozygous females have sufficiently high fraction of affected cells to show haemolysis.

Mutation has survived in its areas of distribution because it confers resistance to malaria.

*Mechanism*

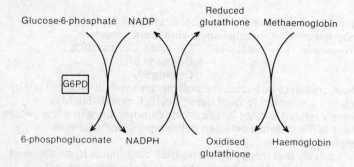

G6PD activity maintains low levels of methaemoglobin in red cells. If methaemoglobin level increases, haemolysis occurs.

*Clinical features*
Over 100 variants G6PD described. Two common types in the UK:
a.  African type A — normal amount of enzyme but rapid decline in activity as red cells age.
— suffer mild enzyme deficiency with 8−20% normal activity. Have haemolysis on drug challenge.
b.  Mediterranean type — severe (0−4% normal) enzyme activity deficit
— mild chronic haemolytic anaemia with severe haemolysis after drug challenge.

## Variants in suxamethonium sensitivity

| Genotype | Phenotype | Prevalence | Response to suxamethonium |
|----------|-----------|------------|----------------------------|
| $E_1^u E_1^u$ | Usual type of esterase | 96% | Normal |
| $E_1^a E_1^u$ | Some decreased sensitivity to inhibitors dibucaine & fluoride | 1/26 | Normal |
| $E_1^a E_1^a$ | Greatly decreased sensitivity to dibucaine and fluoride | 1/2800 | Prolonged |
| $E_1^f E_1^u$ | Some decreased sensitivity to fluoride | 1/280 | Normal |
| $E_1^f E_1^f$ | Greatly decreased sensitivity to fluoride | 1/300 000 | Prolonged |
| $E_1^s E_1^u$ | Some reduction in enzymic activity | 1/190 | Normal or almost normal |
| $E_1^s E_1^s$ | No enzymic activity | 1/140 000 (1% of Eskimos) | Grossly prolonged |
| $E_1^a E_1^f$ | Decreased sensitivity to dibucaine and fluoride | 1/29 000 | Prolonged |
| $E_1^a E_1^s$ | Greatly decreased sensitivity to dibucaine and fluoride | 1/20 000 | Grossly prolonged |
| $E_1^f E_1^s$ | Decreased sensitivity to dibucaine and fluoride | 1/200 000 | Prolonged |
| $E_1^+ E_1^+$ | 30% increase in enzyme activity | 1/10 | Shortened |
| $E_{Cynthiana}$ | 2–3 × increase in enzyme activity | Unknown | Resistant to drug |

## Drug excretion

Dubin-Johnson's syndrome: failure of excretion of bilirubin glucuronide into bile; inherited as autosomal recessive. Jaundice can be precipitated or worsened by oral contraceptives.

*RBC reduced glutathione (GSH) diminished in deficiency of:*
  Glucose 6-phosphate dehydrogenase (G6PD)
  $\gamma$-glutamylcysteine synthetase
  glutathione reductase
  glutathione peroxidase

*and may result in haemolysis when the following are administered:*
  analgesics — aspirin, phenacetin, acetanilide, antipyrine,
              aminopyrine
  antimalarials — primaquine, pamaquine, pentaquine,
              quinacrine, quinine, chloroquine
  antibacterials — sulphonamides, sulphones, nitrofurantoin,
              chloramphenicol, PAS
  miscellaneous — quinidine, probenecid, vitamin K, naphthalene,
              Fava bean

## Porphyrias

Metabolic disorders characterised by tissue accumulation of
porphyrins and/or precursors with characteristic symptoms. Some
types have specific enzyme deficiencies; others as yet of uncertain
mechanism. In general, increased levels of $\delta$-aminolaevulinic acid
(ALA) and porphobilinogen (PBG) associated with acute attacks and
porphyrins with photosensitivity.

Acute attacks bear a superficial resemblance to lead poisoning
and comprise:
  Abdominal symptoms — colic, constipation, nausea, vomiting.
  Tachycardia, raised blood pressure
  Psychiatric abnormalities — restlessness, confusion, psychosis
  Neurological features — peripheral neuropathy, paralysis or
  paresis of limbs, respiratory paralysis (commonest cause of
  death), rarely seizures.
  Pyrexia
  Electrolyte disturbances, inappropriate ADH secretion

Attacks explained on a neurogenic basis and primary lesion is
biochemical.
  Lesions occur at several points of porphyrin metabolism.
  Acute attacks occur intermittently and ascribed to increased ALA
synthetase activity which exacerbates biochemical abnormalities.
Drugs (and endogenous steroids) commonest precipitating factors.
  Acute attacks occur in:
1. Acute intermittent porphyria (Swedish type — commonest in
   UK). Autosomal dominant inheritance of uroporphyrinogen
   synthetase deficiency. Rare before puberty and commoner in
   women often presenting in pregnancy due to increased steroid.
2. Hereditary coproporphyria. Rare. Autosomal dominant
   inheritance of partial deficiency of coproporphyrin oxygenase.

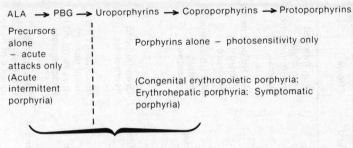

ALA → PBG → Uroporphyrins → Coproporphyrins → Protoporphyrins

Precursors
alone
– acute                         Porphyrins alone – photosensitivity only
attacks only
(Acute
intermittent                    (Congenital erythropoietic porphyria:
porphyria)                      Erythrohepatic porphyria: Symptomatic
                                porphyria)

Precursors + Porphyrins – acute attacks and photosensitivity

(Hereditary coproporphyria. variegate porphyria)

3. Variegate porphyria (South African type — 3/1000 but occurs in
   Europe — George III probably had it). Autosomal dominant but
   deficit obscure — ferrochelatase may be unstable or deficient or
   possibly there is block of coproporphyrin metabolism.

*Drugs which can precipitate acute porphyria attacks*
   *hypnosedatives:* barbiturates (including anaesthetic
                     barbiturates), chlordiazepoxide, glutethimide,
                     dichloralphenazone, ethanol.
   *anticonvulsants:* phenytoin, succinimides, troxidone.
   *oral hypoglycaemics:* chlorpropamide, tolbutamide.
   *antimicrobials:* chloramphenicol, chloroquine, griseofulvin,
                     pyrazinamide, sulphonamides.
   *steroids:* oestrogens, oral contraceptive pill.
   *miscellaneous:* imipramine, pentazocine, ergot.

**Steroid-induced raised intraocular pressure**
Chronic use of steroid eye drops produces raised intraocular
pressure in genetically predisposed.

| | 0–5 | 5–15 | 15+ |
|---|---|---|---|
| Increase in intraocular pressure on exposure to 1% dexamethasone eye drops (mm Hg) | | | |
| Percentage of white population | 66 | 29 | 5 |
| Proposed genotype — autosomal recessive inheritance | $P^LP^L$ | $P^LP^H$ | $P^HP^H$ |
| Chance of ultimate development of open angle glaucoma in later life (compared with $P^LP^L$ individuals) | 1 | 18 | 101 |

**Table 1** Discontinuous variation in drug response

| Pharmacogenetic variation | Mechanism | Inheritance | Occurrence | Drugs involved | Effects |
|---|---|---|---|---|---|
| Haemoglobin H (a form of α-thalassaemia) | HbH is a β chain tetramer, which tends to form Met Hb with oxidising drugs | Autosomal recessive | 1/300 in Thailand | As is G6PD deficiency | Drug-induced haemolytic anaemia. Heinz bodies. |
| HbM | Met HbM is resistant to Met Hb reductase | Autosomal dominant | | Nitrites, nitrates, chlorates, phenacetin, acetanilide, sulphonamides, dapsone, primaquine. | Met Hb cyanosis on drug exposure |
| Hereditary methaemoglobinaemia | reductase deficiency | Autosomal recessive (but heterozygotes show some response) | 1/100 are heterozygotes | | Met Hb cyanosis on drug exposure |
| Hb Zurich / Hb Koln / Hb Hammersmith | Unstable Hb which readily forms Heinz bodies | | Rare | Sulphonamides, primaquine | Drug-induced haemolysis |
| Warfarin resistance | Reduced affinity of vitamin K epoxide reductase for warfarin | Autosomal dominant | Rare | Warfarin, dicoumarol, phenindione | 5–20 times the usual dose of drug required to anticoagulate |
| Chloramphenicol-induced bone marrow depression | Idiosyncratic inhibition of DNA synthesis in marrow cells | Probably genetically determined | Rare | Chloramphenicol | Severe, often irreversible, aplasia of bone marrow |

| | | | | | |
|---|---|---|---|---|---|
| Increased sensitivity to ethanol | Unknown central factors. Increased peripheral autonomic sensitivity. | Racial | Common in Oriental races | Ethanol | Increased flushing, increased intoxication |
| Intravascular clotting with oral contraceptives | Unknown | Strong association with blood groups A and AB | Rare | Oestrogen-containing preparations | Increased risk of venous and arterial thrombosis |
| Atropine sensitivity | Low vagal tone or increased sensitivity to sympathetic effects | Trisomy 21 and other forms of Down's syndrome | Common in Down's syndrome | Atropine and other anticholinergics | Tachycardia and other signs atropine toxicity |
| Malignant hyperthermia | Defect in $Ca^{++}$ storing with muscle fibre | Autosomal dominant | 1/20 000 | Nitrous oxide, halothane, ether, cyclopropane, suxamethonium | Hyperthermia, rigidity, metabolic acidosis, Treat with dantrolene |

**Table 2** Discontinuous variation in drug metabolism

| Pharmacogenetic variation | Mechanism | Inheritance | Occurrence | Drugs involved | Effect |
|---|---|---|---|---|---|
| Acatalasia | Lack of r.b.c. catalase | Autosomal recessive | Up to 1% some Japanese populations | Hydrogen peroxide | Approx 50% suffer recurrent sepsis of mouth and pharynx |
| Slow metabolism of tolbutamide | Impaired metabolic inactivation (possibly same as defective carbon oxidation of debrisoquine) | Autosomal recessive | ? same as defective metabolism of debrisoquine. | Tolbutamide | Increased drug effect with usual doses |
| Unresponsiveness to purine antimetabolites | Lack of hypoxanthine guanine phosphoribosyl transferase (HGPRT), therefore fails to activate drugs to nucleotide analogues | 1. Lesch-Nyhan syndrome: X-linked recessive 2. Some forms of gout: X-linked recessive | | 6-mercaptopurine 6-thioguanine 8-azaguanine azathioprine | Lack of anticancer activity |
| Ethanol: 1. Rapid metabolisers | Variant hyperactive form of ADH 2 | Autosomal | 4-20% Europeans | Ethanol | 40-50% more rapid metabolism |

| | | | | |
|---|---|---|---|---|
| 2. Racial differences | Unknown | ? | Ethanol | Rate of alcohol metabolism: Europeans 0.145 g/kg/h; Eskimos 0.110 g/kg/h; Red Indians 0.101 g/kg/h |
| Impairment of bilirubin conjugation: | Lack of UDP glucuronyl transferase. Failure of drug conjugation and thus impairment of excretion. | | paracetamol tetrahydrocortisol menthol chloral hydrate trichloroethanol salicylamide | Impaired drug glucuronidation |
| 1. Crigler-Najjar syndrome | Complete enzyme lack | Autosomal recessive | | |
| 2. Moderate impairment of conjugation | Inducible enzyme present | Autosomal dominant with incomplete penetration | | |
| 3. Gilbert's syndrome | Inducible enzyme present | Autosomal dominant | | |

# Drugs at the extremes of age

## DRUGS AND INFANTS AND CHILDREN

1/6 newborns in special care nurseries ⎫
3/5 children in hospital       ⎬ receive drug therapy

  Incidence of adverse effects (10–15%) similar to adults in children but higher (25%) in neonates.

  Children not miniature adults in terms of drug handling because of differences in body constitution. For example:

1. Body water (as % body weight)

|  | Neonate | Adult |
|---|---|---|
| Total | 75 | 60 |
| Intracellular | 34 | 41 |
| Extracellular | 40 | 20 |

2 Renal function — changes in clearance (ml/min)

|  | Infant | Adult |
|---|---|---|
| GFR | 10 | 130 |
| Tubular secretion (PAH clearance) | 25 | 650 |

  Adult GFR attained 3–5 months.
  Adult secretory and reabsorptive capacity attained 7 months.

3. Hepatic enzyme activity low in neonates for some systems, e.g. chloramphenicol glucuronyl transferase, but not others, e.g. sulphation of paracetamol.

4. GI function very different in terms of transit time, enzymes etc. in neonates, e.g.

|  | Neonate | Adult |
|---|---|---|
| Gastric emptying time (mins) | 87 | 65 |
| Gastric acid output (mmol/10 kg/hr) | 0.15 | 2 |

5. Ratio of surface area/body weight

|  | Weight (kg) | Surface area ($m^2$) | Ratio (kg/$m^2$) |
|---|---|---|---|
| Neonate | 1.5 | 0.13 | 11.5 |
| Adult | 70 | 1.73 | 40 |

Dosing related to surface area most useful dose adjustment rule

$$\text{Dose} = \frac{\text{Adult Dose}}{1.73} \times \text{Child's surface area}$$

**Pharmacokinetic effects**
1. *Absorption*: Reduced gastric acidity in neonates results in greater oral absorption of ampicillin, flucloxacillin, amoxycillin as compared to adults. Neonates absorb phenobarbitone and vitamin E poorly but digoxin, diazepam and cotrimoxazole normally absorbed.

Generally neonatal GI drug absorption is clinically adequate.

Older infants and children absorb some drugs, e.g. diazepam, clonazepam, sodium valproate more rapidly but with same bioavailability as adults.

Absorption from i.m. injections in neonates may be erratic for some drugs, e.g. gentamicin, digoxin.

Infant skin is thin and percutaneous absorption is good, e.g. steroid creams ($\rightarrow$ Cushing's); topical sulphonamide mafenide ($\rightarrow$ methaemoglobinaemia); hexachlorophane ($\rightarrow$ neurotoxicity).
2. *Distribution*: Fat content is low in children.

|  | Fat as % body weight |
|---|---|
| Premature | 3 |
| Neonate (full term) | 12 |
| Age 1 year | 30 |
| Age 18 years | 18 |

$V_d$ of fat soluble drugs, e.g. diazepam thus lower in babies than adults.

Plasma protein binding of drugs reduced in neonates due to 20% (approx) lower albumin conc and altered capacity so $V_d$ rises.

|  | % binding | | $V_d$ (l/kg) | |
|---|---|---|---|---|
|  | Neonates | Adults | Neonates | Adults |
| Phenylbutazone | 85 | 97 | 0.2 | 0.12 |
| Sulphafurazole | 65 | 84 | 0.4 | 0.16 |
| Phenytoin | 80 | 90 | 1.3 | 0.65 |

Blood-brain barrier more permeable in neonates than older children and adults, e.g. opiates, penicillin.
3 *Metabolism*: Liver volume/kg decreases after birth into adult years. Some (but not all) enzyme systems less active in neonates but many increase (relatively) in children. Examples of plasma $T_{\frac{1}{2}}$ (hours)

|  | Prematures | Neonates | Infants | Children | Adults |
|---|---|---|---|---|---|
| Diazepam | 38–120 | 22–46 | 10–12 | 15–21 | 24–48 |
| Phenobarbitone | 380 | 70–250 | 20–70 | 50–65 | 60–180 |

Previous intrauterine or postnatal drug exposure can affect neonatal metabolism, e.g. phenobarbitone reduces neonatal diazepam $T_{\frac{1}{2}}$ to 12–15 hours. Barbiturates given to mother have been used to reduce neonatal hyperbilirubinaemia by induction of glucuronyl transferase in utero.

Chloramphenicol produces 'grey baby' syndrome in neonates due to high plasma levels as elimination delayed by inefficient glucuronidization.

4. *Excretion*: All renal mechanisms (filtration, secretion, reabsorption) are reduced in babies — filtration is also relatively more important than other mechanisms as compared with adults.

In general, renal excretion of drugs is less in neonates compared to older patients. GFR rapidly increases after a few weeks and doses of drugs excreted this way, e.g. aminoglycosides, penicillins should be increased after first week of life. Examples of changes in $T_{\frac{1}{2}}$ (hours)

|  | Prematures | Neonates | Infants | Adults |
|---|---|---|---|---|
| Carbenicillin | 5–6 | 4 | 2 | 1–1.5 |
| Gentamicin | 5–6 | 4–5 | 3–4 | 2–3 |

## Drug prescribing in infancy

1. Minimum number of drugs for shortest time (as always!).
2. If possible use drugs with high therapeutic index, available kinetic information in children and possibility of drug level monitoring if required.
3. Liquid oral preparations for young children (if available) but can often swallow tablets or capsules. Chronic use of sucrose-containing elixirs may cause caries and gingivitis.
4. Drugs should not be added to milk in infant feeding bottles since interaction could occur or dosage may be reduced if feed not taken completely.
5. In general, rectal administration is erratic and may upset older children so is discouraged but can be useful if child is vomiting or convulsing.
6 Dosage is critical especially in first 30 days (neonate). Use surface area (see above) except for prematures when it is inaccurate. For drugs with a high therapeutic index age can be used according to:

| Age | % adult dose |
|---|---|
| Premature | Not applicable |
| 1 month | 12.5 |
| 2 months | 15 |
| 4 months | 20 |
| 1 year | 25 |
| 3 years | 33 |
| 7 years | 50 |
| 12 years | 75 |

Dosing by weight often useful but in obesity need to dose in terms of ideal body weight (from age and height).

**Most frequent adverse drug effects in infants and children outside neonatal period**

| System | Effect | Drug |
| --- | --- | --- |
| Gastro-intestinal | Nausea and vomiting | Many |
| | Diarrhoea | Ampicillin |
| | Monilial infection | Ampicillin |
| | Stained teeth | Tetracyclines |
| Blood | Marrow suppression | Chloramphenicol; Cytotoxics |
| | Megaloblastic anaemia | Phenytoin; Cotrimoxazole |
| Skin | Macular/Papular rash | Ampicillin; Phenytoin |
| | Urticaria | Penicillin; Aspirin |
| CNS | Drowsiness | Phenobarbitone; Carbamazepine; Antihistamines |
| | Ataxia | Phenytoin; Carbamazepine |
| | Dyskinesia | Metoclopramide; Prochlorperazine |
| | Hyperkinesia | Phenobarbitone |
| Metabolic | Hypokalaemia | Frusemide |
| | Hyperglycaemia | Thiazides; Steroids |
| | Cushingoid syndrome | Steroid (creams) |
| CVS | Bradycardia | Digoxin |
| | Hypertension | Steroids |

**DRUGS DURING PREGNANCY**

Average number of drugs taken during pregnancy – 4.2 (Scotland 1972): not including those taken during labour.

Embryo more susceptible to adverse drug effects than at any other period of life. All drugs can cross placenta if given in sufficient quantity. Effects may be:
  (i)  fetal death and abortion
 (ii)  malformations
(iii)  affect post-natal behaviour or intelligence
(iv)  produce malignancy in later life.

Major risk of malformation is up to 8th week postconception (i.e. often before pregnancy diagnosed) but adverse effects occur after this.

Many adverse effects described in animals but evidence of damage in man less certain.

### Drugs to be avoided during first three months of pregnancy

| Drug | Possible effect on fetus |
| --- | --- |
| Progestogens | Masculinisation of female |
| Oestrogens | Masculinisation of female<br>Vaginal adenocarcinoma 20 years after |
| Androgens | Masculinisation of female |
| Methotrexate | Malformation and abortion |
| Phenytoin | Cleft lip, diaphagmatic hernia, hypoplastic distal phalanges |
| Salicylates | Achondroplasia, hydrocephalus, congenital heart disease, talipes, congenital dislocation of hip |
| Barbiturates | Cleft lip and palate |
| Iron | Congenital malformations increased |
| Antacids | Congenital malformations increased |
| Nicotinamide | Congenital malformations increased |

N.B.  Thalidomide (no longer available) produced malformations in about 25% pregnancies. Few of the above are as dangerous as this and in some cases only minor increases in malformations have been shown.

Rule  Drugs should *only* be used during pregnancy if of proven benefit to mother or fetus and with due consideration of risks. *Any* woman of child-bearing age may become pregnant!

### PERINATAL DRUGS

Birth, from a pharmacologist's viewpoint, is a withdrawal from maternally administered drugs!

Drugs given to mother in pregnancy and labour may affect fetus:

| Class | Drug given to mother | Effects on neonate |
| --- | --- | --- |
| CNS | Opiates | Neonatal depression; seizures; diarrhoea |
| | Ethanol | Congenital defects (fetal alcohol syndrome) |

|  | Barbiturates | Neonatal depression; enzyme induction |
|  | Phenothiazines | Neonatal depression; extrapyramidal effects |
|  | Diazepam, Lorazepam | Neonatal depression; hypothermia |
|  | Lithium | Goitre |
| Antimicrobial agents | Aminoglycosides | Ototoxicity |
|  | Tetracycline | Teeth discolouration; impaired fetal bone growth |
|  | Sulphonamides | Kernicterus; Haemolytic anaemia in G6PD deficiency |
|  | Nitrofurantoin | Haemolytic anaemia in G6PD deficiency |
|  | Quinine | Thrombocytopenia |
|  | Chloroquine | Retinopathy; Ototoxicity |
| CVS | β-blockers | Bradycardia |
|  | Reserpine | Bradycardia; lethargy |
| Hormones etc. | Androgens; some progestogens | Virilisation |
|  | Oestrogens | Feminisation; vaginal adenocarcinoma in teens |
|  | Iodides | Goitre-euthyroid |
|  | Carbimazole; propylthiouracil | Goitre-hypothyroid |

## DRUGS IN BREAST MILK

Many drugs enter breast milk — usually small amounts and not harmful.

Entry depends upon pH and $pK_a$ of drug — lipid soluble drugs diffuse in as their non-ionised form. Milk has lower pH than plasma so concentrates weak bases; weak acids usually at lower concentration than plasma.

Only occasionally do drugs in milk adversely affect infant, examples:

| *Drug given to mother* | *Effect on baby* |
| Phenobarbitone | Drowsiness |
| Chlorpromazine | Drowsiness |
| Lithium | Hypotonia, hypothermia, cyanosis |
| Brompheniramine/Ephedrine | Irritability; disturbed sleep |
| Senna, Cascara, Danthron | Diarrhoea |

## DRUGS AND THE ELDERLY

10% of geriatric admissions are iatrogenic and drug-related. Due to:
1. Elderly receive more drugs than young. Old are about 15% of population but consume over 30% NHS drug expenditure. 75% of people over 75 receive drugs; 2/3 receive 1–3 drugs and 1/3 4–6+ drugs simultaneously.
2. Multiple (and often chronic) illness leads to polypharmacy in frail patients.
3. Non-compliance in elderly is 50–60% of which half is serious (omitting necessary drugs or taking inappropriate drugs). 20% due to lack of knowledge of drug regimen; 20% due to taking drugs not currently prescribed.
4. Increased sensitivity of aged to drugs and adverse effects.

### Increased sensitivity to drugs

*A. Pharmacokinetic effects*
1. *Absorption.* Little evidence of major alteration in absorption. Changes seen with aging are:
 (i) gastric atrophy
 (ii) reduced acid secretion
 (iii) delayed gastric emptying and reduced gut mobility
 (iv) reduced absorption of iron, calcium, thiamine, xylose and galactose (all active transport mechanisms)
 (v) reduction (up to 50%) of gut blood flow
 (vi) increased incidence of duodenal diverticula and bacterial overgrowth resulting in malabsorption.
  None of these significantly influence absorption of those drugs which have been studied; these are passively absorbed.
2. *Distribution* Aging accompanied by relative increase in fat, reduced water, muscle mass and body weight. Ethanol distributes into total body water so higher peak plasma ethanol levels seen in elderly. Lipid soluble drugs, e.g. diazepam, lignocaine, are more extensively distributed (larger $V_d$) in elderly.
  Plasma protein changes may occur with decreased albumin and increased gamma globulin but no defect in drug binding affinity found. Changes in plasma protein mainly reflect illness rather than age itself. Decreased binding in parallel with albumin decrease shown for warfarin, phenytoin, salicylates, sulphonamides, phenylbutazone, pethidine.

| Increased $V_d$ | Decreased $V_d$ |
|---|---|
| Benzodiazepines (Chlordiazepoxide, Diazepam, Oxazepam, Nitrazepam) | Antipyrine Digoxin |
| Chlormethiazole | Ethanol |
| Gentamicin and Kanamycin | Propicillin |
| Hexobarbitone | Quinidine and Quinine |
| Lignocaine | |
| Morphine | |
| Tolbutamide | |

Possibly elderly more susceptible to drug — drug interactions via protein binding displacement — ? due to low albumin.

N.B. Most drug assays measure total drug concentration and this falls if free drug fraction increases although the concentration of free drug (and drug effect) remains constant. Thus for extensively protein bound drugs expect lower ranges of therapeutic and toxic plasma concentrations of total drug.

3 *Metabolism*. Elderly have:

a Altered hepatic metabolism but only in some cases, eg:

| Reduced clearance | Unchanged clearance |
|---|---|
| Diazepam — oxidation | Oxazepam — glucuronidation |
| Desmethyldiazepam — oxidation | Temazepam — glucuronidation |
| Quinidine — oxidation | Nitrazepam — nitroreduction |
| Theophylline — oxidation | Warfarin — oxidation |
| Propranolol — oxidation | Lignocaine — oxidation |
| Nortriptyline — oxidation | Isoniazid — acetylation |

b Decreased hepatic blood flow. Suggests main effect of aging is on Phase I metabolism — 40–50% reduction (mainly due to reduced cardiac output): could affect highly cleared drugs like propranolol.

c. Reduced capacity for microsomal enzyme induction following inducing agents. Also elderly smoke and drink less than young so hepatic enzymes less induced.

No effects found on non-microsomally metabolised drugs like alcohol, isoniazid, aspirin.

Effects complicated by changes in distribution, e.g. increased $V_d$ for diazepam in elderly results in longer $T_{\frac{1}{2}}$ but unchanged clearance.

No obvious rules emerged yet for predicting drug behaviour. Thus aging may (chlordiazepoxide) or may not (oxazepam, lorazepam) impair hepatic drug metabolism. Similarly $V_d$ may be increased (chlordiazepoxide, diazepam) or remain unchanged (lorazepam, oxazepam).

4. *Excretion*. Glomerular filtration rate falls with age. GFR $\simeq$ 153 – 0.96 (Age).

Tubular secretion also declines.

*Reduced renal elimination in aged*

Aminoglycosides e.g. amikacin, gentamicin, streptomycin
Carbenoxolone
Cephazolin
Digoxin
Lithium
Methotrexate
Penicillins e.g. ampicillin, benzylpenicillin
Procainamide
Sulphamethizole
Tetracyclines

*B  Pharmacodynamic effects*
Much of the increased sensitivity of elderly explained by altered
pharmacokinetics but may also show altered response although as
yet little information available. Examples:
  (i) Elderly showed greater and more prolonged CNS depression
      than young after nitrazepam though plasma drug levels and $T_{\frac{1}{2}}$
      similar.
 (ii) Warfarin produces greater inhibition of hepatic clotting factor
      synthesis in the old than in the young.
(iii) Decreased heart rate response to isoprenaline and increased
      sensitivity to β-blockers with age may reflect reduced
      β-adrenoceptor density. Isoprenaline and prostaglandin E, both
      produce less cyclic AMP in lymphocytes of the old: this may
      result from altered cell membrane in old age affecting both
      receptor types or coupling of receptor and adenyl cyclase.
 (iv) Increased frequency and magnitude of drug-induced postural
      hypotension probably results from age-related impairment of
      baroreceptor reflexes.

**Drug usage in the aged**
Many of these rules apply at all ages.
1. Use the fewest drugs and the simplest regime possible.
2  Use the lowest dose.
3. Do not use drugs to treat symptoms without knowing their
   cause.
4. Discontinue a drug if it becomes unnecessary.
5. Do not withhold drugs because of old age but remember drugs
   cannot cure old age.
6. Be especially wary of the following groups of drugs:
     a.  *CNS*: Barbiturates, diazepam, nitrazepam and other long $T_{\frac{1}{2}}$
   benzodiazepines should be avoided. Use temazepam, oxazepam,
   chlormethiazole or chloral.

Phenothiazines often cause hypotension, Parkinsonism and hypothermia in the old and should be used sparingly. Prochloperazine (Stemetil) should be reserved for true vertigo not 'dizziness' which is common in the elderly.

Cerebral and peripheral vasodilators, e.g. cyclandelate, naftidrofuryl, are virtually ineffective and may have serious adverse reaction.

Anti-Parkinsonian drugs should only be used for true Parkinsonian tremors. Anticholinergic drugs are very liable to produce confusion especially in patients with early senile dementia, and may precipitate constipation, urinary retention and glaucoma. Dryness of the mouth and poor oral hygiene encourages oral candidiasis.

Antidepressants should be used cautiously because of their anticholinergic effects: mianserin or trazodone may be useful here; MAOIs are too dangerous.

b. *CVS*: Hypotensive agents should be used cautiously since hypotension can be dangerous. Evidence that control of hypertension helps the over-70's is not yet complete. Hypertension producing encephalopathy or cardiac failure is, however, an indication for therapy. Diuretics can cause hypokalaemia, frequency and incontinence or urinary retention. Centrally acting hypotensives, e.g. methyldopa, clonidine, can cause depression and sedation; β-blockers can exacerbate heart failure, peripheral circulatory problems and occasionally cause confusion, urinary incontinance and airways obstruction. With all treatments watch out for postural hypotension.

Digoxin overdosage is common in the old: many don't need it anyway.

c. *Antidiabetic agents*: avoid long $T_{\frac{1}{2}}$ drugs like chlorpropamide — use tolbutamide or glibenclamide. Try to manage with diet alone and aim only to prevent symptoms, ketosis or hyperosmolality. Insulin injections are very inconvenient for the old and are rarely used. Biguanides have no place.

# Effect of disease on pharmacokinetics

## RENAL IMPAIRMENT

### A. Absorption
Very little information.

Trimethoprim, sulphamethoxazole, cloxacillin, cefazolin — no impairment.

Uraemia may impair drug metabolism and first-pass metabolic fraction can be reduced so drugs are apparently better absorbed (NB Bioavailability = (fraction of dose absorbed) × (fraction of drug metabolised at first pass). Some evidence for this effect for propranolol, pindolol, dextropropoxyphene.

### B. Distribution
Protein binding of many drugs affected.

Generally binding of acidic drugs, e.g. phenytoin, phenylbutazone, phenobarbitone, salicylate, valproic acid, warfarin, is impaired in proportion to degree of renal failure.

Variable effects on basic drugs, usually no change, occasionally decreased, e.g. diazepam, morphine, triamterene.

Binding changes possibly caused by:
a. hypoproteinaemia — usually insufficient to explain all of the decrease
b. different structure of binding protein in uraemia
c. competitive or non-competitive inhibition of drug binding by endogenous ligands, e.g. peptides, organic acids accumulating in plasma of uraemic patients.

Dialysis does not restore binding to normal; transplantation does.

As free drug fraction changed in renal failure, therapeutic range of total drug concentration falls, e.g. phenytoin is 5–10 $\mu$g/ml (c.f. 10–20 $\mu$g/ml in normals).

*Binding reduced in renal failure*
    Azapropazone
    Benzylpenicillin
    Cephalexin
    Cloxacillin
    Diazoxide
    Doxycycline
    Phenytoin
    Prazosin
    Sulphamethoxazole

*Binding unaffected*
    Chloramphenicol
    Desmethylimipramine
    Minocycline
    Nitrofurantoin
    Trimethoprim

## C. Metabolism

*Oxidation* — normal, e.g. lignocaine, barbiturates, pethidine, or accelerated, e.g. phenytoin, propranolol, digitoxin. Exception is quinidine which is slowed.

*Reduction* — ? slowed, e.g. cortisol.

*Hydrolysis* — slowed, e.g. procaine, succinylcholine, cephalothin, insulin, also reduced liberation of active drug from clindamycin phosphate, indanyl carbenicillin.

*Conjugation* with glucuronic acid, sulphate and glycine normal but some acetylations slowed either markedly, e.g. *p*-aminosalicylate or only to a small extent.

## D. Elimination

Overall drug elimination rate (k) is sum of the rates for renal (kr) and non-renal (nr) elimination.

$$k = kr + knr$$

For most drugs kr is also proportional to creatinine clearance ($CL_{cr}$)

$$kr \propto CL_{cr}$$

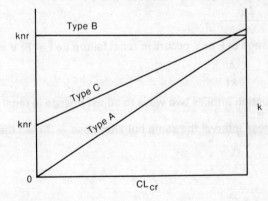

so $k = \alpha \, CL_{cr}$ where $\alpha$ is a proportionality constant and $k = \alpha \, CL_{cr} +$ knr.

If k is plotted against $CL_{cr}$ (the Dettli nomogram) the ordinate intercept will be knr and three classes of drugs can be distinguished.

*Type A*: drugs entirely dependent upon renal function for elimination, e.g. gentamicin, kanamycin and other aminoglycosides; cephaloridine, cephalexin, lithium.

*Type B*: drugs entirely dependent upon non-renal routes (e.g. hepatic) for elimination, e.g. adriamycin, corticosteroids, chloramphenicol, diazepam, propranolol, rifampicin.

*Type C*: drugs dependent upon both renal and non-renal routes of elimination, e.g. digoxin, ethambutol, methyldopa, methotrexate, procainamide.

Type B drugs require no change in regime unless renally excreted active metabolites are involved. Type A and C drugs require dosage modification. This can be done using a Dettli nomogram since k for normal renal function and knr are known for many drugs. (If knr is unknown it can be calculated from knr = k (1 – F) where F = fraction of systemically available drug excreted unchanged in urine.) Using a straight line drawn between k ($CL_{cr}$ = 100 ml/min) and knr ($CL_{cr}$ = 0 ml/min) k for any degree of renal failure can be found by interpolation on this line at the impaired $CL_{cr}$.

In renal failure it is still necessary to maintain the same average steady state concentration $\bar{C}$ during the dosage interval $\tau$ as in normal renal function.

$$\bar{C} = \frac{FA}{Vk\tau}$$

(where A = dose, F = bioavailability fraction).

The analogous equation for renal failure will be

$$\bar{C} = \frac{\hat{F}\hat{A}}{\hat{V}\hat{k}\hat{\tau}}$$

If no change in F or V occurs in renal failure (ie $\hat{F} = F$; $V = \hat{V}$) then

$$\frac{A}{k\tau} = \frac{\hat{A}}{\hat{k}\hat{\tau}}$$

This equation implies two ways to adjust dosage in renal impairment:

(i) keep dose interval the same but alter dose — if $\tau = \hat{\tau}$ then

$$\frac{A}{k} = \frac{\hat{A}}{\hat{k}}$$

and

$$\hat{A} = \frac{A.\hat{k}}{k}$$

(ii)  keep dose the same but alter dose interval — if A = Â then

$$\hat{\tau} = \frac{k.\tau}{\hat{k}}$$

It is thus necessary to determine the ratio of elimination rate constants of normal and renally impaired patients. An estimate of k can be gained by direct measurement or more usually by methods involving creatinine clearance (see above).

These methods assume:
(i)  linear pharmacokinetics
(ii)  no active metabolites whose retention in renal failure could change drug effects
iii  unaltered Vd, e.g. protein binding unaltered
iv  unchanged fraction of dose is absorbed
v  pharmacodynamic response is unchanged in renal failure.
These may not always hold.

*Note on $T_{\frac{1}{2}}$ in renal failure*
Since

$$T_{\frac{1}{2}} = \frac{0.693}{k}$$

the relationship between $T_{\frac{1}{2}}$ and creatinine clearance is

$$T_{\frac{1}{2}} = \frac{0.693}{k_r + k_{nr}}$$

$$= \frac{0.693}{\alpha\, CL_{cr} + k_{nr}}$$

This is the equation of a hyperbola.

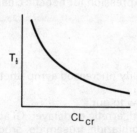

Thus simpler linear relationship between k and $CL_{cr}$ is used to modify dosage regimes.

Because $T_{\frac{1}{2}}$ determines rate at which plateau is approached if it is prolonged a loading dose (L) will be needed to reach steady state quickly. For most drugs L is same as in normals and L = C̄.V.W., where C̄ = desired average plasma drug concentration, V = apparent volume of distribution (l/kg), W = patients weight (kg).

**Pharmacodynamic changes**
Remember some drug effects, without importance in normal renal function, may become significant in renal failure, e.g. tetracycline, glucocorticoids (raise urea due to anti-anabolic effects); carbenoxolone, phenylbutazone and some other NSAIDS (salt and water retention).

Benzodiazepines, barbiturates, phenothiazines and opiates produce greater CNS depression in renal failure.

**Dialysis**
Drugs (like waste products) are removed by diffusion across the artificial dialysis membrane into the dialysis fluid. Factors affecting drug dialyzability are:
1. Molecular weight: MW < 500 easily dialyzed, above this it becomes increasingly less effective.
2. Protein binding: dialysis is passive so tightly bound drugs not removed.
3. Polarity: fat-soluble (polar) drugs, e.g. glutethimide are not dialysed.
4. Apparent volume of distribution: widely distributed drugs, e.g. digoxin, imipramine, dialysed more slowly because rate-limiting factor is rate of entry of blood into dialyzer. Drugs which are concentrated in tissues are difficult to remove by dialysis.

Dialysis clearance = Rate of blood flow to dialyzer

$$= \frac{(Ca - Cv)}{Ca}$$

Ca = arterial drug concentration (entering dialyzer)
Cv = venous drug concentration (leaving dialyzer)
(Note similarly to expression for hepatic clearance)

**CARDIAC FAILURE**

**A. Absorption**
  (i) Reduced gut mobility (increased sympathetic activity)
 (ii) ? Mucosal oedema
(iii) Reduced blood flow to gut.
May result in reduced, erratic or delayed GI absorption of some drugs, e.g. hydrochlorothiazide, frusemide, procainamide.

**B. Distribution**
Reduced tissue blood flow changes distribution; little information on protein binding: prazosin binding decreased.

Apparent volume of distribution (V) reduced for quinidine, lignocaine, procainamide. May result in higher concentration in blood (and, due to preservation of flow, CNS) owing to reduced perfusion of other tissues. May result in higher toxicity. Frusemide

V increased and becomes less effective because lower urine concentration (effect related to urine conc.). Thus variable diuretic efficacy in heart failure.

## C. Metabolism
(i) Blood flow to liver falls in proportion to cardiac output.
(ii) Hepatic metabolic capacity reduced by hepatocellular damage due to hypoperfusion or congestion and hypoxaemia with reduced oxygen supply for microsomal enzymes.

May result in higher levels with increased toxicity of drugs with high extraction ratio, e.g. lignocaine (where toxic metabolites monoethylglycine xylidide and glycine xylidide also accumulate); propranolol; theophylline. N.B. reduced clearance requires a reduced administration rate.

## D. Excretion
Renal clearance affected by
(i) decreased glomerular filtration rate resulting from hypoperfusion.
(ii) increased reabsorption due to altered intrarenal blood flow.

Examples: procainamide (longer $T_{\frac{1}{2}}$ and greater fraction metabolised to active metabolite N-acetylprocainamide which also accumulates since it is largely renally eliminated); digoxin.

## HEPATIC DISEASE

Liver plays central role in drug elimination but liver disease produces effects on drug disposition which are often difficult to interpret. This is because:

a. 'Liver disease' is an assortment of different pathologies with different functional effects e.g.

| Disease | Hepatic blood flow | Hepatocellular mass | Hepatocyte function |
|---|---|---|---|
| Cirrhosis | | | |
| — moderate | ↓ | Unchanged | Unchanged |
| — severe | ↓ ↓ | ↓ | ↓ |
| Viral hepatitis | Unchanged or ↑ | Unchanged or ↓ | ↓ |
| Alcoholic hepatitis | Unchanged or ↓ | Variable | ↓ |

Pathophysiological status varies widely within each diagnostic category and there is no test analogous to creatinine clearance which characterises hepatic performance.

b. Patients usually receive multiple drug therapy which interacts with the hepatic functional state, e.g. enzyme induction may improve hepatic clearance of other drugs.

c. Dysfunction in other organ systems, e.g. hepato-renal syndrome may confound interpretation.

d. Patients may have altered nutritional status either self-generated (alcoholism) or therapeutic (protein-restriction) which alter drug disposition.

Changes in $T_{\frac{1}{2}}$ are particularly difficult to interpret since

$$T_{\frac{1}{2}} = \frac{0.693\ V}{CL_{Hepatic} + CL_{Extrahepatic}}$$

and V is partly determined by plasma protein binding (see p. 50) and $CL_{hepatic}$ depends both on hepatic blood flow and intrinsic clearance (see p. 22). Clearance is more useful because $T_{\frac{1}{2}}$ does not distinguish relative contribution of V and CL also clinically significant changes in V and CL may offset one another and remain unrecognised if only $T_{\frac{1}{2}}$ is measured.

Effects of liver disease may result from:

## A. Changes in intrinsic free drug clearance ($CL_{int}$)
Antipyrine is almost totally metabolised, has E of only 0.07, is essentially unbound to plasma protein, distributes in body water and is a useful marker for hepatic metabolism. Its clearance is reduced in cirrhosis and viral hepatitis. Other examples of reduced intrinsic clearance:

*Cirrhosis*: theophylline, amylobarbitone, diazepam, nordiazepam, chlordiazepoxide (but not lorazepam).
*Hepatitis*: diazepam, chlordiazepoxide (but not lorazepam or oxazepam), hexobarbitone. But no effect on warfarin, phenytoin, tolbutamide.

Thus not all drugs equally affected, i.e. selective impairment of different metabolic routes occurs in different diseases. Some routes, e.g. glucuronidation, apparently less sensitive to pathological changes than others.

## B. Changes in hepatic blood flow
Clearance of highly extracted drugs depends upon hepatic blood flow so changes in hepatic haemodynamics alter their elimination and contribute to impaired lignocaine and propranolol clearance in cirrhosis. Alteration in flow patterns may also occur with *intra- and extra-hepatic shunting* of blood away from metabolising liver cells (so-called 'intact hepatocyte' theory) and 60% or more of portal blood can be diverted from functioning hepatocytes. This can alter hepatic first-pass metabolism (see p. 22) after oral drug administration. Most significant with highly extracted drugs, e.g. reduced first pass extraction from 0.9 to 0.8 doubles the amount of available drug. These effects contribute to increased bioavailability in cirrhosis of chlormethiazole (10 × increase); pethidine, pentazocine, labetalol, propranolol. N.B. since hepatic elimination of these drugs is also impaired, oral administration accentuates this impairment.

### C. Changes in plasma and tissue binding

Albumin and other drug binding plasma proteins are mainly synthesised in the liver, so liver disease can alter the fraction of unbound drug ($f_B$) in the blood. Demonstrated in cirrhosis with diazepam, chlordiazepoxide, lorazepam, phenytoin, propranolol, phenylbutazone, quinidine, tolbutamide. Mainly due to reduced albumin but possibly endogenous ligands increased in liver disease compete for binding.

Cannot also exclude possibility of abnormal binding protein structure.

Protein binding only determines hepatic extraction for drugs with high affinity for plasma proteins (binding > 85% at therapeutic concentrations) and low intrinsic clearance relative to hepatic blood flow ($f_B CL_{int} < Q/4$). Overall effects difficult to predict: if $f_B$ increases without much change in $CL_{int}$ then hepatic clearance increases (since drug metabolism $\propto f_B$), e.g. warfarin, phenytoin. If as well as reduced binding (increased $f_B$) there is simultaneous reduction in $CL_{int}$ the increased free drug concentration compensates for impaired metabolism and plasma concentrations remain virtually unchanged (e.g. diazepam, chlordiazepoxide, tolbutamide in cirrhosis) or exceed the metabolic capacity so the free drug concentration rises (e.g. phenytoin, prednisolone, diazepam have higher incidence of adverse reactions with 'normal' total plasma drug concentrations in cirrhosis). In acute viral hepatitis the free fraction of tolbutamide exceeds the reduction in $CL_{int}$ and $CL_{hepatic}$ is greater than in health with resulting lower plasma levels.

Increased free drug fraction results in increased $V_d$ (see p. 9) which changes $T_{\frac{1}{2}}$ e.g. propranolol ($T_{\frac{1}{2}} \uparrow \times 8$; $V_d \uparrow \times 2$; Cl $\downarrow$ 0.6); chloramphenicol ($T_{\frac{1}{2}} \uparrow \times 2$; $V_d \uparrow$ 0.6; Cl unchanged).

*Ascites* alters drug distribution, e.g. propranolol $V_d$ increased 2-fold in cirrhosis with ascites as compared to cirrhosis without ascites.

### D. Altered drug responsiveness

Changes in cerebral sensitivity to CNS depressant drugs and the need to avoid these and other drugs must be recalled (see p. 233).

*Clinical implications*

Conventional liver function tests have poor predictive function in relation to drug metabolism. Best warning indicators are low serum albumin (< 30 g/l) and/or increased prothrombin time. Fortunately the liver has remarkable functional reserves and damage is usually severe before important changes occur and even then these are usually no greater than 2 or 3-fold. Some individuals may show greater effects but the inter-patient variability in drug effects is often greater than this in the absence of liver disease.

Few generalisations can be made about drug handling in liver disease:
1. Often no need to modify drug regimes specifically because of liver disease: more important to be aware of dangers and to react appropriately using plasma level monitoring and/or clinical skills.
2. Avoid known hepatotoxic drugs.
3. Use drugs eliminated via non-hepatic routes.
4. Avoid drugs requiring hepatic activation, e.g. prednisone.

## RESPIRATORY DISEASE

Changes in plasma protein binding of drugs may occur if $\alpha_1$ acid glycoprotein levels change.

Hypoxia may reduce activity of hepatic oxidative metabolism and also hepatic blood flow. Renal blood flow may also fall, especially in cor pulmonale.

### A. Absorption
Delayed or incomplete oral absorption reported for penicillins in newborns with respiratory distress and for procainamide in adults.

### B. Distribution
Decreased V of antipyrine but little known.

### C. Metabolism and excretion
Increased half-lives reported for some drugs, e.g. antipyrine, theophylline, amikacin, ampicillin. Reduced half-life for tolbutamide in asthma but increased in hypoxic patients with pulmonary fibrosis. Increased clearance of methicillin and dicloxacillin in cystic fibrosis suggests increased renal tubular secretion.

## THYROID DISEASE

### A. Absorption
Intestinal transit time decreased by hyperthyroidism, increased by hypothyroidism, e.g. riboflavine (absorbed by specific, saturable carrier so increased absorption by prolonged contact with absorptive sites) — increased absorption in hypothyroidism, decreased absorption in hyperthyroidism; paracetamol — faster absorption in thyrotoxicosis (absorption rate related to gastric emptying time), reduced in hypothyroidism; digoxin bioavailability sometimes reduced in hyperthyroidism.

### B. Distribution
Little evidence for changes in protein binding in general but propranolol binding reduced in hyperthyroidism. Haemodynamic changes could alter apparent volume of distribution, e.g. V of

propranolol increased in hyperthyroidism. In hyperthyroidism increased tissue $Na^+ K^+$ ATP'ase activity may account for increased V and relative resistance to actions of digoxin and converse effects in hypothyroidism. Hepatic synthesis of sex hormone binding proteins for testosterone and oestrogen is raised. The converse is true in hypothyroidism.

## C. Metabolism

Hepatic microsomal enzyme activity increased by hyperthyroidism and decreased by hypothyroidism; cardiac output and hepatic blood flow raised in hyperthyroidism and reduced in hypothyroidism. Changes in hepatic drug metabolism may thus occur but cannot be predicted, e.g. antipyrine (clearance increased in hyperthyroidism, reduced in hypothyroidism — almost entirely due to changes in enzyme activity); methimazole (increased metabolism in hyperthyroidism); propranolol (increased metabolism in hyperthyroidism — mainly due to changes in hepatic blood flow); corticosteroids (increased clearance in hyperthyroidism).

No effects on phenytoin or propylthiouracil found.

## D. Excretion

Reduced renal blood flow in hypothyroidism; increase in hyperthyroidism, e.g. practolol (reduced elimination rate in hypothyroidism); digoxin (reduced elimination may contribute to digoxin sensitivity of hypothyroidism).

*Note*: Pharmacodynamic changes may be responsible for altered drug sensitivity in thyroid disease, e.g. warfarin potentiated in hyperthyroidism due to increased catabolism of factors II, VII, IX and X.

## GASTRO-INTESTINAL DISEASE

Rarely major effect on absorption, e.g. protein losing enteropathy, other aspects of pharmacokinetics altered. Some examples:

| *Gastro-intestinal factor* | *Drug whose absorption is altered* |
|---|---|
| 1. Achlorhydria (also alters rate of stomach emptying). | ↓ — aspirin, cephalexin<br>↑ — benzylpenicillin |
| 2. Gastrectomy | ↓ — levodopa, quinidine, ethambutol, sulphonamides, iron<br>↑ — digoxin |
| 3. Coeliac disease | ↓ — amoxycillin, pivampicillin, thyroxin<br>↑ — cephalexin, clindamycin, sulphamethoxazole, trimethoprim, propranolol |

4. Crohn's disease          ↑ — sulphamethoxazole
                            — propranolol
                            Delayed peak trimethoprim
                            & lincomycin

5. Pancreatic disease       ↓ — Vitamins A, D, K;
                            cephalexin;
                            phenoxymethylpenicillin

*Note*:  Malabsorption syndromes, coeliac disease etc. have
variable and unpredictable effects on drug absorption. Treatment
may alter response, e.g. phenoxymethylpenicillin absorption
decreased in untreated coeliac disease but normal after 8 months
gluten-free diet.

# Adverse drug reactions & interactions

**Adverse drug reactions**: unintended effects of substances used in prevention, diagnosis or treatment of disease.
Occur in — 10–15% hospital in-patients
— 40% patients in general practice
Responsible for 3–5% hospital admissions.
 1 in 1000 medical in-patients in USA may die as consequence but only 1 in 10 is preventable.
 Rational use of the *minimum number of drugs* per patient is simplest way to avoid adverse drug effects.

## Thompson/Rawlins Classification

|  | Type A | Type B |
|---|---|---|
| Pharmacology | Augmented | Bizarre |
| Predictable | Yes | No |
| Dose-dependent | Yes | No |
| Morbidity | High | Low |
| Mortality | Low | High |

*Examples:*

|  | Type A | Type B |
|---|---|---|
| Phenytoin | Sedation, Cerebellar signs; Enzyme induction. | Rashes; Pseudolymphoma. |
| Amitriptyline | Anticholinergic effects; Sedation; Sensitivity to pressor amines. | Hepatotoxicity. |

*Type A reactions* — in individuals lying at extremes of dose-response curve, occur for 3 reasons:
 (i) Pharmaceutical — differences in bioavailability of preparations produce effects in the predisposed.
 (ii) Pharmacokinetic — individual differences in absorption, distribution, metabolism, excretion result in toxicity.
 (iii) Pharmacodynamic — individual differences in target organ susceptibility.

*Type B reactions* — qualitatively abnormal effects apparently unrelated to drug's known pharmacology occur for 3 reasons:
  (i) Pharmaceutical — idiosyncratic response to non-drug components of drug products, e.g. tartrazine (yellow food dye: asthma), lactose (GI intolerance) or storage degradation products, e.g. of tetracycline (renal tubular damage).
 (ii) Pharmacokinetic — theoretical possibility of formation of novel metabolites or of antigenic complexes.
(iii) Pharmacodynamic — altered target organ responses, e.g. G6PD deficiency, porphyria, allergic responses to drugs which are not intrinsically antigenic.
*Drug interactions* — pharmacological responses which cannot be explained by the action of a single drug but are due to two or more drugs acting simultaneously.
May be harmful by
 (i) increasing toxicity
(ii) decreasing efficacy
OR
beneficial by allowing reduction of dose by enhanced efficacy without increased toxicity.
OR
harmless.

*Incidence*
— increased by number of drugs taken, e.g. with 2–5 drugs 19% incidence of potential interactions; with 6+ drugs incidence is 80+ %.
— occur in 0.5–2% hospital in-patients.
— significance of such figures in clinical practice difficult to determine: not every patient at risk is affected; many isolated case reports exist without validation.

## Mechanisms of interactions
1. *Pharmaceutical incompatibility outside the body.*
2. *Pharmacokinetic*
(i) *Drug absorption* — examples:

| Mixture | Mechanism | Effect |
|---|---|---|
| Tetracycline + $Ca^{++}$, $Fe^{++}$, $Al^{+++}$, $Mg^{++}$ | Chelation | Mutually reduced absorption |
| Griseofulvin + Phenobarbitone | ? | Reduced griseofulvin absorption |
| Anticoagulants } + Cholestyramine Thyroxine | Binding to resin | Reduced drug absorption |

(ii) *Drug distribution* — displacement from protein binding often suggested as cause of interaction but rarely proven. In some cases, e.g. phenylbutazone + warfarin interaction, inhibition of warfarin metabolism seems more likely. Suggested displacement interactions include:

| Bound drug | Displacing drug | Result |
|---|---|---|
| Bilirubin | Sulphonamides | Kernicterus |
| | Vitamin K | |
| Tolbutamide | Salicylates | Hypoglycaemia |
| | Phenylbutazone | |
| Warfarin | Salicylates | Haemorrhage |
| | Trichloroacetic acid | |
| | Clofibrate | |

Altered drug uptake at site of action:

| Primary drug | Inhibiting drug | Effect of interaction |
|---|---|---|
| Guanethidine | Tricyclic | Reduction of |
| Bethanidine | antidepressants; | hypotensive effect |
| Debrisoquine | Phenothiazines, | |
| Clonidine | especially | |
| | Chlorpromazine | |
| Phenylephrine | Tricyclic | Potentiation of |
| Adrenaline | antidepressants; | pressor effect of |
| Noradrenaline | Guanethidine. | catecholamines |

(iii) *Drug metabolism* — enzyme induction by increasing drug inactivation may produce tolerance or completely nullify drug action. Examples include:

| Primary drug | Inducing agent | Effect of interaction |
|---|---|---|
| Oral anticoagulants | Barbiturates | Decreased |
| e.g. warfarin | Glutethimide | anticoagulation |
| | Dichloralphenazone | |
| | Rifampicin | |
| Tolbutamide | Phenytoin | Decreased |
| | Alcohol | hypoglycaemia |
| | Chlorpromazine | |
| Oral contraceptives | Phenobarbitone | Pregnancy |
| Prednisone and | Barbiturates | Reduced steroid levels |
| Dexamethasone | | |
| Doxycycline | Barbiturates | Reduced doxycycline levels |
| Quinidine | Phenytoin | Reduced quinidine levels |
| | Barbiturates | |

Alternatively some drugs may act as enzyme inhibitors and raise the concentration of concurrently administered drugs. Examples:

| Primary drug | Inhibiting drug | Effect of interaction |
|---|---|---|
| Phenytoin | Isoniazid<br>Phenobarbitone<br>Phenylbutazone<br>Chloramphenicol<br>Disulfiram | Phenytoin intoxication |
| Oral anticoagulants<br>e.g. warfarin | Allopurinol<br>Nortriptyline<br>Quinidine | Haemorrhage |
| Tolbutamide<br>Chlorpropamide | Phenylbutazone<br>Chloramphenicol<br>Dicoumarol | Hypoglycaemia |
| 6-mercaptopurine<br>Azathioprine | Allopurinol | Bone marrow suppression |

(iv) *Drug excretion*: may be changed by drugs which alter urinary pH (see Chapter 1).

Alternatively drugs may compete for active renal tubular secretion — examples:

| Primary drug | Competing drug | Effect of interaction |
|---|---|---|
| Penicillin | Probenecid | Increased penicillin blood level |
| Methotrexate | Salicylates<br>Sulphonamides | Bone marrow suppression |
| Salicylate | Probenecid | Salicylate toxicity |
| Indomethacin | Probenecid | Indomethacin toxicity |
| Lithium | Thiazide diuretics | Lithium toxicity |
| Digoxin | Spironolactone | Increased plasma digoxin levels |

3. *Pharmacodynamic interactions* at drug receptor sites or by secondary physiological mechanisms. These may be **synergistic**:

| Primary drug | Interacts with | Resulting in |
|---|---|---|
| Alcohol | Other CNS depressant drugs e.g. barbiturates antihistamines narcotics | CNS depression |
| Tubocurarine | Aminoglycosides<br>Quinidine<br>Procaine | Prolonged paralysis |

| | | |
|---|---|---|
| Oral hypoglycaemic drugs | Salicylates Propranolol | Prolonged or excessive hypoglycaemia |
| Digitalis | Propranolol Guanethidine | Bradycardia due to unopposed vagal effects of glycoside |
| Antihypertensive drugs | Diuretics | Enhanced hypotension |

Or **antagonistic**:

| Primary drug | Interacts with | Resulting in |
|---|---|---|
| β-adrenoceptor agonist bronchodilator, e.g. salbutamol | β-adrenoceptor antagonist, e.g. propranolol | Antagonism of bronchodilator effects |
| Sulphonamides | Local anaesthetics hydrolysed to para-aminobenzoic acid, e.g. procaine | Antagonism of sulphonamide antimicrobial effects |
| Methotrexate | Folinic acid | Antagonism of toxic (and possibly antineoplastic) effects of methotrexate |
| Opiates | Naloxone | Reversal of opiate effects |
| Warfarin | Oestrogens | Warfarin effect antagonised by increased clotting factor synthesis |
| Hypotensive drugs | Non-steroidal anti-inflammatory agents | Antagonism of hypotensive effect due to sodium retention |

**Important drug-drug interactions**
Occur with drugs that have steep dose-response curve, i.e. small changes in dose produce large pharmacological effects:
   Anticoagulants
   Oral hypoglycaemic drugs
   Anticonvulsants
   Antiarrhythmics
   Cardiac glycosides
   Antihypertensives
   Drugs acting on the CNS, e.g. alcohol, MAOI

**Withdrawal reactions**
Adverse effects occurring in absence of causative drug. Examples:
1. Narcotic withdrawal syndrome (see p. 384).
2. Barbiturate, alcohol, benzodiazepine withdrawal syndrome (see p. 381)
3. Acute Addisonian crisis following discontinuation of chronic corticosteroid therapy.
4. Precipitation of angina or even myocardial infarction when β-adrenoceptor blocker abruptly stopped.
5. Paroxysmal hypertension and sympathetic overactivity when clonidine stopped.

**Drugs interacting with diagnostic laboratory tests**

| Test | Method | Drug | Effect on test |
|---|---|---|---|
| Catecholamines | Fluorimetry | Tetracyclines | Raised |
| | | Methyldopa | Raised |
| Cortisol | Sulphuric acid fluorescence | Fenfluramine | Raised |
| | | Spironolactone | Raised |
| Digoxin | Radio-immunoassay | Spironolactone | Reduced |
| Folic acid | Microbiological | Antibiotics | Invalidated |
| Ketones in urine | Ferric chloride | Salicylates | Positive |
| | | Chlorpromazine | |
| | | Sodium valproate | |
| | | Clioquinol | |
| Reducing substances in urine | Benedict's test or Clinitest | Nalidixic acid | Positive |
| | | Salicylates | |
| Vanillylmandelic acid in urine | Fluorescence | Methyldopa | Raised |
| Vitamin B$_{12}$ | Microbiological | Antibiotics | Invalidated |
| Blood grouping & compatibility testing | Agglutination | High molecular weight dextrans; Methyldopa; Mefenamic acid | Invalidated (rouleaux formation) |
| Urate | Spectrophoto-metric | Paracetamol | Raised |

# Drug development and adverse reaction monitoring

## DRUG DEVELOPMENT

Takes up to 10 years.
Costs approximately $30–50 million to develop new drug to marketing stage.

### Pre-clinical development
Research policy decision

↓

Synthesis of new chemical entities (NCE) based on:
  (i) random synthesis of new compounds
 (ii) structural variation of compounds with known pharmacological activity
(iii) biochemical or pharmacological insight
 (iv) chance findings ('serendipity')
                    if active compound found

↓

Animal pharmacology to:
  (i) define pharmacology
 (ii) define toxicity
     (a) short term studies in at least two species, one not being a rodent
     (b) reproductive and teratology studies
     (c) mutagenicity and carcinogenicity studies

### Clinical development
About 1 in 1000 NCE reach this stage
  If decided to proceed with development, studies along several lines:
a. Pharmaceutical — stability
                  — formulation
                  — compatibility with other tablet/infusion ingredients

b.  Pharmacological — further chronic animal toxicity
                    — initial animal metabolic and
                       pharmacokinetic studies
                    — development of assay

c.  Clinical pharmacology studies divided into four phases:

*Phase I* — first time into man to determine actions, pharmacokinetics and toxicology.
 (i) Ethical committee permission required but if in volunteers CSM is not involved.
(ii) Usually fully-informed normal volunteers but if drug likely to be toxic, e.g. anti-cancer agent, then patients with poor prognosis may volunteer.
(iii) Dose ranging single rising dose study beginning with 1/50 to 1/100 the effective dose in animals and increasing until desired effect or toxicity found. Extensive biochemical, haematological and physiological tests conducted.
(iv) If (iii) satisfactory followed by chronic (7–14 day) administration
(v) Usually carried out in only one centre with resuscitation facilities available by clinical pharmacologists with expertise in such studies. Nevertheless procedure in experienced hands is safe: one clinically significant medical event every 9600 days of subject exposure in one 10-year study of Phase I experiments.

*Phase II* — is drug therapeutically useful?
  Requires Clinical Trial Certificate (CTC) or Exemption (CTE) from CSM as well as Ethical Committee permission.
 (i) Initially open, uncontrolled, dose-ranging studies in volunteer patients. Later controlled studies under single-or double-blind conditions with comparisons with inert placebo or standard drugs are included.
(ii) Conducted in several centres by clinical pharmacologists and/or specialists.
(iii) Involve perhaps 100–500 patients only.

*Phase III* — larger trials to compare new drug with existing ones. To establish profile of efficacy and toxicity.
  Requires CTC/CTE and Ethical Committee permission.
 (i) Many centres and/or multi-centre.
(ii) Double-blind, placebo or active drug controlled trials commonly used. Patients must be informed of participation in trial and given full details.
(iii) Mainly conducted by specialists in hospitals or out-patients.
(iv) Involves 250–2000 patients only.

*Phase IV* — information from all studies received by Committee on Safety of Medicines (CSM). If satisfied product licence issued and data sheet (which details licensed indications for use) agreed with manufacturer.

Once product licence issued drug may be advertised and sold for prescription. Until this stage manufacturer cannot do either but in Phase III sometimes possible for doctor to use new drug in specific patient ('named patient basis') notified to CSM. About 1 in 20 drugs entering Phase I reach Phase IV, accounting for cost of drug development.

**Drug regulation in UK**
Ministers of Health and Agriculture (for veterinary products) responsible for administration of Medicines Act (1968) are advised by (amongst others):
a.  Committee on Safety of Medicines (CSM)
b.  Committee on Review of Medicines — to review all marketed
    medicines
c.  British Pharmacopoeia Committee — draw up new editions
The drug regulatory body is part of the Department of Health & Social Security and has the structure:

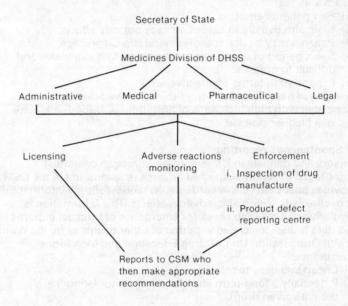

**Adverse reaction monitoring**

Continued surveillance is required even after grant of a product licence since on release of a drug only common, short-term and obvious adverse effects will have been discovered because at most only 2000–5000 individuals will have received the drug. Thus detection of events with incidence < 1 in 1000 unlikely.

Number of patients required to detect 1, 2, or 3 cases of an adverse reaction (assuming no 'background' incidence):

| Incidence of adverse reaction | No. of patients required to detect | | |
|---|---|---|---|
| | 1 case | 2 cases | 3 cases |
| 1 in 200 | 600 | 960 | 1 300 |
| 1 in 2000 | 6 000 | 9 600 | 13 000 |
| 1 in 10 000 | 30 000 | 48 000 | 65 000 |

NB: Chloramphenicol induced bone marrow aplasia occurs about 1 in 20 000.

Mechanisms for discovery of adverse effects include:

## 1. Formal clinical trials

Advantages:
 (i) Close observation of individual patients.
 (ii) Formal protocol for recording effects.
 (iii) Allows assessment of incidence of effects.

Disadvantages:
 (i) Few patients enrolled.
 (ii) Main aim usually to assess efficacy not side effects.
 (iii) Patients may be atypical of general clinical practice.
 (iv) Short period of observation, long-term trials expensive and difficult to organise.
 (v) Expensive in terms of effectiveness.

Example of use: Coronary Drug Project showed clofibrate associated with high incidence of arrhythmias, thrombophlebitis and gall bladder disease.

## 2. Spontaneous reporting

Doctors and dentists in UK (and other European countries) encouraged to report suspected adverse reactions. In UK the CSM provides post-paid yellow cards which request simple information from clinicians concerning adverse effects. This information is regularly scrutinised to check for emergence of unusual patterns and data is also correlated with that of other countries by the World Health Organization Unit of Drug Education and Monitoring.

Advantages:
 (i) Cheap and easy to manage.
 (ii) Potentially a long-term study of a huge population (i.e. all patients given drug).

Disadvantages:
 (i) Under-reporting (much less than 10% of all reactions are detected and reported).
 (ii) Unable to yield incidence estimates since size of population at risk unknown.
 (iii) Not a uniformly sampled population and data may be unrepresentative. Liable to 'band-wagon' effects, i.e.

well-known effects over-reported but unsuspected or bizarre events go unrecorded.
(iv) Not been very successful in reporting previously unsuspected effects.

*Example of use*: Withdrawal of ibufenac from UK after reports of liver damage.

### 3. Vital statistics
Review of epidemiological data from death certificates, hospital discharge summaries etc. to look for unexpected trends or effects.
Advantages:
(i) Potentially a large scale chronic study of drug effects.
(ii) Could be relatively cheap.
(iii) Unbiased by pre-conceived hypotheses.
Disadvantages:
(i) Most of the necessary data (like drug exposure) is not presently accessible.
(ii) Slow and cumbersome in present practice.
(iii) Does not establish causality of relationship.

*Example of use*: Linkage of sudden death with use of isoprenaline bronchodilator aerosol inhalation.

### 4. Case control studies
Drug history of patients with disease compared to that of control population.
Advantage:
(i) Easier and cheaper than following the necessarily much larger population only some of whom will develop reaction.
Disadvantages:
(i) Difficult in practice because danger of bias in selection of control due to a priori hypothesis.
(ii) Gives relative risk but not an incidence of effects.
(iii) Does not establish causal effect of drug.

*Example of use*: Association of lincomycin exposure with pseudomembranous colitis.

### 5. Monitored release and post-marketing surveillance
Aim is to follow a large cohort (say 10 000) patients given new drug for long period (> 1 year). Use mainly confined to new drugs but potentially also for older drugs especially in high risk groups, e.g. old, renal failure.
Advantages:
(i) Acute and chronic effects monitored.
(ii) Cheaper than a long-term clinical trial.
(iii) Gives assessment of incidence.
Disadvantages:
(i) Difficult to maintain integrity of patient group.
(ii) Lacks a control group for comparison since in long-term studies other factors, e.g. nutrition, radiation levels, may also change.

## 6. Intensive monitoring

Can be of variable intensity from analysis of hospital records (e.g. Aberdeen-Dundee Monitoring system) to use of special wards with personnel exclusively for monitoring drug effects and use complementary to usual management team (e.g. Boston Collaborative Drug Surveillance Program). Data collected is stored on computer and regularly examined for trends and associations.

Advantages:

 (i) No a priori hypothesis therefore no bias.

 (ii) Can detect unexpected effects.

 (iii) All possible information stored so incidence, associated factors, e.g. age, sex, electrolyte status, can be extracted.

Disadvantages:

 (i) Expensive

 (ii) Relatively small scale studies so only common reactions will be detected.

 (iii) Only acute effects monitored.

 (iv) Patient sample restricted and could be unrepresentative.

*Example of use*: Link of ethacrynic acid with gastro-intestinal bleeding especially when given i.v. to females, with high blood urea who had previously received heparin.

## General comments

 1. All drugs are dangerous — in general, drugs without side-effects are also without any effects, good or bad.
 2. For most drugs there is insufficient information to provide a risk-benefit analysis. Ask advice from senior doctors if in doubt and build up your experience by getting to know a restricted range of drugs.
 3. Drugs should only be used when there are clear indications and no alternatives.
 4. Always take a drug history.
 5. Restrict the number of drugs prescribed to the minimum.
 6. Regularly review the need for chronic medication.
 7. Clearly record what drugs are prescribed, their dose and frequency for the benefit of others who may look after the patient.
 8. Exercise special care in the use of certain groups of drugs (see earlier) and in the young, the elderly, and patients with organ impairment.
 9. Contribute to knowledge of drugs by reporting on a yellow card cases where an adverse effect occurs on drug therapy.
 10. Keep the patient informed about the treatment and what he may expect from it.

# Drugs for psychiatric and CNS disease

**Antidepressants**

Tricyclics: iminodibenzyls
            dibenzocycloheptenes
            anxiolytic tricyclics
Tetracyclics
Miscellaneous compounds (e.g. viloxazine, nomifensine)
Monoamine oxidase inhibitors (MAOI)
L-tryptophan
Thioxanthines (see p. 93)
Hormones (eg. L-triiodothyronine, TSH)
Lithium (see p. 83)

**Indications for tricyclic and related antidepressants**
endogenous depression — usually good response
neurotic depressive syndromes — usually poor response
schizo-affective syndromes — some patients respond well
phobic anxiety                           ⎫ clomipramine or
depression in obsessive compulsive disorders ⎬ imipramine are
                                             ⎭ used

atypical facial pain — usually good response
enuresis — imipramine used, not very successful

**Indications for specific drugs**
Depression plus:
  (i) CVS disease — use mianserin (or doxepin)
 (ii) Hypertension + adrenergic neurone blocking drugs like
       guanethidine — use mianserin or doxepin
(iii) Prostatism or glaucoma — use mianserin
(iv) Epilepsy — use nomifensine

**Table 3(a)** Tricyclic antidepressants — iminodibenzyls

| Drug | Amine structure | Action (all block NA & 5HT uptake) | Pharmacokinetics | Special clinical features |
|---|---|---|---|---|
| Imipramine (Tofranil, Berkomine) | Tertiary | Equally powerful inhibition of NA and 5HT uptake | $T_{\frac{1}{2}} = 4-8$ h Main metabolite is active — desipramine ($T_{\frac{1}{2}} = 12-25$ h) | Dose 25–300 mg o.n. Little or no sedation. Can cause insomnia. Powerful anticholinergic. |
| Desipramine (= desmethylimipramine = DMI) (Pertofran) | Secondary | Very powerful inhibitor of NA uptake. Little or no action on 5HT. | $T_{\frac{1}{2}} = 12-25$ h | Dose 25–300 mg o.n. Minimal sedation. Minimal anticholinergic. |
| Trimipramine (Surmontil) | Tertiary | Powerful inhibition of 5HT uptake. Some effect on NA and dopamine uptake. Demethyl metabolite mainly acts on NA uptake. | Demethyl metabolite is active | Dose 50–150 mg o.n. Very sedating. Moderate anticholinergic. |
| Clomipramine (Anafranil) | Tertiary | Powerful inhibition of 5HT uptake | Dose dependent kinetics. Steady state attained at 7 days. Active demethyl metabolite (steady state at 14 days). After a single dose detected in blood for 48 hours and in urine for 7 days. | Dose 10–150 mg o.n. Sedating. Postural hypotension. |

**Table 3(b)** Tricyclic antidepressants — dibenzocycloheptenes

| Drug | Amine structure | Action (all block NA & 5HT uptake) | Pharmacokinetics | Special clinical features |
|---|---|---|---|---|
| Amitriptyline (Tryptizol) | Tertiary | Powerful blockade of 5HT uptake. Some action on NA uptake. | $T_{\frac{1}{2}}$ = 8–20 h Active metabolite is nortriptyline ($T_{\frac{1}{2}}$ = 18–93 h) | Dose 25–150 mg o.n. Strongly sedating. Powerful anticholinergic. |
| Nortriptyline (Allegron, Aventyl) | Secondary | Powerful blockade of NA uptake. Some action on 5HT uptake. | $T_{\frac{1}{2}}$ = 18–93 h | Dose 25–150 mg o.n. Less sedating than amitriptyline. Weak anticholinergic. |
| Protriptyline (Concordin) | Secondary | | $T_{\frac{1}{2}}$ = 54–198 h | Dose 15–60 mg o.n. Less sedation, may be stimulant. Moderately anticholinergic. |
| Butriptyline (Evadyne) | Tertiary | Weak inhibitor of NA and 5HT uptake. | $T_{\frac{1}{2}}$ = 65–135 h (mainly metabolites) Much first pass metabolism | Dose 25–50 mg 8 hourly. |

**Table 3(c)** Tricyclic antidepressants — anxiolytic

| Drug | Dose | Pharmacokinetics | Special clinical features |
|---|---|---|---|
| Doxepin (Sinequan) | 50–150 mg o.n. | $T_{\frac{1}{2}}$ = 8–20 h. Active metabolite — desmethyldoxepin ($T_{\frac{1}{2}}$ = 33–81 h). Extensive (55–87%) first pass metabolism, but well absorbed from intestine. | Least adverse effects on CVS of tricyclics. Optimal antidepressant at plasma levels of desmethyldoxepin above 20 ng/ml. |
| Dothiepin (Prothiaden) | 75–200 mg o.n. | $T_{\frac{1}{2}}$ = 46–56 h. | Both these drugs are less powerful antidepressants than amitriptyline, but have a lower incidence of anticholinergic toxic effects. Also have benzodiazepine-like anxiolytic actions. |

**General properties of tricyclic antidepressants**
1. *Mode of action*
block of neuronal uptake$_1$ of NA, 5HT or dopamine (tertiary amines mainly block uptake of 5HT, secondary mainly NA)
2. *Pharmacological*
antagonise effects of reserpine and tetrabenazine
block tyramine induced hypertension
anticholinergic (especially tertiary amines)
receptor blocking (e.g. vasodilation in skin)
sympathomimetic (e.g. produce cardiac arrhythmias)
epileptogenic
slow EEG
3. *Pharmacokinetic*
well absorbed but variable and sometimes extensive 1st pass metabolism
some metabolites are active
relatively long $T_{\frac{1}{2}}$, but much individual variation
large volume of distribution (e.g. imipramine $V_d$ = 28–61 l/kg)
high plasma protein binding
4. *Response*
 (i) Optimal clinical response may occur within a range of plasma concentrations
 (ii) Clinical response usually delayed for 1–3 weeks
5. *A. Common toxic effects*
 (i) *Anticholinergic*: dry mouth, bad taste, blurred vision, glaucoma aggravated, hesitancy of micturition, impotence, delayed orgasm, constipation.
 (ii) *Cardiovascular*: postural hypotension (weak α-adrenergic blockers), palpitations. Overdose: supraventricular tachycardia, ventricular tachycardia, A-V block, bundle branch block, prolonged PR, QRS, QT intervals, T wave flattening, ST depression.
(iii) *CNS*: tremor, sedation (especially tertiary amines), headache, heavy sleep, disturbed sleep, restlessness, choreiform movements, myoclonus, paraesthesiae, driving accidents, withdrawal syndrome (anxiety, restlessness, insomnia, anorexia).
(iv) *Alimentary*: increased appetite, weight gain, anticholinergic effects.
*B. Uncommon toxic effects (important but rare effects italicised)*
 (i) *Anticholinergic*: paralytic ileus, oesophageal reflux, *acute retention.*
 (ii) *Cardiovascular*: *sudden death due to ventricular fibrillation,* cardiomyopathy, hypertension, atrial fibrillation, quinidine-like activity.

(iii) *CNS*: *epileptic seizures* (may alter drug requirement of known epileptics), nightmares, acute confusional psychosis, aggressive behaviour, Parkinsonism, ataxia, dysarthria, orofacial dyskinesia, nystagmus, peripheral neuropathy, tinnitus, hypomania.
(iv) *Alimentary*: cholestatic jaundice, hepatic necrosis, vomiting, diarrhoea, epigastric pain.
(v) *Metabolic & endocrine*: raised or lowered blood glucose, breast enlargement, galactorrhoea, raised plasma aminotransferases and alkaline phosphatase, testicular swelling.
(vi) *Haematological*: eosinophilia, leucopenia, thrombocytopenia.
(vii) *Allergic*: cholestatic jaundice, urticaria, cutaneous vasculitis, angioedema, photosensitivity dermatitis.
  C. *Contraindications*
(i) recent myocardial infarction; arrhythmias; cardiomyopathy
(ii) pregnancy
(iii) prostatic hypertrophy
(iv) glaucoma
(v) epilepsy
(vi) liver failure
(vii) renal failure
  D. *Drug interactions*
(i) increased sedation with central depressants including alcohol
(ii) MAOI: hypertension, hyperpyrexia, excitement, coma, cerebral haemorrhage, death
(iii) lithium: increased tremor
(iv) phenothiazines: increase sedation, hypotension, anticholinergic effects and cardiac arrhythmias
(v) stimulants (e.g. amphetamines): excitement, hypertension, hyperpyrexia, cardiac arrhythmias
(vi) increased anticholinergic effects with anticholinergics
(vii) abolition of hypotensive action of clonidine and adrenergic neurone blockers (e.g. debrisoquine, bethanidine)
(viii) possible rise in blood pressure with directly acting sympathomimetics
(ix) tricyclic plasma levels lowered by inducing agents (e.g. barbiturates)

**Points about newer antidepressants**
1. No claim for greater potency over tricyclics or MAOI.
2. Some have fewer side-effects and therefore may be better compliance.
3. Some (particularly mianserin, nomifensine) are safer in overdose but experience is relatively limited.
4. Generally more expensive than tricyclics or MAOI.

**Table 4** Antidepressants with tetracyclic and miscellaneous structures

| Drug | Structure | Mode of action | Pharmacokinetics | Special clinical features |
|---|---|---|---|---|
| Mianserin (Bolvidon, Norval) | True tetracyclic | Inhibition of prejunctional ($\alpha_2$) noradrenergic receptors. Some post-synaptic blockade of 5HT | $T_{\frac{1}{2}}$ 8–19 h. Well absorbed but bioavailability 30% due to 1st pass metabolism. 4–7% excreted unchanged. | Dose 30–80 mg o.n. Sedating, not sympathomimetic, not anticholinergic, not epileptogenic. Safe in overdose. Hypotension |
| Maprotilene (Ludiomil) | Tricyclic with additional methylene bridge i.e. tetracyclic | Inhibition reuptake NA. Some inhibition reuptake 5HT. | $T_{\frac{1}{2}}$ 27–58 h. Well absorbed Little 1st pass metabolism High protein binding | Dose: 25–75 mg o.n. Like other tricyclics: sympathomimetic, anticholinergic, epileptogenic. |
| Viloxazine (Vivalan) | Bicyclic (a phenoxymethyl tetrahydro-oxazine) | Inhibition of NA and 5HT uptake | $T_{\frac{1}{2}}$ 2–5 h. Rapid and complete absorption. Extensive & rapid metabolism. Not highly protein bound. | Dose: 50–100 mg 8-hourly. Similar actions to tricyclics but also CNS stimulation and nausea. |
| Nomifensine (Merital) | Three rings but is an aminomethylphenyltetrahydro-isoquinoline hydrogen maleinate | Powerful inhibition of NA and dopamine uptake. Some inhibition of 5HT uptake. | $T_{\frac{1}{2}}$ 1.5–2 h (prolonged up to 48 h in renal failure). Rapid and extensive metabolism. Mainly excreted in methoxy form. | Dose: 25–100 mg 8-hourly. Activating. Less cardiotoxic in overdose than tricyclics. Relatively free from anticholinergic and cardiac toxicity. |

| Iprindole (Prondol) | Similar structure to classical tricyclic but has an indole nucleus and cyclooctane ring | Central (but not peripheral) inhibition of NA uptake | $T_{\frac{1}{2}} = 10$ h Extensively metabolised prior to urinary excretion. | Dose: 30–60 mg 8-hourly. Weak sedative, weak anticholinergic. |
| Trazodone (Molipaxin) | Triazolepyridine | Low doses — 5HT antagonist High doses — blocks 5HT uptake and so agonist | $T_{\frac{1}{2}} = 3$–5 h. Complete oral absorption. Extensive metabolism to inactive compounds. | Dose: 50–200 mg 8-hourly. Sedating. Anxiolytic. Very weak anticholinergic and no potentiation of catecholamines so less cardiotoxicity than tricyclics. |

## MONOAMINE OXIDASE INHIBITORS

### General properties
Inhibit MAO and some other oxidases.
Increased intracerebral and peripheral neural stores of amines (including NA). Amine stores discharged by indirectly acting sympathomimetics and by reserpine. Increased $\alpha$ stimulation of the vasomotor centre which results in reflex hypotension.
Clinical response delayed up to 2–6 weeks. MAO is irreversibly inhibited so effects continue for about 2 weeks after stopping treatment.

### Uses
1. Some neurotic depressive syndromes
2. Endogenous depression which has failed to respond to tricyclic
3. Some forms of atypical facial pain
4. Anxiety with depression; phobic anxiety, obsessive–compulsive disorders.

### Toxic effects
1. Food interactions
2. Drug interactions
3. *NS* headaches, aggravation of migraine, drowsiness, stimulation, nightmares, tremor, weakness, paraesthesiae, peripheral neuropathy, muscle spasms, ataxia, fits, confusion, hallucinations, aggravation of schizophrenia and hypomania.
   *Autonomic effects*: dry mouth, hesitancy of micturition, retention of urine, constipation, blurred vision, impotence, impaired orgasm, postural hypotension, sweating.
4. Alimentary: anorexia, vomiting, hepatocellular damage.
5. Haematological: leucopenia.
6. Metabolic: weight gain, oedema, increased ADH secretion, hypoglycaemia.

### Food interactions
Foods containing amines (which can cause a hypertensive reaction): cheeses, meat and yeast extracts (e.g. Marmite), some wines (e.g. Chianti), and beers (e.g. Worthington, Bass), game, banana skins, broad bean pods, pickled herrings, green figs, roe products.

### Drug interactions
*1. Hypertensive reactions:*
 (i) indirectly acting sympathomimetics (e.g. amphetamines, ephedrine, phenylethylamine, metaraminol) and cocaine.
 (ii) less hypertensive reactions from directly acting sympathomimetics, e.g. adrenaline, noradrenaline, phenylephedrine.

**Table 5** Monoamine oxidase inhibitors

| Drug | Clinical features | Particular toxic effects |
|---|---|---|
| **(a) Hydrazines** | | |
| Iproniazid (Marsilid) | Effective, but use limited by toxicity Dose: 25 mg 12- or 8-hourly | High incidence of hepatotoxicity; peripheral neuropathy |
| Phenelzine (Nardil) | Most commonly used MAOI in depression Dose: 15 increasing up to 45 mg twice daily | Drowsiness |
| Isocarboxazid (Marplan) | Dose: 50 mg daily reducing to 10–20 mg daily | |
| **(b) Non-hydrazides** | | |
| Tranylcypromine (Parnate) | Stimulatory The most effective MAOI in depression Dose: 10–20 mg morning and afternoon | Euphoria, insomnia Amphetamine-like effects can lead to dependence and abuse. MAOI most commonly associated with hypertension. |
| Pargyline (Eutonyl) | Dose: 25–27 mg daily. Was used only for refractory hypertension. | Postural hypotension, impotence, insomnia, nightmares |

(iii) Levodopa
(iv) Tricyclics (but such very dangerous combinations used by specialists in small doses for refractory depression).
2. *Effects potentiated of:*
  (i) Narcotics
 (ii) Hypoglycaemics
(iii) Barbiturates and phenytoin
(iv) Ether, chloral, alcohol
 (v) Procaine
(vi) Hypotensives
(vii) Suxamethonium
3. *Excitement or confusion:*
  (i) anticholinergic, antiparkinsonian drugs (e.g. benztropine)
 (ii) reserpine, tetrabenazine, methyldopa

## LITHIUM

### Uses
*Established*:
1. Acute mania (improvement or remission in 70–80% patients)
2. Prophylactic in manic-depressive illness (cyclothymia)
3. Prophylactic in recurrent unipolar affective illness (depression or mania). As effective as tricyclics.
*Not yet established:*
1. Hyperactivity in children
2. Alcoholism
3. Inappropriate ADH secretion
4. Hyperthyroidism
5. Migranous neuralgia
6. To increase neutrophil count during cancer chemotherapy

### Pharmacokinetics
Readily absorbed from gut — peak plasma levels at 3–5 hours. $T_{\frac{1}{2}}$ = 18–20 h (up to 36 h in elderly) – becomes longer (50 + h) with prolonged therapy.
Not bound to plasma proteins.
Renal elimination: readily filtered at glomerulus; 75% reabsorbed in proximal tubules in competition with $Na^+$; no distal reabsorption.
Elimination accelerated by sodium; impaired by sodium deficiency and by diuretics because of competitive effects in proximal tubule.

## Administration

Oral only: as lithium carbonate once or twice daily (300 mg tablet = 8 mmol/l). Usually start at 600–900 mg daily, then adjust dose by weekly (up to 3600 mg) monitoring of plasma levels.

Response starts after 2–4 weeks in prophylaxis and 10 days in hypomania. Full benefit in 6–12 months.

(Slow release preparation (Priadel) 400 mg/tablet — peak level at 5–7 h).

## Therapeutic plasma levels

Mania 0.8–1.4 mmol/l 12 h after dose. Prophylaxis 0.4–0.8 mmol/l 12 h after dose. Check levels every 3 months.

## Toxic effects

*Dose dependent:*
0.8–1.2 mmol/l: mild tremor
1.5–3 mmol/l: tremor, ataxia, weakness, drowsiness, thirst, diarrhoea.
3–5 mmol/l: severe tremor, confusion, spasticity, convulsions, dehydration, coma, death.
Chronic renal damage related to high chronic dosage.

*Dose independent:*
1. Goitre, hypothyroidism (10%), hyperthyroidism (rare).
2. Nephrogenic diabetes insipidus (? Li inhibits ADH stimulation of adenyl cyclase), hyperaldosteronism.
3. Reversible ECG changes; cardiac arrhythmias.
4. Loss of bone calcium.
5. Weight gain.

*Drug interactions*
1. Thiazides, loop diuretics enhance lithium retention and toxicity.
2. Tardive dyskinesias and other extrapyramidal syndromes due to neuroleptics made commoner. (Lithium can be used with tricyclics & MAOI)
3. Earlier lithium plasma peak with metoclopramide
4. Delayed lithium plasma peak with anticholinergics

*Pregnancy*
1. ?Increased incidence of cardiovascular malformations particularly if given in first trimester.
2. Breast feeding contraindicated — Li excreted in milk.

## Miscellaneous substances used in depression

| Drug | Clinical use |
|------|-------------|
| L tryptophan (Optimax) | Not proved to be anti-depressive, but probably potentiates activity of MAOI and of tricyclics. $T_{\frac{1}{2}}$ = 2.7 h. Mildly sedating. Low toxicity. Dose 5–9 g daily. |
| L triiodothyronine, thyroxine & TSH | Possibly potentiates tricyclic antidepressants |
| Oestrogens | Efficacy not proven in intractable depression in women. |
| Pyridoxal phosphate (vitamin $B_6$) | Efficacy not proven in depression associated with taking contraceptive pill. |

## NEUROLEPTICS (MAJOR TRANQUILLISERS)

1. Reduce stimulation of dopamine receptors usually by receptor blockade.
2. Effective in excited psychotic states, hallucinations and delirium. Clinical potency correlates well with ability to block central dopamine receptors.

## Main actions of phenothiazine neuroleptics

*1. Central*
Anti-hallucinatory and anti-psychotic
Reduction in emotional responsiveness (ataractic state)
Sedation and reduction in attention span with slower learning
Anti-emetic, anti-hiccough
Produces extrapyramidal syndromes, but can reduce chorea
Aggravation of epilepsy
Hypothalamic inhibition:   reduced sympathetic outflow
                            loss of temperature control
                            increased prolactin release

*2. Peripheral*
α-adrenoceptor blockade
Anticholinergic
Local anaesthetic
Quinidine-like action on heart
Weak antihistamine ($H_1$)

## Role of dopamine in actions of neuroleptics

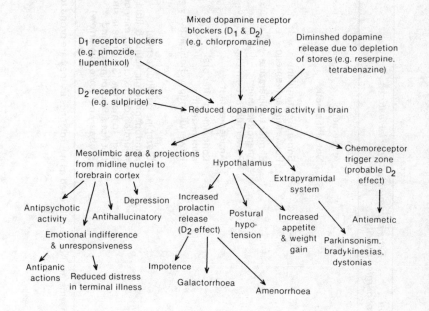

(Dopamine $D_1$ receptors: adenyl cyclase linked (like ß receptors)
Dopamine $D_2$ receptors: not linked with adenyl cyclase)

## Toxicity of the phenothiazine neuroleptics

1. Postural hypotension
2. Dry mouth, nasal stuffiness, failure of ejaculation, constipation, urinary retention, blurred vision
3. Sedation, drowsiness, confusion, depression, emotional inertia
4. Convulsions
5. Tremor, Parkinsonism, dystonia, dyskinesia, akathisia (motor restlessness), tardive dyskinesias
6. Cholestatic jaundice (2–4% of patients of chlorpromazine, especially during 2nd–4th week of treatment) — often associated with eosinophilia
7. Corneal and lens opacities, pigmentary retinopathy
8. Light sensitivity dermatitis and pigmentation, urticaria, oedema, maculopapular and petechial rashes
9. Raised cholesterol, impaired glucose tolerance
10. Leucopenia, thrombocytopenia (both very rare)
11. Cardiac arrhythmias, cardiac arrest
12. Oligomenorrhoea, amenorrhoea, gynaecomastia, galactorrhoea
13. Malignant syndrome (coma, autonomic disturbances)

Main types of neuroleptics

| Group | Sedation | α-blockade | Anti-cholinergic | Extra pyramidal toxicity | Special features |
|---|---|---|---|---|---|
| 1. Phenothiazines | | | | | |
|    a aliphatic side chains | ++ | ++ | ++ | ++ | Anti-emetic |
|    b. piperidine side chains | +++ | +++ | +++ | + | Not anti-emetic |
|    c piperazine side chains | + | + | + | +++ | Some are stimulant Powerfully anti-emetic |
| 2. Butyrophenones | + | + | + | +++ | Similar to piperazine phenothiazines Powerfully anti-emetic |
| 3. Thioxanthines | + → +++ | ++ | ++ | ++ | Antidepressant |
| 4. Diphenylbutylpiperidines | + | ± → + | ± | + | Long acting after oral administration Powerful antipsychotic activity |
| 5. Dihydroindoles | ++ | ± | | + | |
| 6. Dibenzodiazepines | + | | ++ | ± | Clozapine has little central antidopaminergic action & little neurological toxicity, but may be toxic to marrow (Sulpiride is similar but not anti-cholinergic and probably not toxic to marrow) |

(Depletors of cerebral amines such as reserpine and tetrabenazine are not usually used as neuroleptics as they are prone to produce depression)

    ± = very little
    + = mild
  ++ = moderate
+++ = considerable

**Table 6** Individual neuroleptic drugs

| Drug | Dose | Pharmacokinetics | Special uses apart from in psychoses |
|---|---|---|---|
| **1. Phenothiazines** **a. Aliphatic side chain** | | | |
| Chlorpromazine (cpz) (Largactil, Chloractil) | 100–2000 mg daily oral (can also be given i.m. and i.v. 25–100 mg). 100 mg p.r. | $T_{\frac{1}{2}} = 2-24$ h. $V_d = 22$ l/kg 30% bioavailability after oral administration. Incompletely absorbed. Completely absorbed after i.m. injection. 70 metabolites. Cpz and 7-OH are active, Cpz sulphoxide is inactive. | Anti-emetic, sedation in elderly and violent patients without causing stupor. Narcotic withdrawal. Anti-hiccough. |
| Promazine (Sparine) | 100–1500 mg daily oral 50 mg i.m. | | Not sufficiently active to be used in psychosis but useful tranquilliser — especially in old. |
| **b. Piperidine side chain** | | | |
| Thioridazine (Melleril) | 100–800 mg daily oral | $T_{\frac{1}{2}} = 10-36$ h. Active metabolite is mesoridazine. Prolonged $T_{\frac{1}{2}}$ in elderly. Metabolism slowed during sleep. | Useful for agitated old patients — maybe less extrapyramidal effects. |
| **c. Piperazine side chain** | | | |
| Trifluoperazine (Stelazine) | 2–6 mg daily oral 1–3 mg daily i.m. | | Tranquilliser in behavioural disturbance and psychoneuroses. |

**Table 6** (continued)

| Drug | Dose | Pharmacokinetics | Special uses apart from in psychoses |
|---|---|---|---|
| Prochlorperazine (Stemetil) | 5–50 mg daily oral 1–2 ml i.m. of 1.25% solution of mesylate. 5–25 mg p.r. | | Menieres disease Anti-emetic |
| Perphenazine (Fentazin) | 12 mg daily oral 5 mg 6-hourly i.m. | $T_{\frac{1}{2}} = 9$ h | Anti-emetic Anti-hiccough |
| 2. Butyrophenones | | | |
| Haloperidol (Haldol, Serenace) | 0.5–5 mg oral 8–12-hourly Up to 30 mg i.m. 6-hourly. | $T_{\frac{1}{2}} = 12$–38 h. Well absorbed, but 60% bioavailability. Metabolised to inactive products. 1st order elimination. Metabolism slowed during sleep. | Anaesthetic premed, withdrawal of narcotics, Gilles de la Tourette syndrome. Tranquillisation in acute behavioural disturbances, especially mania. |
| Benperidol (Angril, Anquil) | 0.25–1.5 mg daily oral. | | Deviant & antisocial sexual behaviour. |
| Droperidol (Droleptan) | 2–20 mg daily oral, 5–10 mg i.m. 5–15 mg i.v. | | Anaesthetic premed, antiemetic, given with narcotic for neuroleptanalgesia. |
| Trifluoperidol (Triperidol) | 0.5–2.5 mg daily oral. | | Tranquillisation in acute behavioural disturbances, especially mania. |

| Drug | Dose | | Indication |
|---|---|---|---|
| **3. Thioxanthines** | | | |
| Chlorprothixene (Taractan) | 50–100 mg daily oral. | | |
| Flupenthixol (Depixol) | Oral and i.m. | | Depression. |
| Clopenthixol (Clopixol) | i.m. | | |
| **4. Diphenylbutylpiperidines** | | | |
| Pimozide (Orap) | 2–20 mg daily oral. | $T_{\frac{1}{2}} = ?18$ h | |
| Fluspirilene (Redeptin) | Oral and i.m. | | |

N.B.
An analgesic phenothiazine, not used as an antipsychotic:

| | | |
|---|---|---|
| Methotrimeprazine (Nozinan) | 15–100 mg s.c., i.m., oral. | Severe pain including terminal illness. Anti-emetic. |

**Drug interactions with the phenothiazines**
1. Anticholinergic effects on gastro-intestinal tract affect absorption of paracetamol, levodopa, digoxin, lithium
2. Alcohol potentiates sedation
3. Effects of hypnotics and anxiolytics potentiated
4. Sedative, respiratory depressant and 'cortical' effects of narcotic analgesics potentiated
5. Potentiation of hypotensive drugs
6. Chlorpromazine is moderate enzyme inducer, but also inhibits the metabolism of tricyclic antidepressants

**Clinical uses of phenothiazines**
*Psychiatry*:
— schizophrenia
— hypomania
— delirium
— drug withdrawal (but not alcohol and hypnotics)
— panic attacks
*α-blockade:*
— shock
— hypertension — reactions with MAOI
Terminal illness
Anti-emetic, antihiccough, Meniere's disease
*Surgery:*
— premedication
— hypothermic techniques
— neuroleptanalgesia
     *N.B. In schizophrenia*:  schizomanics may respond to lithium better than neuroleptics
     long-term use of drugs minimised
     good prognosis cases identified and drugs withdrawn early
     recognise possible physical and social precipitating factors and treat these

**Depot neuroleptics**

| Approved name | Trade name | Administration |
| --- | --- | --- |
| Fluphenazine decanoate | Modecate | 2.5–500 mg i.m. every 2–3 weeks (average 25 mg every 3 weeks) |
| Fluphenazine enanthate | Moditen enanthate | |
| Flupenthixol decanoate | Depixol | 20–200 mg i.m. every 2–4 weeks |
| Clopenthixol decanoate | Clopixol | 200–400 mg i.m. every 2–4 weeks |
| Fluspirilene | Redeptin | 1.25–10 mg i.m. every 6–15 days (usually weekly) |

An initial test dose is usually given to determine susceptibility to extrapyramidal reactions. May need concurrent anti-Parkinsonian drugs but dosage reduction may be more effective in minimising these reactions with long-term therapy.

*Advantages*
1. Avoids high GI and hepatic first-pass metabolism giving reliable absorption.
2. Oily ester slowly hydrolysed and absorbed from muscle giving constant blood levels.
3. Improves patient compliance with medication.
4. No evidence that hypersensitivity more common than with oral phenothiazines.

**Management of acutely disturbed patients**
1. Establish cause
   — system failure? (cardiac, respiratory, hepatic, renal failure)
   — infection?
   — drug-induced? for delirium tremens see p. 381
   — silent myocardial infarction?
   — nutritional?
   — pneumonia?
   — post-operative?
   — acute psychosis?
2. Provide stable comforting environment: side room with night lights; reassure; infrequent changes of nurses; enlist relatives and friends to be with patient.
3. Sedate only when necessary because masks physical signs. Use oral drugs (syrups useful) if possible (injections can be difficult to give and encourage paranoia).

*Use*
a. chlorpomazine   100 mg p.o. or 100–200 mg i.m. or
                              50 mg p.o. 6-hourly.
b. *or* haloperidol   5–10 mg p.o. 6-hourly or
                              2.5–10 mg i.m. every hour until 4 injections
                              given
4. Treat cause and if appropriate obtain psychiatric opinion.

**ANXIOLYTIC DRUGS**

Anxiolytic = minor tranquilliser = a drug which ameliorates feelings of tension and anxiety. All hypnotics have anxiolytic actions and all anxiolytics have hypnotic properties at the appropriate dose.

**Table 7** Drug-induced extrapyramidal disorders

| Syndrome | Mechanism | Causative drugs | Treatment |
|---|---|---|---|
| *Parkinsonism*: complete syndrome or single features: tremor, akinesia, rigidity, oculogyric crises | Blockade of extrapyramidal dopamine receptors or depletion of dopamine stores | Neuroleptics Reserpine Tetrabenazine Methyldopa (Metoclopramide — very rarely) | Anticholinergics, e.g. benzhexol 5–15 mg orally daily (modest improvement) |
| *Acute dystonic reactions*: within 48 h of start of treatment abrupt onset of retrocollis, torticollis, facial grimacing, dysarthria, laboured breathing, involuntary movements, scoliosis, lordosis, opisthotonus, dystonic gait. Children and adolescents most susceptible. | ? Increase in transmitter turnover | Neuroleptics Metoclopramide Levodopa | i.v. diazepam 5–20 mg i.v. benztropine 2 mg |
| *Akathisia*: motor restlessness after days, weeks or months of treatment | Overstimulation or increased sensitivity of central dopamine receptors | Neuroleptics Levodopa | Reduction in drug therapy, drug holiday, benzodiazepines. But no change in treatment and akathisia may resolve spontaneously |
| *Chronic tardive dyskinesias*: oro-facial chewing & sucking movements, accompanied by distal limb chorea and dystonia of trunk. 15% of patients treated with neuroleptics for more than 2 years develop this. Often persists or worsens on stopping drug. Stop during sleep, reduced by distraction, worsened by emotion. | Structural injury in extrapyramidal system. Denervation hypersensitivity with increase in the number of dopamine receptors in affected neurones. | Neuroleptics | No known satisfactory treatment. Perhaps some benefit from haloperidol, pimozide or thiopropazate. (block dopamine receptors); reserpine or tetrabenazine (depletes amines); lithium (?decreases amine release); choline or lecithin (?increases acetylcholine) |

## Benzodiazepines
Powerfully anxiolytic drugs which act in the CNS by potentiating the action of the inhibitory transmitter, GABA, possibly by stimulating specific benzodiazepine receptors which are associated with post-synaptic GABA receptors. Ro 15–1788 can bind to these benzodiazepine receptors and block the sedative, psychomotor and subjective effects of diazepam.

### Actions
1. anxiolytic; sedative (not analgesic, not antidepressive, not antipsychotic)
2. muscle relaxant
3. anticonvulsant
4. increase appetite
5. anterograde amnesia (high blood levels)

### Adverse effects
1. CNS
a. *mainly dose dependent*: sedation, fatigue, somnolence, muscle weakness, diplopia, blurring of vision, ataxia, dysarthria, incoordination, apathy, impaired memory, prolonged reaction time (& traffic accidents).
b. *rare paradoxical effects*: excitement, rage, hostility, aggression, antisocial behaviour, depression (& suicide). Such effects may depend upon patient's previous personality.
c. *other rare effects*: Korsakoff-type amnesic syndrome, hypnagogic hallucinations
2. Relatively little CVS and respiratory depression (but large doses lethal if taken with other central depressants or in lung disease). Apnoea if large i.v. dose given rapidly.
3. Allergy uncommon; acute anaphylaxis; urticaria; angioedema; maculopapular eruptions; light sensitivity dermatitis; fixed drug eruptions; non-thrombocytopenic purpura.
4. Dependence (physical and psychic): withdrawal state (1–10 days delay) lasts 1–2 weeks, characterised by anxiety, panic, agitated depression, insomnia, anorexia and weight loss, delirium tremens-like syndrome and rarely fits. Abrupt discontinuation produces temporary withdrawal reactions in some patients on high therapeutic doses for 4 months or longer, worst effects seen after excessive doses over extended periods. Thus gradual withdrawal advisable.
5. Drug interactions: potentiation by other CNS depressants; weak inducer — may increase or decrease phenytoin activity.
Rare: increased activity of coumarin anticoagulation.
Rare: aggravation of Parkinsonism in patients on levodopa.

6. Local:
   (i) Intravenous: pain, thrombophlebitis (at least 6% of injections) especially in elderly, smokers, women on pill, repeated injections using a small vein; Also: peripheral neuropathy, carpal tunnel syndrome (due to extravascular leaking).
   (ii) Intra-arterial: spasm, pain, ischaemia, gangrene. No evidence of toxicity on liver, kidney, marrow or fetus.
   *Diazemuls* is a lipid suspension of diazepam for i.v. injection with reduced tendency to produce thrombophlebitis.

## Metabolic interrelationships of some benzodiazepines

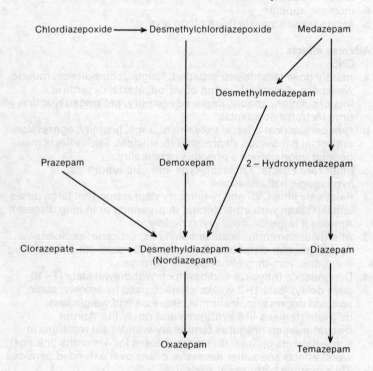

## Uses of benzodiazepines

| Indication or use | Recommended drugs |
|---|---|
| Sustained anxiety | Any. e.g. diazepam, chlordiazepoxide, |
| Panic attacks | Any, esp. those which can be injected i.v. e.g. diazepam. |
| Hypnotic | Temazepam |
| Psychosedative for surgical and investigative techniques | Diazepam |
| Abreaction and flooding techniques in psychotherapy | Diazepam |
| Epilepsy | Diazepam, clonazepam, nitrazepam, lorazepam (see p. 102) |
| Withdrawal from alcohol and other drugs of dependence | Any, e.g. diazepam. |
| Muscle relaxant in spasticity and painful musculoskeletal disease. | Any, e.g. diazepam |

## Other anxiolytic drugs

| Drug | Main problems | Special features |
|---|---|---|
| Barbiturates e.g. amylobarbitone phenobarbitone | Dependence, respiratory depression, enzyme induction, paradoxical excitement and confusion, rashes, rebound fits on withdrawal, profound sedation in anxiolytic doses | None |
| Propanediols e.g. meprobamate | Dependence, rashes, nausea. Profound sedation in anxiolytic doses. Rebound fits on withdrawal. | Minor muscular relaxing effect |
| Benzoctamine | Dependence, sedation. | Minor muscular relaxing effect. Short $T_{\frac{1}{2}}$ (2–3 h) |

## Treatment of anxiety
1. Treatment is undesirable if anxiety is acting on drive and productivity.
2. Treatment only appropriate if the anxiety is so pronounced as to interfere with useful activity.
3. Drugs should not be used to suppress symptoms which are likely to persist for an indefinite period.
4. Dependence on anxiolytic drugs is most likely to develop in patients who use alcohol to relieve anxiety.
5. Exclude symptoms as sole manifestation of other diseases (e.g. schizophrenia, dementia, depression, thyrotoxicosis, tuberculosis).
6. Drug therapy after 1–5 have been considered, and reassurance, psychotherapy, relaxation techniques, meditation, have been tried, or found to be impracticable.
7. Benzodiazepines are the usual drugs of choice for as short a time as possible, intermittently and with a flexible dosage (i.e. symptoms matching the treatment to the severity of the symptoms).
8. β blockers if peripheral symptoms are somatic (tremor, palpitations)
9. Some forms of anxiety respond to antidepressant drugs.
10. Small doses of neuroleptics (given for limited periods of minimise the risk of tardive dyskinesias) may be effective in anxiety and carry a negligible risk of dependence.
11. Barbiturates, meprobamate, alcohol not used.

## Benzodiazepine pharmacokinetics
A useful classification of benzodiazepines subdivides according to ranges of half-life (see Table 8). Note that:
1. Many form active metabolites with long $T_{\frac{1}{2}}$. Therapeutic effect of several is due to same metabolite and so these may not offer real alternatives.
2. Accumulation of parent drug and metabolites with multiple dose therapy occurs over $5 \times T_{\frac{1}{2}}$ (see Chapter 1) and a slow accumulation rate is paralleled by a slow 'washout' rate so hangover effects common but reappearance of pre-treatment symptoms (anxiety, insomnia etc.) is correspondingly slow. Long $T_{\frac{1}{2}}$ may allow once daily dosing and omission of a dose makes little difference.
4. Metabolism of long acting benzodiazepines involves hepatic oxidation and efficiency of this is influenced by age and liver function; intermediate and short-acting benzodiazepines involves non-oxidative pathways (glucuronidation; nitroreduction) relatively unaffected by old age or liver disease.
5. Rapid oral absorption useful if hypnotic or acute anxiolytic effect required but may produce dysphoria (diazepam, clorazepate most rapidly absorbed; oxazepam least rapid).

6. Distribution from blood into fat occurs rapidly after i.v. diazepam and accounts for its short duration of action in status epilepticus or as neuroleptanalgesic in endoscopy.
7. No change in dose required for benzodiazepines in renal failure.

## HYPNOTICS

Greatly over-prescribed (over 45's: 45% women & 15% men take them!) Commonest reason for 'insomnia' is reduced physiological need with age. Also exclude common primary causes of insomnia:

anxiety
breathlessness
cough
depression
eczema and other itching
  conditions
full bladder and/or rectum

cold
noise
tea and other stimulating drugs
alcohol
chronic hypnotic use
pain

### General problems of hypnotics
Suppression of REM and slow wave sleep, thus suppression of dreaming and GH release & rebound dreaming.
Rapid production of dependence; rebound insomnia and anxiety.
Possibility of more severe withdrawal syndromes.
Rapid production of tolerance.
CVS and respiratory depression.
Hangover.
Confusion and falls in the elderly.
Ataxia, motor and other accidents.
Drug interactions

### Hypnotic drugs
a. Recommended for use as hypnotics
   1. benzodiazepines
   2. chlormethiazole
   3. chloral derivatives
b. Not recommended for use as hypnotics
   4. barbiturates
   5. piperidinediones (e.g. glutethimide)
   6. antihistamines (e.g. promethazine)
   7. alcohols
   8. quinazolines (methaqualone)
Uses Only for short periods, e.g. preoperatively, emotional crises.
Certainly not routinely in hospital or for difficult children.

**Table 8** Benzodiazepines

| Drug | Therapeutic dose | Active metabolites | $T_{\frac{1}{2}}$ (h) of parent compound | Special features |
|------|------------------|--------------------|------------------------------------------|------------------|
| *Longer acting* | | | | |
| Diazepam (Valium, Atensine) | 2–10 mg | Desmethyldiazepam ($T_{\frac{1}{2}}$ 36–200 h) Oxazepam | 20–50 | General 'all purpose' benzodiazepine but also useful i.v. in status epilepticus. i.m. injection poorly absorbed. |
| Chlordiazepoxide (Librium, Calmoden) | 10–25 mg | Desmethylchlordiazepoxide Desmethyldiazepam Oxazepam | 3–30 | i.m. injection poorly absorbed (precipitates at injection site) |
| Clorazepate (Tranxene) | 15 mg | Desmethyldiazepam Oxazepam | 30–60 | Parent drug completely metabolised to desmethyl diazepam (i.e. is a pro-drug) |
| Nitrazepam (Mogadon, Nitrados, Somnite, Remnos) | 5–10 mg | None | 24 | Hypnotic use but also anticonvulsant |
| Flurazepam (Dalmane) | 15–30 mg | Desalkylflurazepam ($T_{\frac{1}{2}}$ = 40–250 h) Hydroxethylflurazepam | 2 | Hypnotic |
| Medazepam (Nobrium) | 5–15 mg | Desmethylmedazepam Desmethyldiazepam | Probably about 24 h | |
| Clobazam (Frisium) | 10–20 mg | N-desmethyl-clobazam | 24 | Claimed to produce no psychomotor impairment. Less hypnotic & muscle relaxant effects than diazepam |

| Drug (name) | $T_{\frac{1}{2}}$ (h) | Dose | Active metabolites | Comments |
|---|---|---|---|---|
| Clonazepam (Rivotril) | 30 | 1–8 mg | None | Mainly used as an anticonvulsant |
| *Shorter acting with no active metabolites* | | | | |
| Oxazepam (Serenid) | 5–20 | 15–60 mg | None | |
| Lorazepam (Ativan) | 10–20 | 1–2.5 mg | None | Useful i.v. in status epilepticus. Well absorbed by i.m. injection — thus useful in delirium tremens |
| Temazepam (Euhypnos, Normison) | 5–20 | 10–30 mg | None | |
| *Ultra-short acting* | | | | |
| Triazolam (Halcion) | 2–4 | 125–250 µg | Hydroxytriazolam | Used only as hypnotic. Psychotic reactions have been reported |
| Midazolam (Hypnovel) | 2 | 2.5–7.5 mg | Hydroxymidazolam ($T_{\frac{1}{2}}$ 1–1½ h) | Used i.v. for profound psychosedation, e.g. endoscopy |

**HYPNOTICS** (continued)

**1. Benzodiazepines** (see page 102)

| Drug | Trade name | Dose | $T_\frac{1}{2}$ (h) | Active metabolites |
|------|------------|------|------|--------------------|
| Nitrazepam | Remnos Surem Nitrados Somnased Mogadon Somnite | 5–10 mg | 24 (20–30) | No major active product |
| Flurazepam | Dalmane | 15–30 mg | 2 | N-hydroxyethyl flurazepam ($T_\frac{1}{2}$ short — no accumulation) N-desalkyl flurazepam ($T_\frac{1}{2}$ = 40–250 h) |
| Triazolam | Halcion | 125–250 $\mu$g | 2–4 | $\alpha$-hydroxy triazolam ($T_\frac{1}{2}$ = 7 h) |
| Temazepam | Euhypnos Normison | 10–30 mg | 8 (5–20) | No major active product |

(Length of sleep does not closely correspond with blood levels of benzodiazepines. Long acting drugs, e.g. diazepam, clorazepate, chlordiazepoxide, may be satisfactory hypnotics).

**2. Chlormethiazole (Heminevrin)**
*Dose*: 400 mg o.n.
*Pharmacokinetics*: $T_\frac{1}{2}$ = 1 h; time to peak = 1 h; Extensive (85%) first pass metabolism; (bioavailability increased to nearly 100% in liver disease).
*Toxicity*:
1. nasal, conjunctival and bronchial discomfort
2. gastric irritation
3. respiratory and CVS depression
4. 2% solution IV can cause thrombophlebitis and haemolysis
5. dependence
*Uses*:
1. hypnotic (especially in elderly)
2. anxiolytic
3. acute withdrawal from alcohol, barbiturates, narcotic analgesics
4. i.v. in status epilepticus

### 3. Chloral

| Derivative | Trade name | Dose | Preparations |
|---|---|---|---|
| Chloral hydrate | Noctec | 0.5–2.0 g (adult) 30–50 mg/ kg (child) | Chloral mixture 500 mg/5 ml. Paediatric chloral elixir 200 mg/5 ml. Noctec is a capsule containing 500 mg. |
| Dichloralphenazone | Welldorm | 1.3–195 g (adult) | Welldorm tablets contain 650 mg. Welldorm elixir 225 mg/5 ml |

*Pharmacokinetics*: Well absorbed, rapidly metabolised (reduced) to more active trichlorethanol ($T_{\frac{1}{2}} = 8$ h).
*Toxicity*:
1. respiratory and CVS depression
2. gastric irritation
3. rashes: erythematous, scarlatiniform, urticarial, scaling
4. jaundice
5. proteinuria
6. interactions: alcohol ('Mickey Finn'), warfarin (see chapter 6)

### Hypnotic drugs — not recommended

| Drug | Enzyme induction | CVS & respiratory depression | Problems Dependence | Other |
|---|---|---|---|---|
| Barbiturates | +++ | +++ | +++ | Paradoxical excitement Confusion in the elderly Rebound CNS hyperexcitability. Severe withdrawal problems. |

**Hypnotic drugs — not recommended** (continued)

| Drug | Enzyme induction | CVS & respiratory depression | Problems Dependence | Other |
|---|---|---|---|---|
| Glutethimide | ++ | +++ | +++ | Cerebral oedema Papilloedema Anticholinergic effect Rebound CNS hyperexcitability |
| Promethazine | ? | +++ | ? | Great variability in response Vertigo, delirium, excitement, anticholinergic. |
| Alcohols: Ethyl alcohol | + | +++ | +++ | CNS and other organ damage Delirium tremens, etc. |
| Ethchlorvynol | + | +++ | +++ | Delirium tremens Dizziness, nausea Long $T_{\frac{1}{2}}$ (24 h) |
| Methaqualone | Similar in toxicity to barbiturates | | | |

# EPILEPSY

Before treating, ask:
1. Are the fits epileptic rather than another disorder (e.g. syncope, cardiac arrhythmia, sleep paralysis, hypoglycaemia, hyperventilation)?
2. Is the epilepsy secondary to a treatable condition (e.g. tumour)?
3. Are there treatable factors which precipitate the epilepsy (e.g. flashing light, hangover, hunger)?
4. Is there a significant risk of further fits if the patient is left untreated?

If treatment is decided on:
1. The type of epilepsy suggests a choice of drug (see table below).
2. Initially a single drug at a time is tried — if necessary with the help of plasma levels.
3. Changes in drug treatment must not be sudden and gradual reduction of dose of one drug must accompany introduction of new drug.

N.B. Important to treat epilepsy as soon as possible: repeated seizure episodes worsen prognosis for control.

## Main drugs in the treatment of epilepsy

| Type of epilepsy | Drugs |
|---|---|
| Petit mal. 3 Hz spike & wave. | Ethosuximide, sodium valproate, clonazepam, (troxidone) |
| Myoclonic epilepsy ⎫<br>Akinetic seizures ⎬ | Sodium valproate, clonazepam |
| Salaam attacks with hypsarrhythmia | Corticotrophin nitrazepam |
| Grand mal ⎫<br>Temporal lobe epilepsy ⎬<br>Other forms of focal epilepsy ⎭ | Phenytoin, carbamazepine, sodium valproate, (phenobarbitone, primidone) |

## Toxic effects of phenytoin

A. 1. *Nervous system*:
      Cerebellar syndrome (ataxia, tremor, nystagmus, dysarthria)
      Sedation
      Depression, psychotic excitement, paranoia
      Peripheral neuropathy
      Increased frequency of fits (rare consequence of high levels)
   2. *Immune diseases & skin disorders*:
      Allergic rashes
      Acne
      Hypersensitivity hepatitis
      Drug fever
      Systemic lupus erythematosus-like syndrome
   3. *Mesodermal changes*:
      Coarsening of facial features
      Gum hypertrophy (usually resolves on improved periodontal care)
      Dupuytren's contracture
      Lymphadenopathy (very rarely lymphoma develops)
   4. *Haematological*:
      Folate deficiency (common)
      Megaloblastic anaemia (uncommon)
      Aplastic anaemia (rare)
   5. *Endocrine*:
      Inhibition of ADH release
      Aggravation of diabetes mellitus

B.  *Possible effects on fetus*: (but may be partly due to maternal fits)
Increased perinatal mortality
Raised frequency of cleft palate and hare lip
Microcephaly
Congenital heart disease
C.  *Drug interactions*:
The following impair phenytoin metabolism:
sulthiame
pheneturide
isoniazid
chloramphenicol
dicoumarol
The following accelerate phenytoin metabolism:
ethanol
carbamazepine
Phenytoin effects potentiated due to displacement from protein binding by:
phenylbutazone
diazoxide
sulphonamides
Phenytoin is an inducer and potentiates the metabolism of:
oral contraceptives
oral anticoagulants
dexamethasone
vitamin D
folic acid

**Management of status epilepticus**
Medical emergency, admit to intensive care unit.
1.  Set up intravenous line, taking blood for levels of anticonvulsant drugs.
Terminate fits as soon as possible with:
i.v. benzodiazepines:
diazepam 10 mg
clonazepam 1 mg
lorazepam 5 mg
given over 2 minutes. Repeated if necessary. Alternatively i.v. chlormethiazole 0.8% (up to 500 mg in 6 h).
If fits not controlled rapidly by above:
i.v. thiopentone 150–750 mg
intubation + muscle relaxant + artificial respiration
2.  Determine cause of status and treat if possible.
3.  Recommence normal drug therapy as soon as possible. If patient not on drugs, a loading dose of phenytoin (15 mg/kg) via nasogastric tube.

**Table 9(a)** Drugs used in petit mal

| Drug | Effective plasma level | Usual oral dosage range | $T_{\frac{1}{2}}$ | Pharmacokinetics | Toxicity | Clinical use |
|---|---|---|---|---|---|---|
| Ethosuximide (Zarontin) | 40–120 µg/ml | 0.5–2 g daily | 70 h adults 30 h children | Extensive metabolism to inactive products. Very little plasma protein binding | Non-toxic apart from mild giddiness, nausea & abdominal discomfort | Drug of first choice in petit mal (ineffective in grand mal, but can be used with phenytoin) |
| Trimethadione Troxidone (Tridione) | 300–600 µg/ml | 0.6–1.2 g daily | 16 h (for active substances) | Main metabolite, dimethadione, is pharmacologically active dimeth: trimeth = 20 : 1. | Toxic: hemeralopia, sedation, scotomata (stop drug), rashes, agranulocytosis (rare), nephrosis, hepatitis | Almost obsolete |
| Sodium valproate (Epilim) | 40–80 µg/ml | 200–700 mg b.d. | 7–10 h | Well absorbed. High plasma protein binding. Metabolites not yet identified, but effect persists beyond elimination from plasma | GI disturbances, enhancement of sedatives, temporary hair loss, false +ve ketone test in urine, weight gain, liver failure (rare), pancreatitis (rare) | Possible second line drug in petit mal. Also may be useful in grand mal, TLE, akinetic attacks and myoclonic epilepsy |
| Clonazepam (Rivotril) | | 4–8 mg (adults) | 30 h | No active metabolites | Sedation, incoordination, hypotonia, dysphoria, paradoxical excitement | Possible second line drug in petit mal. Also used in grand mal status and in akinetic and myoclonic epilepsy |

**Table 9(b)** Drugs recommended in grand mal and focal epilepsy

| Drug | Effective plasma level | Usual oral dose range | $T_{\frac{1}{2}}$ | Pharmacokinetics | Toxicity | Clinical use |
|---|---|---|---|---|---|---|
| Phenytoin (Epanutin) | 10–20 $\mu$g/ml (some patients well controlled with lower levels) | 100–500 mg daily | No single $T_{\frac{1}{2}}$ because zero order kinetics. Usually 12–120 h. | Well absorbed, but bioavailability reduced if $Ca^{++}$ given simultaneously. Great individual variation rate of metabolism. | See page 107 | Drug of first choice in grand mal and focal epilepsy (ineffective in petit mal, but can be used with ethosuximide). Used in trigeminal neuralgia. |
| Sodium valproate (Epilim) | See Table 9(a) | | | | | One of the second drugs of choice in grand mal and focal epilepsy. |
| Carbamazepine (Tegretol) | 4–10 $\mu$g/ml | 100–1200 mg 12-hourly | Initially 25–60 h. 10 h on chronic administration. | Well absorbed. Partly metabolised to carbamazepine -10, 11 expoxide (active; $T_{\frac{1}{2}}$ = 2 h). 75% plasma protein bound. | Sedation, ataxia, giddiness, nystagmus, slurred speech, hyponatraemia & water intoxication. Enzyme inducer. Mild, reversible leucopenia common. | One of the second drugs of choice in grand mal and focal epilepsy. Drug of first choice in trigeminal neuralgia; may help diabetes insipidus. |

| | Plasma concentration | Dose | Half-life | Pharmacokinetics | Unwanted effects | Notes |
|---|---|---|---|---|---|---|
| Phenobarbitone | 10–25 $\mu$g/ml | 60–180 mg daily | 100 h adults 40 h children | Well absorbed. 50% bound to plasma proteins. Half is metabolised to inactive derivatives. | Sedation, nystagmus, enzyme induction, paradoxical excitement, rebound fits on withdrawal, folate deficiency | Only a reserve drug in refractory epilepsy |
| Primidone (Mysoline) | | 125–250 mg daily | 10 h (but long lived active metabolites) | 2 active metabolites: phenobarbitone ($T_{\frac{1}{2}}$ = 100 h) & phenylethylmalonamide ($T_{\frac{1}{2}}$ = 30 h) | Sedation, nystagmus, enzyme induction, parodoxical excitement, rebound fits on withdrawal, folate deficiency. | As phenobarbitone. |

## PARKINSONISM

Drug-induced (see p. 96) mediated via altered dopamine receptor activation.

Idiopathic and other aetiologies cause degeneration of striatonigral pathway. Changes occur in thalamus, pigmented brain stem nuclei, and diffusely, resulting in disorders of balance and intellectual deficits. Although changes in GABA, noradrenaline, 5-HT may be demonstrated the most important changes are in disturbances of acetycholine (excitatory) and dopamine (inhibitory) *receptor balance*:

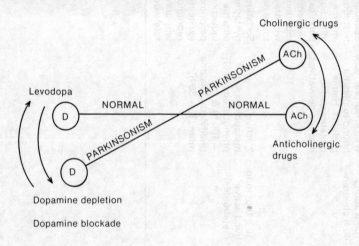

Parkinsonism produced by:
  (i)  blocking dopamine receptors (e.g. phenothiazines, butyrophenones)
 (ii)  depleting dopamine stores (e.g. reserpine)
(iii)  interfering with dopamine synthesis (e.g. methyldopa)

### Levodopa = 1-dihydroxyphenylalanine (Berkdopa; Brocadopa; Larodopa)

Dopamine does not cross the blood-brain barrier but its precursor levodopa can and is metabolised to dopamine in situ by dopa decarboxylase thence to noradrenaline and adrenaline. Effective on akinesia, rigidity and tremor also helps associated symptoms like speech disturbance, dysphagia and sialorrhoea. Ineffective in drug-induced Parkinsonism.

**Table 10** Drug induced movement disorders

| Involuntary movement | Causative drugs | Clinical features | Onset after beginning therapy | Effect of drug withdrawal | Treatment |
|---|---|---|---|---|---|
| Parkinsonism | Phenothiazines Butyrophenones Reserpine Tetrabenazine Methyldopa (rare) | Dose dependent High incidence (~50%) | Gradual: several months | Reversible but slow to disappear | Anticholinergic drugs (levodopa useless) |
| Tremor | β-agonists Lithium Tricyclic antidepressants | Dose dependent High incidence (~30%) | Rapid | Rapid reversal | None |
| Acute dystonia | Phenothiazines Butyrophenones Metoclopramide Diazoxide | Usually children or adolescents Low incidence (1–2%) | Rapid | Rapid reversal | Anticholinergic drugs Diazepam |
| Akathisia | Phenothiazines Butyrophenones | High incidence (~30%) | Gradual: several months | Reversal over several days | Anticholinergic drugs |
| Tardive Dyskinesias | Phenothiazines Butyrophenones | High incidence (~30%) especially in elderly | Slow: several months to years | May worsen Persists in over 40% | Discontinue drug Tetrabenazine Pimozide Baclofen Choline |

*Pharmacokinetics*
About 40% of an oral dose absorbed by active transport utilising the carrier for aromatic amino acids. High protein diet reduces absorption by competition for the carrier by dietary amino acids. Dopa decarboxylase of gastric mucosa degrades levodopa so levodopa absorption dependent upon gastric emptying rate: delayed emptying, e.g. due to anticholinergic drugs, reduces absorption. 95% of absorbed levodopa metabolised not in brain but peripherally (mainly heart, blood vessels, gut, liver and kidneys). Peripheral decarboxylation enhanced by enzyme co-factor pyridoxine which should be avoided in tonics, vitamin pills etc. $T_\frac{1}{2}$ is 1–2.5 h.

*Dose*
Begin with 125 mg 6 hourly and increase total daily dose by 250–500 mg on alternate days until side-effects occur. When a mild side-effect occurs the next increment is withheld for a few days until tolerance gained. Next increment added until intolerable side-effect reached. Wide variation in final tolerable dose: some patients can take 6–8 g/day.

Levodopa is being superceded by levodopa + decarboxylase inhibitor preparations (see below).

*Adverse effects*
1. Gastro-intestinal: nausea almost universal, usually subsides spontaneously at low doses but occasionally becomes dose-limiting.
2. Cardiovascular: mainly postural hypotension (due to central $\alpha$-adrenergic receptor stimulation by noradrenaline, similar to action of clonidine, also peripheral inhibition of baroreceptor reflexes). Arrhythmias, mainly in patients with underlying heart disease so contraindicated in such patients and after myocardial infarction.
3. Involuntary movements — commonest dose-limiting reactions: facial grimacing, tongue movements, restlessness, jerking of the limbs.
4. Psychological: agitation, paranoia, confusion, depression, vivid nightmares may also limit dose.
5. Patients may become anxious about acidic urinary levodopa metabolites which stain clothing black or brown.
6. Contraindicated by narrow-angle glaucoma, severe psychosis and malignant melanoma.
7. MAOI must be withdrawn 14 days before levodopa and should never be used concurrently since severe hypertension occurs.

## Dopa decarboxylase inhibitors
Peripheral dopa decarboxylase inhibition reduces:
 (i)  levodopa dose to produce optimum therapeutic benefit by 80%
(ii)  incidence of nausea and vomiting
(iii)  time to reach optimum dose
(iv)  risk of cardiac arrhythmias and postural hypotension
*But* involuntary movements and psychiatric side effects are same
as for levodopa alone.

Two preparations available:
 4 : 1 ratio levodopa : benserazide (Madopar)
10 : 1 ratio levodopa : carbidopa (Sinemet)

Benserazide combination causes less nausea and vomiting and
may therefore be more effective peripheral decarboxylase inhibitor
combination.

*Dose*
Various sizes of capsule of Madopar and Sinemet available. Start
with one capsule and increase dose every 3–4 days until full
therapeutic effect gained or side-effects supervene. Some patients
only tolerate slower rate of dose increase.

Useful benefit occurs after 1–3 weeks but rarely necessary to
exceed dose of 1 g levodopa when combined with decarboxylase
inhibitor to achieve maximum effects. Continue treatment for 6
months before failure concluded from the absence of clinical
response.

## Problems of chronic levodopa treatment
1. Involuntary movements (chorea is commonest but also
   dystonia, myoclonus and ballistic movements). May occur at
   times related to dose:
   a. Peak dose
   b. Onset and end-of-dose
   c. Nocturnal myoclonus
   d. Early morning muscle cramps with dystonia
2. Oscillation in performance
   a.  Wearing-off effect — progressive reduction in duration of
       benefit from each dose.
   b.  On-off effect — unpredictable swings from relative mobility
       to bradykinesia and hypotonia.
3. Toxic confusional states with nightmares and visual
   hallucinations.
4. ?Dementia is commoner.
   Life expectancy is almost normal for patients who can tolerate
levodopa.

## Anticholinergic drugs

 (i) Block striatal muscarinic cholinergic receptors *but* also
      peripherally (responsible for most adverse effects, e.g.
      glaucoma, urinary retention, constipation. N.B. Mental
      confusion and excitement although antihistamine compounds
      are sedative).
 (ii) Rigidity and tremor respond best — akinesia unaffected (80%
      patients get 30% overall improvement).
(iii) Slowly increase from starting dose every 2–5 days until benefit
      or side effects occur.
 (iv) No evidence for superiority of one drug.
  (v) May help Parkinsonism due to phenothiazines etc. but never
      give prophylactically.
 (vi) Given i.v. (e.g. benztropine 2 mg; procyclidine 10 mg) for acute
      drug-induced dystonia and oculogyric crises.
N.B.  Tardive dyskinesia is not improved, may worsen.

## Amantadine (Symmetrel)

Developed as antiviral against Influenza A2, by chance found to
improve Parkinsonism. Probably releases stored neuronal
dopamine (acts similarly to amphetamine on adrenergic neurone).
   Akinesia, tremor and rigidity all respond but improvement
considerably less (75–50%) than with levodopa and benefit may
not be sustained. Can be used with levodopa or anticholinergics.
Drug-induced Parkinsonism refractory.

### Dose

100 mg/day for one week then 100 mg twice daily if no adverse
effects. Response usually occurs within 2 weeks.

### Adverse effects

Usually well tolerated but dry mouth, tremor, restlessness,
confusion, hallucinations, nightmare, myoclonic jerks (rare) and
livido reticularis. Caution necessary in epileptics or in patients
given central stimulants like amphetamine because fits can occur.

## Bromocriptine (Parlodel) (see also page 262)

At high doses a dopaminergic agonist but less effective than
levodopa. Usually ineffective in patients not responsive to
levodopa. Akinesia, rigidity and tremor all improve but may take 3
months to get optimum dose and response.
   No evidence that bromocriptine changes natural history and
deterioration of basal ganglia in Parkinsonism but 'on-off'
phenomena and response swings not reported in patients given
bromocriptine without levodopa.

**Some anticholinergic drugs used in parkinsonism**

| Approved name | Proprietary name | Starting dose | Maximum daily dose (mg) | Comments |
|---|---|---|---|---|
| Benzhexol | Artane | 1 mg 12-hourly | 15 | Sustained release (Artane Sustets) available |
| Benztropine | Cogentin | 0.5 mg 12-hourly | 4 | Anti-histamine: sedative and potentiates CNS depressants, e.g. alcohol. |
| Orphenadrine | Disipal | 50 mg 8-hourly | 400 | More euphoriant than benzhexol, may cause insomnia and less effective on tremor. Injection (i.m. only) available. |
| Procyclidine | Kemadrin | 2.5 mg 8-hourly | 60 | Sedative — injection available (i.m. or i.v.) |

*Dose*
Initially 1.25 mg at night with food, gradually increased to
40–200 mg/day. Duration of action 8–12 h (cf 1–3 h for levodopa).
Can be given with levodopa.

*Indications*
a. levodopa intolerance: bromocriptine does not usually cause
   vomiting so useful with levodopa induced nausea.
b. response-swings with levodopa may stabilise on bromocriptine
   (? because longer $T_{\frac{1}{2}}$ of effects of latter).
   *Major dose-limiting side effects* are psychiatric disturbances
(25–30% suffer hallucinations, altered behaviour and/or awareness)
— may last 2–6 weeks after stopping drug. Like levodopa it causes
involuntary movements but nausea and vomiting (unlike levodopa)
are rare.
   **Selegiline** (Eldepryl) is an inhibitor of MAO B used with
levodopa. Hypertensive reactions do not occur.


## DRUG TREATMENT OF MIGRAINE

ACUTE ATTACK

**1. Anti-emetics**
a. Metoclopramide anti-emetic of choice in migraine — improves
   absorption of other drugs by accelerating gastric emptying
   10 mg, tablet taken 10 minutes before other drugs (can also be
   given i.m.).
b. Cyclizine hydrochloride 50 mg oral (Valoid).
c. Cyclizine lactate 50 mg injection.
d. Triethylperazine maleate (Torcean) tablet (10 mg) injection
   (6.5 mg) and suppository.

**2. Analgesics**
Most attacks controlled by 900 mg aspirin or 1 g paracetamol or
125 mg flufenamic acid.

**3. Anxiolytics**
(e.g. diazepam 5 mg) may be helpful if given with analgesics.
Useful if patient can sleep during an attack.

**4. Ergotamine**
Used only if analgesics plus metoclopramide have failed. Most
patients with classical migraine will respond to analgesics plus
metoclopramide plus ergotamine.

*Dose*
(Older recommended doses are too high)
Dose per attack limited to
1–2 mg oral
or 1.08 mg inhaled
or 0.25 mg injected.
(ergotamine tartrate injection has been withdrawn, but
dihydroergotamine mesylate (Dihydergot) 1 mg/ml injection is
available).

**Some available preparations**:

| *Name* | *Content per tablet* | *Suggested dose per attack* |
|---|---|---|
| Effergot | ergotamine tartrate 2 mg<br>caffeine 50 mg | ½ tablet |
| Femergin | ergotamine tartrate 1 mg | 1 tablet |
| Cafergot | ergotamine tartrate 1 mg<br>caffeine 100 mg | 1 tablet |
| Migril | ergotamine tartrate 2 mg<br>cyclizine hydrochloride 50 mg<br>caffeine hydrate 100 mg | ½ tablet |

OR   half a cafergot suppository (1 mg ergotamine)
OR   3 puffs of Riker Medihaler Ergotamine (1.08 mg ergotamine)

*Toxicity*
1. Nausea, vomiting, headache, malaise.
2. Cold extremeties, Raynaud's phenomena, claudication,
   paraesthesiae, gangrene (some of these vasospastic
   complications reversed by IV sodium nitroprusside).
3. Contraindicated in pregnancy.

**5. Cyproheptadine (Periactin)**
Antihistamine and anti-5-HT. Given orally 4–8 mg for acute attack
or prophylaxis.

*Toxicity*
Sedation, anticholinergic, increased appetite.

PROPHYLAXIS

Not undertaken unless 2 attacks/month.
Not usually given to children.
Usually only necessary for months (not years).

## 1. Anxiolytics
Small doses e.g. diazepam 2–4 mg at night.

## 2. Antidepressants
Imipramine 50–150 mg at night or (more sedating) amitriptylline 50–150 mg at night.

1 and 2 may be effective especially if anxiety and/or depression present. N.B. anxiety or depression may accompany serious CNS disorders.

## 3. Anticonvulsants
Sometimes useful (especially if abnormal EEG in attack), phenytoin 100–200 mg at night, carbamazepine 100 mg twice daily.

## 4. β-blockers
Propranolol 80 mg twice daily; atenolol 150 mg daily effective in most patients (but up to 240 mg propranolol daily may be required). In the rare instances when prophylaxis needed in children these are drugs of choice.
N.B.  Never used with ergotamine because of increased risk of vascular disease.

## 5. Pizotifen (Sanomigran)
A 5-HT antagonist.

*Dose*
0.5–2 mg 2 to 3 times daily.

*Toxicity*
Sedation, increased appetite and weight gain. Sometimes effective, but has not been formally compared with β-blockers.

## 6. Clonidine (Dixarit)
Low doses of clonidine reduce sensitivity of vessels to vasoactive amines. 25–50 μg 2 or 3 times daily is most likely to succeed in patients who have a dietary precipitating factor; useful in $\frac{1}{3}$ of patients.

*Toxicity*
Not severe with these doses but can produce dry mouth, drowsiness and depression.

**7. Ergotamine derivatives**
a. Dihydroergotamine (Dihydergot): 1–2 mg 2 or 3 times daily is an effective prophylactic. Toxicity is unusual.
b. Methyserzide (Deseril): 5-HT antagonist and nonadrenaline potentiator. Reduces 80% of headaches in 80% of patients. Rarely used because of toxicity: retroperitoneal and intrathoracic fibrosis (rare if dose kept low and used for not more than 6 consecutive months); GI disturbances; euphoria; hyperaesthesia; weight gain and oedema; constriction of large and small arteries.
N.B. Ergotamine tartrate should never be used in classical migraine as a prophylactic.

## Cluster headache (migraineous neuralgia)
1. Ergotamine tartrate 1–2 mg may terminate an attack but attacks usually too short lived for acute treatment. This is the only indication for prophylactic ergotamine tartrate (1–2 mg daily).
2. Prophylactic lithium carbonate (perhaps a lower plasma level than depression: 0.6–0.7 mmol/l may be effective).
3. A single oral dose of prednisolone (30 mg) may prevent a cluster of headaches from continuing.

## MYASTHENIA GRAVIS

Associated with serum IgG antibody binding to acetylcholine receptors in post-synaptic membrane with reduced receptor population.

### Diagnosis
Edrophonium chloride (Tensilon) test: Inject 1–2 mg i.v. of this short-acting anticholinesterase. If no side effects occur then 5–8 mg is given. Positive test is clinical improvement: wears off after 5 mins.

### Treatment
1. Anticholinesterases: do not repair basic deficiency of receptors but allow acetylcholine released by nerve to act for longer. Individual requirements for drug vary so dose needs titration.
   a. Pyridostigmine (Mestinon) 60 mg 6–8-hourly increasing to 120 mg 3-hourly. Mild GI effect. Contains quaternary nitrogen and is charged at all pH so poorly and slowly absorbed: may be usefully combined with faster absorbed neostigmine for patients weak on waking.
   b. Neostigmine (Prostigmin) 15 mg 6–8-hourly but often more frequently (300 mg/day; up to 2-hourly intervals). Short (2–6 h) duration of action. Pronounced muscarinic activity so needs atropine or propantheline to prevent colic and salivation.

*Others*: Ambenonium (Mytelase); Distigmine (Ubretid).
*Side effects* due to parasympathetic stimulation include colic, diarrhoea, miosis and increased sweating, salivation, lachrimation and bronchial secretion. Atropine or propantheline (Pro-Banthine) control gut side-effects.
2. Steroid: Immunosuppression but needs continued therapy and so high incidence of side effects (see p. 265). Steroids indicated if (a) poor response to anticholinergic drugs and/or thymectomy; (b) in older males.

   Begin with low dose (or weakness worsens), e.g. prednisolone 10 mg; increase by 5–10 mg/week until symptoms controlled or 120 mg maximum reached. Try to use alternate day treatment to minimise side-effects. Anticholinergics usually reduced during steroid therapy. Steroids can be combined with azathioprine
3. Other immunosuppressants: azathioprine; 6-mercaptopurine.
4. Thymectomy.
5. Plasmapheresis — removes antibody.

*Myasthenic crisis*: deterioration in myasthenia can be due to infection, drugs, surgery or exertion (e.g. childbirth) or spontaneous. Responds to edrophonium (see above).
*Cholinergic crisis*: deterioration caused by excess anticholinesterase treatment. Worsened by edrophonium. Treated by withdrawal of anticholinesterase and administration of cholinesterase reactivator pralidoxime (1–2 g i.v. over 2–4 mins). Atropine used to block excessive muscarinic effect.

**Drugs which interfere with neuromuscular transmission (myasthenics therefore more sensitive)**
1. Aminoglycosides  — Streptomycin
                    — Gentamicin
                    — Neomycin
                    — Kanamycin
2. Other antibiotics  — Viomycin
                      — Colistin
                      — Polymyxin
3. Antiarrhythmics  — Quinidine & Quinine
                    — Procainamide
                    — Lignocaine
4. Muscle relaxants  — Curare
                     — Gallamine
                     — Pancuronium
   (but less sensitive to succinylcholine)
5. Respiratory depressants, e.g. barbiturates

# Analgesics — including terminal care

## NARCOTIC ANALGESICS

Narcotic analgesics act by binding to opiate receptors in CNS.
Opiate receptors found in:
pulvinar of thalamus
limbic system and connections
substantia gelatinosa of cord
Receptor agonists are stereospecific (I-isomers are active) and competively antagonised by naloxone.
*Endogenous analgesic peptides* also bind to these receptors:
leucine encephalin
methionine encephalin } — released from brain and adrenal medulla
β-endorphin — released from pituitary of brain simultaneously with ACTH.

### Opium
Dried juice of seed capsule of Papaver somniferum.
Contains:
morphine   9–17%
codeine    0.5–4%      total opium alkaloids
noscapine
2–9%                   = Papaveretum (Omnopon)
papaverine   0.5–1%
thebaine   0.1–0.8%

*Actions of morphine*
A.  CNS
Relief of pain — esp prolonged. Raises pain threshold and reduces emotional reaction to pain.
Euphoria — not seen in normal individuals, but occurs on relief of pain or removal of withdrawal state.
Drowsiness, sleep, coma
Respiratory depression, cough suppression
Vomiting
Convulsions
Pupillary constriction (direct action on Edinger-Westphal nucleus)
Increases release of ADH
Inhibits release of ACTH, FSH, LH

B. Peripheral
   Histamine release. Bronchoconstriction in asthmatics.
   Hypotension
   Increased smooth muscle tone
   Constipation

*Pharmacokinetics*
i.m. injection : peak 1 hour, effect lasts 3–4 hours. Oral absorption
irregular and greater doses needed due to 70% first pass
metabolism. Peak effect at 2 hours.
Plasma $T_{\frac{1}{2}} = 2–3$ h.
Relatively small amounts cross placental barrier but fetus is highly
sensitive (cf diamorphine crosses placental barrier readily).

*Uses*
Pain from 10–20 mg s.c. or i.m. 4–6–hourly, orally in elixir
Premedication
Left ventricular failure
(Diarrhoea — not recommended)
Symptomatic suppression of cough
Suppression of respiratory effort during assisted ventilation
Suppression of withdrawal state in narcotic dependence
(methadone mainly used for this)

*Toxicity*
Vomiting, nausea, giddiness
Sedation, confusion
Respiratory depression
Constipation
Hypotension
Aggravation of epilepsy
True allergy (rare) but histamine release (bronchospasm, skin
flushing and itching) is common
Retention of urine
Dependance
Drug interactions: with phenothiazines and tricyclic
anti-depressants-enhanced sedation and orthostatic hypotension

**Papaveretum (Omnopon)**
A preparation of total opium alkaloids standardised to equivalent of
50% anhydrous morphine.

*Dose*
10–20 mg oral or injected.
*Not recommended* because of risk of confusing dose with that of
morphine.

## DRUGS IN TERMINAL CARE
(Based on drugs most commonly used at St Christopher's Hospice.)

During terminal illness 60% of patients experience pain. Most terminal pain is potentially relieved by drugs. Major analgesic drugs must be given at such intervals (usually 4-hourly) that the effect of the previous dose has not worn off. *Never* prescribe the drugs PRN. Pain itself is hyperalgesic (if necessary the patient must be woken up to be given an analgesic). Analgesics should be given orally whenever possible. Dose increased until patient pain free and memory and fear of pain erased. Constant pain of this type tends to get progressively worse, isolates the patient, demands his whole attention and produces anxiety, depression and fear which themselves potentiate the pain. Treating the isolation, pain, anxiety and depression can break this vicious circle.

PAIN CONTROL

### Mild pain
1. *Soluble aspirin*   2–3 × 300 mg tablets 4-hourly.
2. *Paracetamol*   2 × 500 mg tablets 4-hourly.
3. *Distalgesic*   (dextropropoxyphene 32.5 mg plus paracetamol 325 mg) 2 tablets 4-hourly.

### Moderate pain
1. Diconal (dipipanone 10 mg plus cyclizine 30 mg) 1–2 tablets 4-hourly. Very useful. Can be given on an outpatient basis.
2. Analgesic elixirs of diamorphine and morphine appear in the NF. Are suitable for oral use and usually given with a neuroleptic (e.g. prochlorperazine syrup (5 mg/5 ml); chlorpromazine 6.25 mg/2 ml or 25 mg). The NF suggests that cocaine should not be added, but the following is still used in some centres:

      | | | |
      |---|---|---|
      | diamorphine HCl | 2.5–40 mg | |
      | cocaine | 10 mg | |
      | 95% ethyl alcohol | 2.5 ml | 'Brompton mixture' |
      | syrup | 5 ml | |
      | chloroform water up to | 20 ml | |

3. Phenazocine (Narphen) 5 mg tablets × 1–3, 4-hourly.

### Severe pain
1. Morphine or diamorphine orally 4-hourly. St Christopher's use a diamorphine and cocaine elixir giving 10–80 mg 4-hourly. If this does not control the pain then chlorpromazine and/or other analgesics (e.g. aspirin, phenylbutazone, distalgesic) are added. If this is not effective then diamorphine s.c. injections (not morphine because this is bulky to inject).

2. Neuroleptics given with the narcotic analgesic to potentiate anguish-relieving properties of latter and as anti-emetics.
3. Oxycodone pectinate (Proladone) suppositories (30–60 mg 8 hourly if vomiting).

## Vomiting
Phenothiazines e.g. prochlorperazine 5–10 mg orally or i.m. 4-hourly if necessary with:
1. metoclopramide 10 mg orally or i.m. OR
2. cyclizine (Valoid) 50 mg orally or i.m.

## Anorexia
Prednisolone (enteric coated) 5–15 mg daily.

## Malignant large bowel obstruction
Analgesics plus docusate sodium (Dioctyl forte 1–2 tablets 8 hourly) until obstruction is complete. Lomotil (see Table 30) 2 tablets 6-hourly.

## Dyspnoea
1. Bronchodilators : salbutamol tablets
                     aminophylline suppositories.
2. Steroids : start at 45 mg prednisolone daily and reduce to 15 mg daily.
3. Antibacterials : cotrimoxazole or ampicillin if dyspnoea accompanied by cough or other evidence of infection.
4. If large effusions or neoplastic invasion of lung narcotic analgesics must be used to relieve distress.
5. If excessive secretions and noisy breathing, hyoscine 0.4–0.6 mg i.m. (with a narcotic analgesic) will often dry secretions and quieten breathing.

## Depression and anxiety
1. Prednisolone 5–15 mg daily may greatly improve mood.
2. Relief of physical distress
3. Tricyclic antidepressants, e.g. amitriptyline 25–100 mg daily
4. If anxiety is dominant : dothiepin 75–100 mg at night. i.v. diazepam 5–20 mg for panic states.

## Skeletal metastases
Add prednisolone 15–45 mg, with phenylbutazone 600–800 mg, daily if necessary to narcotic analgesic treatment. Other measures may be required (e.g. radiotherapy, phenol nerve block).

## Cough
1. Linctus methadone 5–10 ml (2 mg/5 ml) at night
2. Antibacterials

3. Bromhexine 8 mg tds to liquify tenacious sputum
4. Diamorphine if the above are not effective

**Itch**
1. Chlorpheniramine 4 mg 8-hourly
2. Local or systemic steroids
3. Cholestyramine if biliary obstruction

**Hiccough**
1. Metoclopramide 10 mg oral or i.m.
2. Chlorpromazine 25 mg oral or i.m.

## NON-STEROIDAL ANTI-INFLAMMATORY ANALGESICS (NSAIA)

Act peripherally and centrally on prostaglandin synthesis:

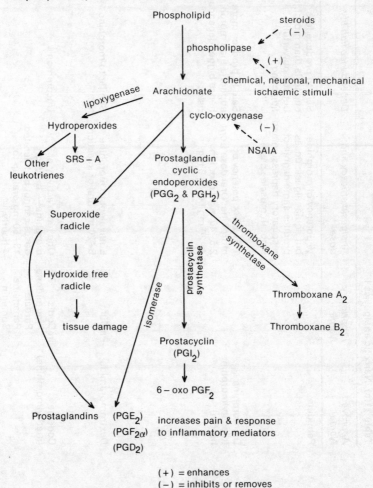

Phospholipid

steroids
(−)

phospholipase

(+)

chemical, neuronal, mechanical
ischaemic stimuli

lipoxygenase     Arachidonate

cyclo-oxygenase
(−)

Hydroperoxides                              NSAIA

Other          SRS – A          Prostaglandin
leukotrienes                     cyclic
                                 endoperoxides
                                 ($PGG_2$ & $PGH_2$)

Superoxide                                      thromboxane
radicle                                         synthetase

Hydroxide free                                  Thromboxane $A_2$
radicle

tissue damage                                   Thromboxane $B_2$

isomerase   prostacyclin
            synthetase

            Prostacyclin
            ($PGI_2$)

            6 – oxo $PGF_2$

Prostaglandins   ($PGE_2$)     increases pain & response
                 ($PGF_{2\alpha}$)  to inflammatory mediators
                 ($PGD_2$)

(+) = enhances
(−) = inhibits or removes

**Table 11(a)** Narcotic analgesics I

| Approved Name | Proprietary Name | Analgesic efficacy and dose | Dependance liability | Special features |
|---|---|---|---|---|
| Pethidine | | ½ potency of morphine but equianalgesic doses produce same degree of respiratory depression and smooth muscle spasm | Said to produce less euphoria than morphine but still powerfully addicting | Absorbed well from gut but 50% first pass metabolism. Can produce vomiting but no constriction of pupil and less cough suppression than morphine. |
| Diamorphine (diacetylmorphine heroin) | | 1·5–2·5 × potency of morphine. Oral dose from 2·5–40 mg s.c. or i.m. 4–20 mg i.v. 1–5 mg. | Said to produce more euphoria than morphine hence bigger dependance risk. | More active than morphine because enters brain more rapidly. In CNS converted to monoacetylmorphine and morphine. Action lasts ~ 3 hours (but $T_{\frac{1}{2}} = 3$ mins). Possibly less vomiting than morphine. Enters fetus more readily than morphine. |
| Dextromoramide | Palfium | Equivalent to morphine 5–20 mg oral or injection | Similar to morphine | Duration of action 3–4 hours. Useful oral drug for moderate pain. |
| Codeine (methylmorphine) | in Codis Pharmidone Pardale Panadeine Sonalgin Solpadeine Veganin | One tenth activity of morphine — but high doses cannot be tolerated. 15–50 mg oral, up to 4-hourly. Injection : 15–60 mg. | Uncommon | Used for mild pain, cough suppression and symptomatic control of diarrhoea. Releases low levels of morphine into plasma and brain ($T_{\frac{1}{2}} = 2\frac{1}{2}$ h). Injection may be useful in moderate pain. |

| | | | | |
|---|---|---|---|---|
| Dihydrocodeine | DF 118 | Similar to or more potent than codeine. | Uncommon | Mild to moderate pain and cough suppression |
| Diphenoxylate | Contained in Lomotil with atropine | 2.5 mg/tablet Lomotil 4 tablets initially, then 2, 6-hourly | Can occur with prolonged use. May produce euphoria. | Use limited to symptomatic treatment of acute self-limiting diarrhoea |
| Methadone | | Similar to morphine oral or injection 5–15 mg (45 min delay in onset after oral). | Less euphoria than morphine. Less severe withdrawal syndrome. | Similar analgesic to morphine and used to replace morphine and diamorphine in addicts |

**Table 11(b)** Narcotic analgesics II

| Approved Name | Proprietary name | Analgesic efficacy and dose | Dependance liability | Special features |
|---|---|---|---|---|
| Dipipanone | Diconal (10 mg dipipanone + 30 mg cyclizine) | $2\frac{1}{2} \times$ activity of morphine. 10–25 mg i.m. injection. Diconal given orally | Similar to morphine | Powerful orally active analgesic |
| Ethoheptazine | Equagesic 75 mg Ethoheptazine + 150 mg meprobamate + 250 mg aspirin. | 2 Equagesic tablets 3 or 4 times daily similar efficacy to codeine. | Not reported | For mild pain |
| Levorphanol | Dromoran | $3–4 \times$ activity of morphine. 1.5–3 mg oral. 2–4 mg injection. | Similar to morphine | Similar analgesic to morphine |
| Oxycodone | Proladone | 30 mg suppository at night (equivalent to 20 mg morphine orally). | Similar to morphine | Useful for night-long analgesia |
| Phenazocine | Prinadol Narphen | $3–4 \times$ activity of morphine. 5 mg orally or sublingually 4–6-hourly. | Similar to morphine | Similar analgesic to morphine |
| Pentazocine | Fortral | $\frac{1}{2}$ activity of morphine 25–100 mg oral 3–4 hourly. 30–60 mg i.m., s.c. or i.v. injection. | Less dependence than morphine | Partial opiate agonist. Usefulness limited by frequent dysphoric reactions. Not for myocardial infarction. |
| Buprenorphine | Temgesic | 15 × activity of morphine. 0.3–0.6 i.m. or slow i.v. injection 6–8-hourly. | Less dependence than morphine | Partial opiate agonist. Powerful analgesic not readily reversed by naloxone. Can also be given by sublingual tablet. |

a. *All* the NSAIAs inhibit cyclo-oxygenase
   Three types of cyclo-oxygenase inhibitors
   1. *Irreversible* (e.g. aspirin) effects persist beyond removal of drug
   2. *Non-competitive reversible* (e.g. phenacetin) — trap free radicles. Removal of lipid peroxides, hydrogen peroxide and superoxide blocks prostaglandin synthesis.
   3. *Rapid and reversible* (e.g. propionic acid derivatives) (Dietary eicosapentanoic acid is also a reversible inhibitor and accounts for reduced prostaglandin synthesis, proneness to bleeding and low incidence of thrombosis in Eskimos)
b. Other actions of *some* NSAIAs
   1. Inhibition of phosphodiesterase (e.g. indomethacin) → raised cAMP → reduced lysosomal activity → reduced generation of superoxides
   2. Removal of hydroxyl radicles (e.g. aspirin)
   3. Inhibition of leucocyte migration (e.g. indomethacin)
c. Other shared properties of NSAIAs
   1. Anti-inflammatory, antipyretic, analgesic
   2. Inhibition of platelet aggregation
   3. Gastric irritation, ulceration and haemorrhage. Aggravate peptic ulcer.
   4. Hypersensitivity reactions are common
   5. (Probable) renal damage on prolonged use; transient rise in blood urea and shedding of epithelial cells in urine after brief drug exposure
   6. (Probable) hepatic damage
   7. Prolongation of labour
   8. Potentiation of effects of anticoagulants (esp. phenylbutazone, azapropazone and aspirin. Naproxen and ibuprofen do not prolong prothrombin time.)

## ASPIRIN

*Pharmacokinetics*
1. Low doses: First order elimination, 80% converted to salicylurate.
2. High doses saturate this conjugation reaction and thus eliminated by zero order kinetics, so $T_{\frac{1}{2}}$ changes with dose.
3. $V_d$ reduced in patients with R.A.
4. 80–85% bound to plasma protein.

*Toxicity*
1. Asymptomatic blood loss, haematemesis and malaena, nausea, vomiting, exacerbation of peptic ulceration.

**Table 12** NSAIA: aspirin group

| Drug | Proprietary names | Dose | Tolerability | Special uses |
|---|---|---|---|---|
| Aspirin<br>Soluble aspirin | Disprin<br>Solprin | Adult: 300–900 mg<br>4–6-hourly, up to 4 g daily.<br>Not used in children under 1 year. | Excellent in acute illness. Gastric irritation with full doses on prolonged use. | Long term prophylaxis of occlusive vascular disease (dose 100 mg/day). |
| Aloxiprin (buffered aspirin) | Palaprin | | | |
| Enteric-coated aspirin | Nu-Seals | | Better tolerated than plain aspirin on prolonged use.<br>Additional paracetamol should not be given with benorylate. | |
| Slow release aspirin | Levius<br>Caprin<br>Breoprin | | | |
| Choline magnesium trisalicylate | Trisilate | | | |
| Benorylate (aspirin-paracetamol ester which dissociates after absorption) | Benoral | 1–1.5 g 8–12–hourly | | |
| Salsalate | Disalcid | | Little gastric bleeding because insoluble in gastric secretions | |
| Diflunisal | Dolobid | For acute pain: 250–500 mg twice daily | Better tolerated than aspirin but avoid in peptic ulceration | May be useful in treating night pain & morning stiffness |

2. Hypersensitivity:
   a. asthmatic attacks in patients with nasal polyps
   b. urticaria and angioedema
3. Salicylism: tinnitus, deafness, nausea, vomiting and abdominal pain
4. Gout (urate retention with low doses, urate elimination with high doses)
5. Transient decrease in renal function
6. Aggravation of bleeding disorders
7. Hepatotoxicity uncommon; abnormal LFT common.
8. Delayed onset of labour. ?Small for dates babies associated with aspirin use in pregnancy.
9. Drug interactions:
   potentiation of gastric irritants
   potentiation of hypoglycaemics
   potentiation of anticoagulants
   reduces effects of steroids
   reduces effects of spironolactone

*Uses*
1. Non-specific musculo-skeletal pain and soft tissue rheumatism
2. Febrile illnesses and mild/moderate pain
3. Rheumatoid arthritis
4. Acute rheumatism
5. Osteoarthritis
6. Long term prevention of thrombotic disease
7. Control of radiation-induced diarrhoea

**Table 13** NSAIA: some alternative agents

| Approved name | Proprietary names | $T_{\frac{1}{2}}$ (h) | Pharmacokinetics | Tolerability | Clinical features |
|---|---|---|---|---|---|
| *Phenylacetic acid derivatives* | | | | | |
| diclofenac | Voltarol | 1–2 | Can depress plasma salicylate levels | Rashes less common than with fenclofenac but more GI disturbances. | Oral dose: 25–50 mg 8-hourly; also 100 mg suppositories |
| fenclofenac | Flenac | 12–20 | | Rashes common (8–15% in first three weeks) | 0.6–1.2 g/day in 2 divided doses. |
| *Phenylpropionic acid derivatives* | | | | | |
| ibuprofen | Brufen Ebufac | 2 | | Low incidence of side effects | Dose 200–400 mg 3–4 times daily. Unsuitable for gout, ankylosing spondylitis or acute inflammatory processes. |
| ketoprofen | Alrheumat Orudis | 2 | | | Slow release & suppository preparations available. Dose 50 mg 2–4 times daily. |
| naproxen | Naprosyn | 12–15 | Non-linear protein binding in high doses | Low incidence of side effects | Useful in acute gout: 750 mg initial dose then 250 mg 12-hourly. Usual dose 0.5–1 g/day in 2 divided doses. |
| flurbiprofen | Froben | 3–6 | | Little gastric irritation Occasional rashes | Single daily dose (600 mg at night) increasing to 900 mg/day in divided doses. |
| fenbufen | Lederfen | | Prodrug: at least 2 active metabolites with long half-lives are produced in the liver. No accumulation in moderate renal failure. | | |

| Oxicam piroxicam | Feldene | 36–100 | No evidence of altered metabolism in elderly | Well tolerated | Single daily dose (20 mg) Can be used in acute gout (40 mg initially then 40 mg/day for 1 week). |

N.B. May need to try several drugs to suit a particular patient

**Table 14** NSAIA: Pyrazolone group

| Drug | Proprietary names | Dose | Pharmacokinetics | Toxicity | Clinical features |
|---|---|---|---|---|---|
| phenylbutazone | Butazolidin Butacote | 100–200 mg orally 8–12-hourly. Also PR & IM. | Completely absorbed orally. Small $V_d$; 98% protein bound. 99% metabolised to oxyphenbutazone & to the C-glucuronide. $T_{\frac{1}{2}} = 2$–4 days. | Rashes & GI disturbances common. Agranulocytosis rare. Salt & water retention. Jaundice. Drug interactions. | Highly effective anti-inflammatory agents, but reserved for acute gout & intractable ankylosing spondylitis because of toxicity. |
| oxyphenbutazone | Tanderil Tandacote | 100 mg 8–12-hourly. 250 mg suppositories. | $T_{\frac{1}{2}} = 1$–2 days. | | Oxyphenbutazone eye ointment used in episcleritis, scleritis & anterior uveitis. |
| azapropazone | Rheumox | 1–2 g daily in divided doses. | Well absorbed orally. Not extensively metabolised. $T_{\frac{1}{2}} = 1$ day. 98% protein bound. | Not yet adequately assessed, but can cause rashes and GI disturbances. | Effective analgesics & anti-inflammatory agents. Azaprazone used in acute gout. |
| feprazone | Methrazone | 200–600 mg daily in divided doses | | | |

**Table 15** NSAIA: anthranilic acid derivatives

| Approved name | Proprietary name | Dose | Pharmacokinetics | Toxicity | Clinical features |
|---|---|---|---|---|---|
| mefenamic acid | Ponstan | 500 mg 8-hourly | Slow absorption from gut (peak at 2–3 h) 99% bound to plasma proteins. | Diarrhoea is common. Less common: dizziness, rashes, leucopenia, autoimmune haemolysis. | Analgesic, weak anti-inflammatory |
| flufenamic acid | Meralen | 200 mg 8-hourly | Perhaps more rapidly absorbed than mefenamic acid. $T_{\frac{1}{2}} = $ 3 h. | | |

**Table 16** NSAIA: indoleacetic acid derivatives

| Approved name | Proprietary names | Dose | Pharmacokinetics | Tolerability | Clinical usefulness |
|---|---|---|---|---|---|
| indomethacin | Artracin Imbrilon Indocid Mobilan Tannex | Oral: 25–250 mg 8–12-hourly. Slow release 75 mg tablets. PR: 100 mg suppositories. | Rapidly absorbed from intestinal & rectal mucosa. High protein binding. Partly metabolised by demethylation and deacetylation. Some excreted unchanged in urine & bile. $T_{\frac{1}{2}} = 7$ h, but action is much more prolonged than this. | *Frequent*: headache (20–50%), giddiness, GI disturbance, esp. dyspepsia; exacerbation of PU. *Uncommon*: drowsiness; confusion; depression; hypersensitivity; thrombocytopenia. | Powerful anti-inflammatory, useful in RA & acute gout & other musculoskeletal disorders: bursitis, tendonitis, trauma, ankylosing spondylitis; Reiter's syndrome; psoriatic arthritis; enteropathic enteropathies; useful in OA hip; may alleviate fever of lymphoma & post-cardiotomy syndrome. |
| sulindac | Clinoril | 100–200 mg 12-hourly. | Given as sulphoxide (inactive) is rapidly absorbed. Metabolised to sulphide (active). $T_{\frac{1}{2}} = 16$ h. Enterohepatic circulation | Less gastric irritation, less CNS toxicity than indomethacin. Constipation common. | Similar effectiveness to indomethacin |
| tolmetin | Tolectin | 100–200 mg 8-hourly. | Well & rapidly absorbed. Highly protein bound. $T_{\frac{1}{2}} = 1$ h. Excreted in urine partly unchanged, partly metabolised and conjugated. Metabolism accelerated when given with aspirin. | Less gastric irritation than indomethacin. Less CNS toxicity than indomethacin but GI disturbances common. Headache & dizziness can | Similar effectiveness to indomethacin in RA |

# Drugs for cardiovascular disease

### ANGINA PECTORIS

*Angina pectoris*:  referred pain from an ischaemic myocardium. Much (but not all) angina is due to atherosclerotic coronary artery disease.

### Scheme of factors producing angina

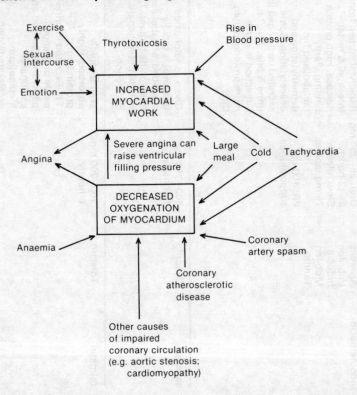

MANAGEMENT OF ANGINA

**A. Risk factors which can be manipulated**
1. insufficient exercise
2. hypertension
3. smoking
4. plasma lipid changes
5. obesity
6. abnormal glucose tolerance

1. Physical activity must not be curtailed and a graded exercise program recommended. Exercise raises plasma high density lipoprotein, increases plasma fibrinolytic activity and improves myocardial efficiency. Development of collateral vessels may be encouraged.
2. Even minimal hypertension must be controlled — rapid falls in blood pressure should be avoided.
3. Stop smoking. Nicotine has sympathomimetic activity: stimulates sympathetic autonomic ganglia, and indirectly stimulates noradrenergic nerve terminals (like cocaine) raising peripheral resistance, heart rate and blood pressure. Arrhythmias and increased platelet stickiness also occur and plasma high density lipoprotein concentration probably falls. Atherosclerosis is accelerated by raised blood pressure and deposition of platelet thrombi on the arterial intima.
4. Raised low density lipoprotein fractions (LDL and VLDL) cholesterol and reduced concentrations in the high density fraction (HDL) are associated with accelerated atheroma formation. A diet with reduced animal fat and relatively raised vegetable oils increases HDL/total cholesterol ratio.
    One-third of angina patients have abnormal fasting plasma lipids but no evidence that diet or lipid-lowering drugs influence anginal symptoms or prognosis once ischaemic heart disease has become established.
5. Obesity does not itself accelerate coronary atherosclerosis, but may be associated with other risk factors. Weight loss is often accompanied by a reduction in angina.
6. Diabetes mellitus associated with raised incidence of occlusive arterial disease (? due to abnormal plasma lipids). No evidence that minor reductions in glucose tolerance linked with ischaemic heart disease.

**B. Treat factors which increase myocardial oxygen demand or supply**
1. hypertension
2. cardiac failure
3. left ventricular outflow obstruction
4. tachyarrhythmias

5. thyrotoxicosis
6. smoking (increases carboxyhaemoglobin and constricts arteries)
7. anaemia

**C. Drug treatment:**
1. nitrates — to treat attack or prophylactically
2. β-adrenergic blocking
3. calcium antagonists.
Can be used in combination but some restrictions.

NITRATES

a. **Glyceryl trinitrate** — sublingually during attack
                          — prophylactically before exercise.
Directly acting vasodilator — mainly veins.
Plasma $T_{\frac{1}{2}} \sim 2-3$ min. Action begins within 2 min and lasts up to 30 min.
Given *sublingually* because:
1. High first-pass hepatic metabolism ($\sim 80-90\%$) to active metabolites when given orally.
2. Rapid buccal absorption.
Tell patient:
 (i) about possible side effects (see below).
 (ii) not to put tablets in sunlight, in bottles with other tablets or cotton wool (glyceryl trinitrate is volatile and absorbs on to other materials from tablet).
 (iii) to check expiry date of tablets.
 (iv) use prophylactically.
 (v) effect terminated by swallowing or spitting out tablet.
   Glyceryl trinitrate *ointment* (Percutol) also avoids hepatic first-pass inactivation. Acts for at least 2–3 up to 6 hours. Skin must be covered after ointment applied. Dose 2–5 gm every 2–6 hours. Role in angina prevention undecided.

*Transdermal glyceryl trinitrate* (Transderm-Nitro)
Self-adhesive plastic patch which is applied to the skin (usually applied to the lateral chest) once every 24 h. During this time it releases trinitrin (5 mg/24 h) which is systemically absorbed via the dilated veins and arteries in the skin at a controlled rate. Several days should elapse before a fresh patch is applied to the same area of skin.

## ACTION OF NITRATES IN ANGINA PECTORIS

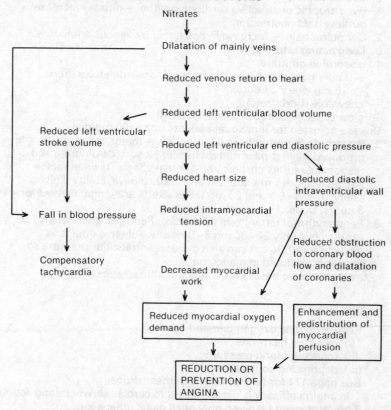

**Sustained-action glyceryl trinitrate tablets** (Sustac; Nitrocontin)
Evidence of beneficial effect used at maximum dosage. Start at low
doses and increase as tolerated over period of weeks to maximum
(6.4 mg 8-hourly).

*Adverse effects*
Headache — tolerance occurs in 1–2 weeks
Palpitations and tachycardia — may exacerbate angina
Postural hypotension and dizziness — patient may need to sit or lie
   down
Flushing
Chronic high doses rarely cause methaemoglobinaemia
Tolerance probably rare but rebound coronary vasoconstriction on
   withdrawal could occur and nitrates should not be abruptly
   discontinued. No evidence of cross-tolerance between chronic
   prophylactic doses and acute dosing for anginal attacks.

*Contraindications*
1. Hypertrophic obstructive cardiomyopathy — nitrates increase outflow tract obstruction.
2. Cor pulmonale — increase hypoxaemia by venous admixture.
b. **Long acting nitrates**:
1. Isosorbide dinitrate
   — sublingual (Isordil) — can be used for acute attack (max. 10 mg every 2 hours)
— chewable (Sorbitrate)
— slow release (Cedocard, Isoket Retard).
Dosage adjusted for individual patients up to 120 mg/day.
2. Isosorbide 5-mononitrate (Elantan 20) — major active metabolite produced by first-pass metabolism of isosorbide dinitrate and responsible for its chronic anti-anginal effect. This metabolite has no first-pass metabolism and 100% bioavailability if given orally. $T_{\frac{1}{2}} = 4-5$ h and 20 mg tablet exerts anti-anginal effect for 8 hours. Dose: 1–2 tablets 8-hourly.
3. Pentaerythritol tetranitrate (Mycardol; Peritrate) given orally for prophylaxis only 20–60 mg 6–8-hourly. Adverse effects as glyceryl trinitrate but can also increase intraocular pressure so not recommended in glaucoma.
Cross-tolerance between nitrates theoretically possible.


## β-BLOCKERS

Reduce cardiac oxygen demand by:
  (i) reducing heart rate
 (ii) reducing blood pressure
(iii) depressing contractility
See page 171 for further details of these drugs.
   In angina efficacy is partly related to cardiac slowing: long acting β-blockers need be given only once daily, otherwise pharmacological differences between drugs unimportant. Aim for a resting heart rate 55–60/min.
   Can use in combination with nitrates.
   Atypical (Prinzmetal) angina rarely responds, and may worsen, with β-blockers (probably due to unopposed coronary vasoconstrictor α-activity).
N.B.
  (i) Sudden withdrawal of β-blockers may increase angina or precipitate myocardial infarction.
 (ii) β-blockers probably prevent myocardial re-infarction (? also prevent primary infarction).

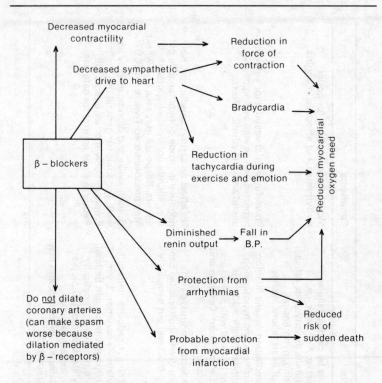

## CALCIUM ANTAGONISTS

Blockade of calcium entry into the cells of the heart and blood vessels results in:
 (i)   decreased speed and force of cardiac contraction
 (ii)  reduced activity in pacemaker nodal tissue in the atria
(iii)  coronary artery vasodilation
(iv)   peripheral arteriolar dilation
   Particularly useful for:
 (i)   Atypical (Prinzmetal) angina and coronary spasm.
(ii)   With nitrates when β-blocker contraindicated.
   Can be used with β-blockers (care!) when pain difficult to control.
   **Nifedipine** is liquid (in capsule) — can bite open capsule for immediate treatment of angina — others only for prophylaxis.

## SECONDARY PREVENTION IN SURVIVORS OF MYOCARDIAL INFARCTION

1. Stopping smoking of proven benefit.
2. Regular physical activity probably effective.
3. Control hypertension, obesity, diabetes mellitus.

**Table 17** Some calcium antagonists used in angina

| Drug | Dose | Adverse effects | Comments |
|---|---|---|---|
| Verapamil (Cordilox) | 80–120 mg, 6–8-hourly | Contraindicated by cardiac failure, sino-atrial disease, A-V block, i.v. β-blockers, digitalis toxicity. Side effects: nausea, vomiting, hypotension, exacerbation of heart failure, rashes. | Most commonly used for nodal arrhythmias, but effective in angina. |
| Nifedipine (Adalat) | 30–120 mg, 4–8-hourly | Peripheral vasodilation causes flushing, headaches, dizziness and hypotension. This may precipitate angina 30 mins after dose. Can be used with β-blockers but heart failure can occur. Oedema and hepatitis also occur. | Powerful arterial vasodilator valuable in hypertension as well as angina. No useful anti-arrhythmic effects. |
| Lidoflazine (Clinium) | 12 mg daily week 1, 120 mg 12-hourly week 2, 120 mg 8-hourly thereafter | Dizziness, headache, tinnitus, gastric upsets. Not negatively inotropic (so can be used with β-blockers) but negatively chronotropic. | No effect on cardiac conduction, not negative inotrope or hypotensive, but may slightly potentiate hypotensive agents. Response may take 6–8 weeks. May produce broad T-wave on ECG. |
| Perhexiline (Pexid) | 50–100 mg 12-hourly | Dizziness, flushing, headache, nausea, weight loss relatively common. Liver damage and hypoglycaemia can be fatal. Neuropathy (commoner in genetically 'poor hydroxylators' of drug). Diplopia, papilloedema, extrapyramidal syndromes, seizures, impotence and loss of libido also reported. | Quinidine-like and diuretic activity as well. Too toxic for general use. Employed only if other agents fail. Requires close control for safe use. |

4. Evidence that reduction of plasma lipids is beneficial is limited. Probably prudent to reduce saturated fats intake to 8–10% of food energy and cholesterol to < 300 mg/day; have a polyunsaturated/saturated fatty acid ratio of 0.75; take increased proportion of vegetable protein. Antihyperlipidaemic drugs not of proven benefit.
5. Drug treatment
   a. β-blockers — substantial reduction in rate of sudden death shown especially if begun as soon as possible (within four hours) of infarction.
      (i) Propranolol, timolol, metoprolol, oxprenolol all shown to have varying degrees of efficacy.
   b. Platelet active drugs. Evidence of efficacy, especially if begun as soon as possible.
      (i) Aspirin
      (ii) Sulphinpyrazone
      (iii) Dipyridamole + Aspirin

## CARDIAC FAILURE

Occurs when heart unable to pump blood at the rate required for systemic metabolic requirements at rest and during normal activity. Mortality akin to some malignancies: 5 year survival about 50%.

$$\text{Cardiac Output} = \text{Heart Rate} \times \text{Stroke Volume}$$

Stroke Volume determined by:
1. *Filling pressure* ('Pre-load'). Frank-Starling ventricular function curve shows that stroke volume increases with increasing LV filling pressure.

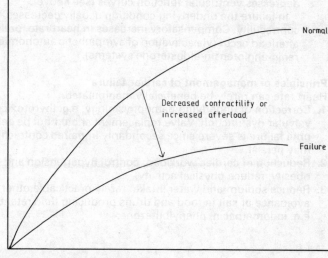

Stroke Volume

Normal

Decreased contractility or increased afterload.

Failure

LV filling pressure

2. *Afterload* depends on intraventricular pressure and ventricular volume and is equivalent to tension in ventricular wall during contraction. Ventricular volume determined by aortic impedance (roughly equivalent to peripheral resistance). Myocardial disease depresses the ventricular function curve.

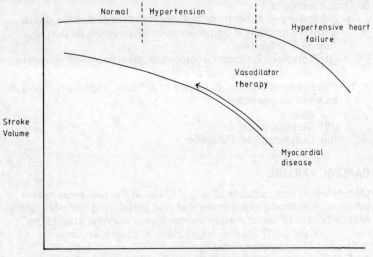

3. *Contractility (inotropic state) of myocardium* — decrease depresses ventricular function curves (see above).
   In failure the underlying condition usually decreases contractility. Compensatory increases in heart rate, preload and afterload occur (via activation of sympathetic autonomic and renin-angiotensin-aldosterone systems).

## Principles of management of cardiac failure
Heart rate can rarely be beneficially manipulated.
1. Correction of underlying pathophysiology, e.g. thyrotoxicosis, valvular dysfunction. Valve replacement should not be delayed until failure is severe since secondarily impaired contractility may persist.
2. Reduction of cardiac workload: control hypertension and obesity, reduce physical activity.
3. Reduce sodium and water intake: rarely practicable other than avoidance of salt in food and drugs producing fluid retention, e.g. indomethacin, phenylbutazone.

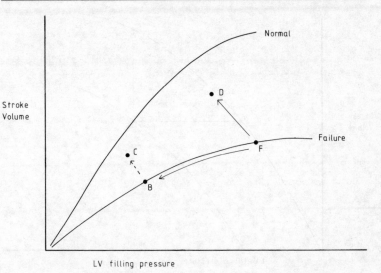

LV filling pressure

4. Diuretics: reduce overexpanded extracellular fluid volume: reduce filling pressure without increased output (F → B) but stroke volume may later rise due to slowly improving ventricular function (→ C).
5. Inotropic agents increase contractility, e.g. digitalis, catecholamines, aminophylline, and shift ventricular function curves up and to right (→ D).
6. Vasodilators. Venous dilators reduce filling pressure (F → V) and
   a. Reduce pulmonary capillary pressure thus decreasing pulmonary oedema, improving oxygenation so catecholamine drive falls.
   b. Decrease LV volume, ventricular diameter and so wall tension and thus oxygen demand (large hearts consume more oxygen).
   c. Reduce valve ring dilation and improves muscular anatomy and dynamics.
   d. Decrease risks of dysrhythmias and conduction defects.
   e. Reduce LV diastolic pressure allowing better coronary perfusion during diastole.

*Arterial dilators*
a. Reduce impedance so cardiac output increases see above and shift Frank-Starling curve (F → A).
b. Reduce myocardial oxygen consumption because reduced LV wall tension.
c. Increase forward flow by reducing regurgitation in aortic or mitral insufficiency.

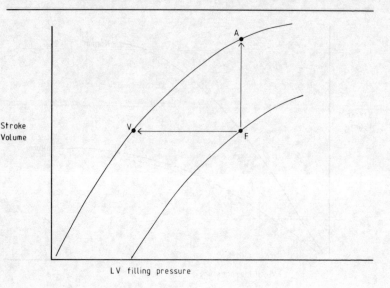

DIGITALIS GLYCOSIDES

Digoxin and digitoxin most commonly used.

*Uses*
1. Fast atrial fibrillation to control ventricular rate.
2. Atrial flutter — favours return to sinus rhythm or converts to fibrillation when ventricular rate easier to control.
3. Supraventricular tachycardia — long term oral prophylaxis for regular tachycardias but avoid in Wolff-Parkinson-White syndrome.
4. Congestive heart failure
   (i) with atrial fibrillation — benefit due to rate control.
   (ii) with sinus rhythm benefit controversial. Short-lived acute changes shown in many studies, although some showed chronic beneficial effects. One study showed no benefit from adding digoxin to adequate diuretic therapy and in several studies digoxin withdrawal was achieved without deterioration. Thus to treat failure, first achieve optimal diuretic response before adding digoxin and try to withdraw digitalis after about a month's therapy (? risks of toxicity then greater than benefit).
5. No evidence that digitalis useful in acute failure and may cause arrhythmias.

## Mode of action

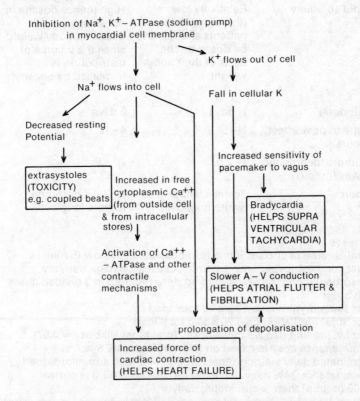

Inhibition of Na$^+$, K$^+$ – ATPase (sodium pump)
in myocardial cell membrane

K$^+$ flows out of cell

Na$^+$ flows into cell

Fall in cellular K

Decreased resting
Potential

Increased sensitivity of
pacemaker to vagus

extrasystoles
(TOXICITY)
e.g. coupled beats

Increased in free
cytoplasmic Ca$^{++}$
(from outside cell
& from intracellular
stores)

Bradycardia
(HELPS SUPRA
VENTRICULAR
TACHYCARDIA)

Activation of Ca$^{++}$
– ATPase and other
contractile
mechanisms

Slower A – V conduction
(HELPS ATRIAL FLUTTER &
FIBRILLATION)

prolongation of depolarisation

Increased force of
cardiac contraction
(HELPS HEART FAILURE)

## PHARMACOKINETICS OF CARDIAC GLYCOSIDES

|  | Digoxin | Digitoxin |
|---|---|---|
| Absorption from gut | Variable 20–80% (bioavailability may be a therapeutic problem) | 100% |
| Hepatic metabolism | Minimal | 90% (thus sensitive to induction of mixed function oxidase by other drugs) |
| Renal excretion | 80% (a relatively water-soluble drug) | Minimal (therefore safer than digoxin in renal failure) |

| | | |
|---|---|---|
| Protein binding | 25% | 95% |
| Lipid solubility | Relatively low (therefore obese patients should not be dosed on the basis of their body weight) | High (hence dosage in obese patients is based on body weight since the volume of distribution is increased by obesity) |
| $T_\frac{1}{2}$ (hours) | 1½ days | 6 days |
| Time to peak effect (hours) | 1½–5 | 4–12 |
| Approx. therapeutic levels (nmol/1) | 1–2.5 | 20–35 |
| Source | digitalis lanata (white foxglove) | digitalis purpurea (purple foxglove) |

*Dosage*
Oral is route of choice; if this is impossible then slow (5 min) i.v. injection best (avoid i.m. — painful, causes necrosis, variably absorbed). Long $T_\frac{1}{2}$ means *loading dose* required in 3 divided doses 5 h apart:
For sinus rhythm give 12 μg/kg total load
For atrial fibrillation give 20 μg/kg total load
For i.v. loading use 2/3 these doses (oral bioavailability = 0.67)
*Maintenance dose* is based on this loading dose. Since % eliminated daily via non-renal route = 14% load and total % load eliminated = 34% daily. If creatinine clearance ($Cl_{cr}$) is normal (100 ml/min) then % eliminated daily =

$$14 + \frac{100}{5} = 14 + 20 = 34\%$$

Thus for renal impairment % eliminated daily = $14 + \frac{Cl_{cr}}{5}$

Daily maintenance dose = loading dose × % eliminated each day.
   In renal failure the loading dose is reduced by 1/3. Dialysis removes very little digoxin and need not be considered in deciding the maintenance dose.
   Always monitor clinical response and toxicity in patients treated with digoxin.

## TOXICITY OF CARDIAC GLYCOSIDES

Narrow therapeutic range: toxicity seen in 15–20% unselected patients and is potentially fatal.

Optimal dose must be sought for each patient. In atrial fibrillation slowing of pulse rate especially on exercise is best guide as there is poor correlation between plasma level and ventricular rate. In heart failure control is more difficult as toxicity can occur when plasma concentration in 'therapeutic range'. Diagnosis of toxicity is a clinical decision not a laboratory diagnosis.

### A. Gastrointestinal

Common — anorexia, nausea, vomiting — probably via central effect on chemoreceptor trigger zone in medulla.
Uncommon — diarrhoea, constipation, abdominal pain.
Rare — haemorrhagic bowel necrosis.

### B. Cardiovascular

May not be preceded by GI effects.
First degree heart block is sometimes premonitory of more serious arrhythmias. Commonest effects are sinus bradycardia; bigeminal rhythm (paired ventricular extrasystoles), but any type of arrhythmia or conduction defect may occur.
Less commonly — cardiac arrest, increasing cardiac failure.

### C. Neurological

Common — headache, drowsiness, fatigue, acute confusional state, blurred vision, altered colour vision, visual aberrations.
Rare — neuralgia, paraesthesiae, coma, optic neuritis producing scotomata or blindness, paresis of ocular muscles, muscular weakness.

### D. Others

Rare — skin rashes due to allergy, gynaecomastia.

## PREDISPOSING FACTORS TO DIGITALIS INTOXICATION

1. *Electrolyte disturbance*
Hypokalaemia
Hypercalcaemia
Hypernatraemia
Hypomagnesaemia
Alkalosis

*2. Drugs*
a. Potassium depletion
   (i) Potassium depleting diuretics
   (ii) Carbenoxolone
   (iii) Mineralocorticosteroids, corticosteroids and ACTH.
b. Increased myocardial excitability
   (i) Catecholamines
   (ii) Reserpine (catecholamine release).
c. Increased danger of conduction block
   (i) β-blockers
   (ii) Verapamil
d. Unknown mechanism (all described for digoxin)
   (i) Quinidine (? decreased renal clearance; ? reduced non-renal clearance; ? reduced tissue binding)
   (ii) Verapamil (probably decreased renal clearance)
   (iii) Amiodarone
   (iv) Nifedipine
   (v) Possibly broad-spectrum antibiotics, e.g. tetracycline (increased reabsorption of drug from large bowel because gut flora killed so don't metabolise drug)

*3. Disease states*
Hypothyroidism — prolonged $T_{\frac{1}{2}}$, reduced $V_d$
Hypoxia — sensitises to arrhythmias
Renal failure (digoxin) — impaired excretion
Myocarditis
Severe heart disease $\Big\}$ impaired intracellular $Ca^{++}$ release
Severe pulmonary disease — hypoxia, acid-base changes
Acute rheumatic carditis — increased risk of heart block

*4. Old age*
(reduced renal function also decreased muscle mass reduces ATPase binding sites thus reducing apparent volume of distribution).

*5. DC cardioversion*

**Contraindications to Digitalis**
1. Heart block
2. Hypertrophic obstructive cardiomyopathy (inotropic effect increases outflow obstruction).
3. Wolff-Parkinson-White syndrome (accelerated anterograde conduction down anomalous pathway in atrial flutter or fibrillation may precipitate ventricular fibrillation).
4. Patients likely to require cardioversion.

**Table 18** Vasodilators used for treatment of heart failure

| Venous | Venous and arterial | Arterial |
|---|---|---|
| *Nitrates:*<br>Glyceryl trinitrate: oral (Sustac) ointment<br><br>Isosorbide dinitrate:<br>oral (Isoket; Isordil)<br>i.v. (Cedocard IV; Isoket) | Sodium Nitroprusside i.v. (Nipride)<br><br>*α-blockers:*<br>Prazosin: oral (Hypovase)<br>Phentolamine: i.v. (Rogitine)<br>Phenoxybenzamine: oral (Dibenyline)<br><br>Captopril: oral (Capoten)<br><br>*Ganglion-blockers:*<br>Trimetophan: i.v. (Arfonad) | *Directly acting smooth muscle relaxants:*<br>Hydralazine: i.v. and oral (Apresoline)<br>Minoxidil: oral (Loniten)<br><br>$\beta_2$-Agonists<br>Salbutamol: i.v. and oral (Ventolin)<br>Terbutaline: i.v. and oral (Bricanyl)<br>Nifedipine: oral (Adalat) |

## Management of acute pulmonary oedema
1. Sit patient up.
2. Oxygen — up to 30% can be used and 100% is safe if no lung disease present.
3. IV loop diuretic, e.g. frusemide 20 mg — acts as venodilator and produces prompt diuresis.
4. Morphine (10 mg) or Diamorphine (2.5–5 mg) i.v. if obstructive airways disease is excluded — reduces afterload, acts as venodilator, relieves bronchospasm and reduces tachypnoea (but can excessively depress respiratory centre).
5. Alternative to opiates (useful in obstructive airways disease) is 250–350 mg aminophylline slowly i.v. over 5–10 mins. Relieves bronchospasm, improves myocardial contractility, mild diuretic.
6. In refractory cases incubate and use positive pressure ventilation — raised intrathoracic pressure reduces venous return, allows suction to clear airways and reduces cardiac work load by artificial ventilation.

## Management of chronic heart failure
1. Rest, but remember dangers of venous thrombosis so exercise legs etc. Patients needing prolonged rest require minidose heparin prophylaxis.
2. Diuretic therapy to reduce patient's weight and oedema. Aim at loss of about 0.5 kg/day. $K^+$ supplements required; avoid added salt and salty foods. Loop diuretics usually required initially: occasionally milder thiazide diuretics substituted later. If large doses of powerful diuretics required to clear oedema in hospital similar doses probably needed at home as well.
3. Digoxin — see comments above.
4. Large pleural effusions should be drained to help breathing but ascites usually clears with diuretics.
5. Vasodilators — nitroprusside or i.v. nitrates offer relative flexibility in dosage; hydralazine or prazosin useful in ambulant patients. Some patients become refractory on chronic treatment (increase dose; increase diuretic; change to another vasodilator). Not clear if prognosis improved but quality of life is better.

## Failure of treatment in heart failure
1. Poor compliance.
2. Inadequate dosage.
3. Concurrent use of drugs producing heart failure (see below).
4. Severe splanchnic venous congestion reducing bioavailability of oral diuretics — try parenteral administration.
5. Secondary hyperaldosteronism — try concurrent spironolactone, amiloride or triamterine.
6. Water retention with hyponatraemia — try water restriction or osmotic diuretic. If disease potentially reversible consider dialysis to remove excess sodium and water.

7. Excessive salt intake.
8. Try small doses of corticosteroids in diuretic-refractory cases: works after 3–4 days but not due to increased GFR.
9. Complications: pulmonary emboli, arrhythmias, bacterial endocarditis, cardiomyopathy, infarction, progression of underlying disease.

**Drug-induced heart failure**
1. Myocardial depression
   a. Reversible
      (i) β-adrenergic blockers (non-selective blockers raise peripheral resistance as well as having negative inotropic effects so $β_1$-blockers or those having ISA theoretically perferable — in practice all can produce failure. Digoxin and diuretics protect against failure if β-blockers needed).
      (ii) Disopyramide — other antiarrhythmics (lignocaine, mexilitine, quinidine, procainamide) only rarely cause failure in usual dosage.
      (iii) Calcium ion antagonists (nifedipine, verapamil) occasionally cause failure, especially if β-blockers used.
      (iv) Tricyclic antidepressants.
   b. Irreversible
      (i) Cytotoxic agents — anthracyclines (related to cumulative dose); cyclophosphamide (high doses).
      (ii) Alcohol (cardiomyopathy).
      (iii) Emetine.
      (iv) Chloroquine.
2. Salt and water retention (also aggravate hypertension).
   1. Corticosteroids and ACTH.
   2. Oestrogens.
   3. Carbenoxolone.
   4. Non-steroidal anti-inflammatory drugs expecially phenylbutazone, indomethacin.
   5. Chlorpropamide.
   6. Sodium containing drugs — some antacids, carbenicillin sodium, some X-ray contrast media (e.g. Conray 420).

**CARDIAC ARRHYTHMIAS**

**Vaughan Williams classification**
Based on micro-electrode studies of isolated myocardium.
Most agents non-specifically inhibit phase 4 depolarisation and increase effective refractory period.

*Class I* ('membrane stabilising action' — a local anaesthetic property)
Reduce rate of rise (dV/dt) of phase 0 by inhibiting $Na^+$ entry through fast channel.

a. increase duration of action potential
   — Quinidine
   — Procainamide
   — Disopyramide
b. decrease duration of action potential
   — Lignocaine
   — Mexiletine
   — Phenytoin
   — Tocainide
c. no effect on duration of action potential
   — Lorcainide

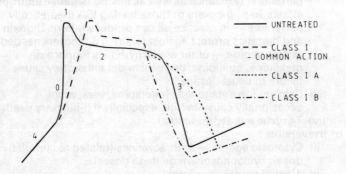

*Class II*
Drugs which prevent release of catecholamines (e.g. bretylium) or block β-adrenoreceptors (e.g. propranolol, practolol, sotalol, metoprolol). A few at exceedingly high concentrations (e.g. propranolol) have Class I actions.
   No direct effect on catecholamine untreated action potential. Probably acts because cyclic AMP (catecholamine second messenger) is arrhythmogenic.

*Class III*
Prolong duration of action potential without much effect on dV/dt of phase 0, e.g. Amiodarone, Disopyramide (minor effect); Sotalol (minor effect)

*Class IV*
Block slow inward $Ca^{++}$ current. A-V node (where this current produces major depolarisation) particularly sensitive. N.B. A-V node is part of re-entry circuit for many paroxysmal supraventricular tachycardias, e.g. Verapamil; Diltiazem.

*Class V*
Inhibit $Cl^-$ flux, e.g. alinidine (related to clonidine). None safe enough for clinical use.

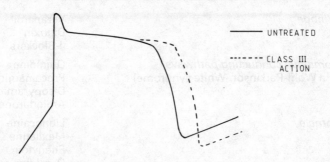

UNTREATED

CLASS III
ACTION

**Electrophysiological (Touboul) classification**
Based on His-bundle recording in patients but usually only acute
effects considered.

*Class 1*
Depress A-V node conduction and increase its refractory period,
e.g. propranolol and other β-blockers; verapamil; digoxin.
*Effects*:  Prolong ventricular response to atrial tachycardia; control
re-entry tachycardia if A-V node in circuit.

*Class 2*
Act on His-Purkinje system but not A-V node. 2A: affect conduction
in His-Purkinje system (comparable to V-W class I A actions), e.g.
quinidine, procainamide, disopyramide.
*Effects*:  Control ventricular and atrial tachyarrhythmias;
Wolff-Parkinson-White syndrome.
2B effect on His-Purkinje system but do not slow conduction
although refractory periods altered (e.g. decreased by lignocaine,
mexiletine, phenytoin — i.e. like V-W I B; increased by bretylium).
*Effects*:  Limited to ventricular tachyarrhythmias.

*Class 3*
Have mixture of class 1 and 2 actions and some other properties,
e.g. amiodarone also increases refractory periods of atrium,
ventricle and accessary pathways.
*Effects*:  atrial and ventricular tachyarrhythmias and tachycardia of
Wolff-Parkinson-White syndrome.

**Clinical classification**
Effects on type of cardiac tissue supporting arrhythmia.

| | |
|---|---|
| *Sinus node* | β-blockers |
| | Verapamil |
| | Digoxin |
| *Atrium* | Quinidine |
| | Procainamide |
| | Disopyramide |
| | Amiodarone |

| | |
|---|---|
| *A-V node* | Verapamil |
| | Digoxin |
| | β-Blockers |
| *Anomalous conducting pathways* | Quinidine |
| (as in Wolff-Parkinson-White syndrome) | Procainamide |
| | Disopyramide |
| | Amiodarone |
| *Ventricle* | Lignocaine |
| | Mexiletine |
| | Phenytoin |
| | Quinidine |
| | Procainamide |
| | Disopyramide |
| | Amiodarone |

*Note*:  No classification is completely successful in correlation of clinical utility and pharmacological properties.

ARRHYTHMIA TREATMENT

**Atrial tachyarrhythmias**
Exclude remediable causes, e.g. thyrotoxicosis, drugs.

*1. Conversion to sinus rhythm*
Usually pointless in untreated thyrotoxicosis, cardiomyopathy, hypertension, rheumatic heart disease because early recurrence likely.

Vagal stimulation, e.g. carotid sinus massage, Valsalva manoeuvre, rarely successful in atrial fibrillation or flutter but may terminate paroxysmal atrial tachycardia.

*If circulation compromised* by arrhythmia (systolic BP < 80 mmHg; cold extremities; clouded consciousness; sweating; oliguria; pulmonary oedema) proceed to DC cardioversion immediately. Synchronised DC shocks (50–400 J) necessary (unsynchronised shock may produce ventricular fibrillation); start with small charge 25–30 J and increase by 100 J until several 400 J shocks given. Best performed under short-acting i.v. anaesthetic or diazepam 5–20 mg i.v. Relative contraindications: previous digoxin therapy; hypo and hyper-kalaemia.

Cardioversion usually works for atrial tachycardia and flutter but fibrillation may be very resistant. Cardioversion more likely if cardiac failure, hypoxaemia, metabolic acidosis and potassium imbalances are corrected. Avoid digoxin in these cases. Resistant SVT is a serious problem: all drugs except amiodarone are negative inotropes and may exacerbate the situation if they fail to control the rate. Transvenous cardiac pacing should thus be considered.

**Table 19** Antiarrhythmic drugs

| Drug | Dosage | Pharmacokinetics | Adverse effects | Comments |
|---|---|---|---|---|
| Lignocaine (Xylocard; Lidothesin) | Slow i.v. bolus 50–100 mg then 4 mg/min for 30 min, 2 mg/min for 2 hrs then 1 mg/min thereafter. | Rapid distribution so effect of bolus lasts only a few mins. $T_{\frac{1}{2}}$ 1.5–2 h in normals but increased several-fold by heart or hepatic failure. High hepatic extraction with metabolism to toxic metabolites. Therapeutic plasma level 2–5 $\mu$g/ml. Clearance decreased (with elevation of plasma levels) on prolonged (48+ hours) infusion. | Paraesthesiae, giddiness, somnolence confusion, fits, myocardial depression. | Reduce infusion (not bolus dose) by half in shock, cirrhosis, β-blockade, heart failure (because liver blood flow is low in these cases so lignocaine clearance impaired). |
| Mexiletine (Mexitil) | Slow iv bolus 3 mg/kg (max 250 mg) then 3.5 mg/kg over 30 min then 1–2 mg/min depending on response. Oral: loading dose 400–600 mg then 200–300 mg 8-hourly. | Hepatic metabolism (~ 90%) $T_{\frac{1}{2}}$ 10–13h, longer in heart failure. Therapeutic plasma level 0.5–2 $\mu$g/ml. | Nausea (relatively common), nystagmus, tremor, confusion, dysarthria, bradycardia, hypotension. | Most often used orally after lignocaine discontinued but relatively low therapeutic index. |
| Tocainide (Tonocard) | 500–750 mg slowly iv over 15–30 mins then 600–800 mg orally. After 8 hrs begin maintenance of 600 mg 8-or 12-hourly. | Complete oral absorption without hepatic first pass metabolism. Renal (~ 40%) and hepatic (~ 60%) elimination — latter to inactive metabolites. $T_{\frac{1}{2}}$ ~ 15 h. Therapeutic plasma level 4–10 ~g/ml. | Paraesthesiae, tremor, dizziness, nausea. | In renal failure — 25% dose reduction if $Cl_{cr}$ < 30 ml/min — 50% reduction in anuria. Only in severe hepatic failure is dose reduction needed. Probably less negatively inotropic than lignocaine. |

**Table 19** (continued)

| Drug | Dosage | Pharmacokinetics | Adverse effects | Comments |
|---|---|---|---|---|
| Quinidine | Too dangerous i.v.; PO as sulphate — 0.2–0.3 g 3-hourly up to 4 g/day. Long acting bisulphate (Kinidin durules; Kiditard) given ~ 500 mg 12 hourly — 1st dose preceded by loading dose 0.6–0.8 g sulphate to give therapeutic levels in 3 hours. | Plasma levels useful to control dosage and toxicity. (Therapeutic 2.5–5 μg/ml). Hepatic metabolism, $T_{\frac{1}{2}}$ 7–9 h, increased by hepatic and cardiac failure; old age but not renal failure. | Depresses intracardiac conduction (stop if QRS > 140 secs). Paroxysmal ventricular arrhythmias = quinidine syncope. Diarrhoea and GI upset; vertigo; tinnitus; thrombocytopenic purpura; agranulocytosis. Anticholinergic so usually sinus rate ↑ | Dangerous drug. d-isomer of quinine so causes cinchonism. Increases plasma digoxin levels (→ toxicity); enhances hypotensive agents and coumarins; exacerbates myasthesia. |
| Procainamide (Pronestyl) | i.v. 100 mg bolus over 2 mins then up to 20 mg/min to max 1 g in 24 hours — usual maintenance 2–6 mg/min. p.o. 1 g stat then 500 mg 3-hourly or 1–1.5 g 8-hourly as Procainamide durules. | Polymorphic acetylation but ~ 60% renal excretion. $T_{\frac{1}{2}}$ 2.5–3.5 hours, prolonged in renal and cardiac failure. Therapeutic plasma level 4–10 μg/ml. | Hypotension after i.v. dose (vasodilator effect). Systemic lupus syndrome. Anticholinergic, so ventricular rate may increase as sinus rate slows. | Continuous monitoring BP and ECG essential if used i.v. Limited oral use to 6 months because risk SLE (especially in slow acetylators). |
| Disopyramide (Norpace; Rythmodan) | i.v. 2 mg/kg over 5 min to 150 mg max then 0.4 mg/kg. PO 300 mg loading dose then 100–150 mg 6-hourly. Max 200 mg 6-hourly. Sustained | 50% hepatic metabolism; 50% excreted unchanged in urine. Therapeutic plasma level 2–6 μg/ml. | Pronounced anticholinergic effects (dry mouth; urinary retention; glaucoma etc). Occasionally ventricular fibrillation (like quinidine). | Avoid in heart failure; glaucoma; enlarged prostate. |

| | | | |
|---|---|---|---|
| | release (Rythmodan Retard) 250–375 mg 12-hourly. | Negative inotrope — may precipitate cardiac failure. | Increased bioavailability in cirrhosis (shunting across liver allows higher oral absorption). Cannot give i.v. with β-blocker or digitalis toxicity. Avoid in heart failure; A-V block, sick-sinus syndrome, cardiomegaly. |
| Verapamil (Cordilox) | 5–10 mg i.v. stat slowly or 5–10 mg by slow infusion over 1 h (max 100 mg/24 h). Orally 40–120 mg 8-hourly. | Hypotensive effect disappears by 20 mins but effect on A-V node onset at 10–15 mins and lasts up to 6 h. Oral drug takes 2 h to act. Complete absorption but 80–90% first pass metabolism to norverapamil which has some activity $T_\frac{1}{2}$ 3–7 h. | Heart block, asystole, bradycardia, negatively inotropic, hypotension. Side effects rare with oral verapamil (nausea, dizziness, flushing). | Not negatively inotropic. Important drug interactions — potentiates warfarin; increases digoxin levels; potentiates bradycardia with β-blockers and verapamil. Contraindicated in sino-atrial and A-V block. |
| Amiodarone (Cardarone-X) | 200 mg p.o. 8-hourly for at least 1 week — when desired effect occurs dose reduced weekly to minimum dose (usually 200 mg daily). | Very long $T_\frac{1}{2} \sim$ 28 days so takes long time to reach steady state. Blood levels very low because highly concentrated in tissues. Plasma levels of little clinical value as not clearly related to efficacy. Response begins after 3–7 days treatment and increases over several weeks. | Sinus bradycardia common. Corneal microdeposits (only visible with slit lamp) reversible, no effect on vision. T wave becomes notched, lengthened and flattened. Photosensitive rashes. Contains iodine so alters PBI — can cause hypo- and rarely hyperthyroidism Headaches, nightmares and rarely peripheral neuropathy, tremor. | |

If control not urgent consider anti-arrhythmic drugs:
V-W Class IA and III
— Disopyramide i.v.
— Procainamide i.v.      first choices
— Amiodarone p.o. — use limited at present
   Important to determine if A-V block present since slowing atrial focus with anticholinergic drugs (like disopyramide) paradoxically results in faster ventricular rate because of conduction of greater proportion of atrial impulses. Pre-treatment with A-V node blocking drugs (e.g. Verapamil, Practolol) prevents this.
   Occasional unpredictable reversion occurs with digoxin, verapamil and β-blockers.
   Once reversion to sinus rhythm obtained, *recurrence* prevented by suppression of atrial ectopics (usually responsible for initiation of further attacks) using:
disopyramide
quinidine (slow-release form only suitable for prophylaxis)
amiodarone.
N.B.  Procainamide could be used but chronic use may produce systemic lupus erythematosus.


2.  Control of ventricular rate
Symptomatic improvement occurs when ventricular rate controlled if conversion to sinus rhythm impossible, i.e. atrial arrythmia continues but fewer impulses conducted to ventricles so heart rate slows and output increases.
   If possible, determine AV conduction pathway.
 (i) Commonly AV node to His-Purkinje system with normal QRS or aberrant conduction. AV node refractoriness increased with verapamil, β-blockers or digoxin so reducing number of impulses transmitted to ventricles. Digoxin still drug of choice for atrial fibrillation (has added effect on conduction down bundle of His). Can add verapamil or β-blocker to initial digoxin therapy if control inadequate. Verapamil and β-blockers should not be mixed.
(ii) Anomalous conduction pathway present (Wolff-Parkinson-White syndrome). Refractoriness of anomalous pathway unaffected by verapamil or β-Blockers. Digoxin may dangerously accelerate conduction in pathway and precipitate tachycardia. It should be avoided in Wolff-Parkinson-White syndrome. Drugs of choice impair atrial and anomalous pathway conduction: disopyramide; quinidine; procainamide; amiodarone.

### Junctional tachycardias
The majority of these are paroxysmal and are caused by
re-entry circuits which include the A-V node.

Abnormal atrial junctional tissue or anomalous bypass tracts,
e.g. bundles of Kent and James are usually part of the circuit.

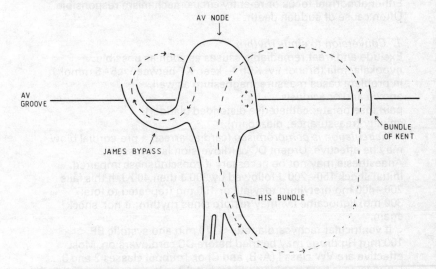

*1. Conversion to sinus rhythm*
Vagotonic manoevres more likely to succeed than in other SVTs
but unreliable.

VW Class IV agent drug of choice because of effect on node:
verapamil 10 mg i.v. usually terminates tachycardia: response
virtually diagnostic of junctional tachycardia.

VW Class IA drugs also useful because prolong refractory
period of bypass and break re-entry cycle: disopyramide i.v. is
best.

DC cardioversion effective but rarely needed because drugs
so effective.

*Recurrence* prevented by:
a. prevention of premature beats occuring when only one AV
   conduction pathway is available for conduction. These initiate
   re-entry cycles.
b. control of sinus tachycardia which can produce unidirectional
   block and dissociation of the two AV pathways.
c. equalisation of recovery times of both pathways.
d. complete block of one of the pathways.
e. prolongation of recovery time of part of the circuit.

   a, c, d, e, achieved using a VW class IV drug, e.g. verapamil or
class IA: disopyramide, procainamide or quinidine or class III
amiodarone.

b achieved using β-blocker.

A few patients have serious attacks resistant to prophylaxis and surgery to sever the anomalous bundle is necessary.

**Ventricular tachyarrhythmias in acute myocardial infarction**
Either abnormal focus or re-entry circus mechanism responsible. Often cause of sudden death.

*1. Conversion to sinus rhythm*
Exclude and treat remediable causes as soon as possible:
hypokalaemia (oral or i.v. KCl) — keep $K^+$ between 4.5–5 mmol/1.
In problem cases measure magnesium as well.
anoxia and/or acidosis.
pain (use opiate; catheterise distended bladder).
anxiety (reassurance; diazepam).

*If circulation is compromised* (cardiac arrest) a pre-cordial blow may be effective. Urgent DC cardioversion is necessary. Anaesthesia may not be necessary if consciousness impaired. Initial shock 150–200 J followed by 300 J then 400 J. If this fails 200–400 mg bretylium tosylate or 100 mg (repeated to total 300 mg) lignocaine i.v. may restore sinus rhythm; if not, shock again.

If ventricular tachycardia rate < 170/min and systolic BP < 100 mm Hg drugs may be tried before DC cardioversion. Most effective are VW class I (A, B, and C) or Touboul classes 2 and 3. Lignocaine is commonly used first but there is presently no rational way to select a drug. If one fails try another from a different class.

*2. Prophylaxis*
Heart rate < 60/min with ventricular ectopies — use atropine 0.3–0.6 mg i.v. to increase sinus rate.

Evidence that warning arrhythmias (excepting the rare 'R or T' phenomena) predict primary ventricular fibrillation is poor therefore either:
 (i)  monitor only for ventricular fibrillation and then treat as above, or
(ii)  use lignocaine prophylactically (controversial).

**Bradycardia after myocardial infarction**
Due to excessive vagal activity; hypotensive/syncopal response to opiates; A-V block. Aim to keep rate > 50/min (higher if ventricular ectopics occur frequently).

Try effect of increased venous return by raising legs. If this fails give atropine 0.3 mg i.v. every 5 mins to maximum 2.4 mg/h and titrate for desired effect. Digoxin, β-blockers and verapamil should be withheld or dosage reduced.

Pacing required if bradycardia unresponsive to atropine and severe (extending infarct; complete A-V block due to extensive anterior infarct or inferior on background of old anterior infarct). Temporary demand pacing at rate 65–75/min should prevent escape ventricular arrhythmias but with severe myocardial damage output becomes rate dependent and pacing rate should be titrated for optimum haemodynamic response.

N.B. isoprenaline is now rarely needed in heart block.

### Extrasystoles
1. Explanation and reassurance — in absence of organic heart disease extrasystoles usually benign.
2. Discourage smoking; restriction of alcohol, tea and coffee may sometimes be effective.
3. Complex ventricular extrasystoles (multifocal, R on T etc) occur even in normal hearts but may indicate increased risk of sudden death in patients with serious myocardial disease. No evidence that treatment reduces risk but may need symptomatic treatment if patient distressed by them:
   (i) β-blockers — but can increase frequency of ventricular extrasystoles if sinus rate falls too low.
   (ii) disopyramide.
   (iii) mexiletine.

## TREATMENT OF SHOCK

Reduced perfusion of essential organs produces tissue hypoxia and derangement of function. Three main types of shock which involve dysfunction of the heart, blood volume and blood flow distribution to varying degree:
a. Hypovolaemic — loss of whole blood, plasma or electrolytes
b. Cardiogenic — cardiac infarction, tamponade or pulmonary embolism
c. Septic — complicates many infections including postoperative.
Main principles are:
1. *Optimise pre-load*: replace lost blood volume; in postoperative and myocardial infarction optimal blood volume may be 250–500 ml greater than normal to get maximum effect from Frank-Starling curve. According to circumstances blood, plasma, crystalloids (usually large volumes needed to replace blood loss) or plasma substitutes needed. Substitutes currently available:
   (i) Dextrans (polysaccharides produced enzymically from starch with MWs of 40 000; 70 000; 110 000 and 150 000 — Dextran 40, 70, 110 and 150 respectively). May cause bleeding (interfere with platelets), make blood cross matching difficult (red cell rouleaux form easily), prolong bleeding time (Dextran 110). Dextran 40 causes renal failure. All cause anaphylactoid reactions ranging from minor skin eruptions to hypotension and oedema.
   (i) Gelatin (degraded to MW of 30 000), e.g. Haemacel.

(iii)  Albumin — every expensive.
2. *Improve myocardial contractility* if output still inadequate when
pre-load optimum.
  (i)  Catecholamines with varying properties (see table).

| | $\beta_1$ | $\beta_2$ | $\alpha$ | Dopaminergic | Useful dosage range ($\mu g/kg/min$) |
|---|---|---|---|---|---|
| Dopamine | ++ | 0 | + → ++ | ++ | 1–30 |
| Dobutamine | ++ | + | + | 0 | 2–40 |
| Adrenaline | ++ | ++ | + → ++ | 0 | 0.06–0.18 |
| Noradrenaline | ++ | 0 | ++ | 0 | 0.01–0.07 |
| Isoprenaline | ++ | ++ | 0 | 0 | 0.02–0.18 |
| Prenalterol | ++ | 0 | 0 | 0 | 0.5 mg/min up to total dose of 20 mg |

*Notes*
1. All have short $T\frac{1}{2}$ (minutes) except prenalterol — $T_\frac{1}{2} = 2$h.
2. All extensively metabolised except prenalterol — excreted 60%
   unchanged in urine.
3. Dopaminergic receptors produce vasodilatation of renal and mesenteric
   beds.
4. Dopamine
   — 0.5–2 $\mu$g/kg/min — renal vasodilatation ↑ GFR, ↑ renal $Na^+$ exc
     etion, diuresis
   — 2–10 $\mu$g/kg/min — $\beta_1$ effects predominate — ↑ heart rate, ↑ cardiac
     output.
   — > 10 $\mu$g/kg/min — partly indirect (due to noradrenaline release) —
     $\alpha$-adrenergic effects predominant — ↓ renal blood flow, ↓ peripheral
     perfusion.
5. Adrenaline
   — low doses, $\beta$ effects predominate — ↑ cardiac output, ↑ heart rate,
     ↓ peripheral resistance.
   — High doses, $\alpha$ effects predominate — ↑ peripheral resistance.
   — All doses reduce renal blood flow and urine output.
6. Noradrenaline
   — ↑ cardiac output ↑.peripheral resistance
   — ↓ renal blood flow.
7. Isoprenaline
   — ↑ cardiac output, ↓ peripheral resistance so ↓ renal fraction of
     cardiac output and much of increased output is to muscles.
Dopamine preferred agent except if bradycardia (use isoprenaline) or
severe hypotension (use noradrenaline).
 (ii)  Digitalis — unsuitable for this purpose.
(iii)  Glucagon — only indicated if catecholamines ineffective or
       contraindicated by arrhythmia. Dose 4–12 mg/h. Causes
       hyperglycaemia, nausea, vomiting.
3. *Reduce afterload* (see above)
 (i)  direct acting agents, e.g. nitroprusside, nitroglycerine, phentolamine.
(ii)  $\beta_2$-agonists — salbutamol 0.5–1.6 $\mu$g/min i.v., also has some positive
      inotropic ($\beta_1$) effect.

*4. Correct metabolic disturbances*
— oxygen
— if arterial blood pH persistently < 7.2 give small (50 mmol) doses of sodium bicarbonate but remember dangers of sodium overload and overcorrection.
*5. Steroids* e.g. dexamethasone 3 mg/kg. No objective evidence of benefit but often used.
*6. Antibiotics* in septic cases.

## Treatment of anaphylactic shock

1a  Adrenaline 0.5–1 mg (0.5–1 ml of 1 : 1000 adrenaline) given intramuscularly. NB: not subcutaneously because absorption slow in shock. Repeat every 15 minutes until improvement occurs. Rationale:
$\alpha$ effects cause vasoconstriction and raise B.P.
$\beta$ effects cause
  (i)  bronchodilatation
  (ii) reduce mediator release.
1b  i.v. hydrocortisone 300 mg
2.  $H_1$-antagonist e.g. chlorpheniramine (Piriton) 10–20 mg slowly i.v. Rationale: histamine is one mediator involved — blood histamine levels raised in anaphylaxis and correlate with hypotension.
3.  General measures:
raise foot of bed
volume replacement with i.v. fluids.
4.  In severe cases:
oxygen and possibly intubation and ventilation
aminophylline and/or a nebulised $\beta_2$-agonist (e.g. salbutamol) for resistant bronchospasm.

## HYPERTENSION

### Decision to treat hypertension
Based on:
1.  Level of BP — systolic hypertension as significant as diastolic. At least 3 recordings of raised BP desirable.
2.  Age — BP rises with age in our society so must be considered.
3.  Sex — women do as badly as men with hypertension.
4.  Family history of stroke or sudden death — no evidence that patients do worse than others with similar BP.
5.  Fundus appearance — papilloedema, exudates or haemorrhages — treatment mandatory.
6.  ECG — left ventricular hypertrophy — treatment essential.

### Treatment of hypertension

*A. General*
1.  Reduce obesity
2.  Look for and control diabetes mellitus

3. Stop smoking
4. Treat hyperlipidaemias if present
5. Exclude treatable causes, e.g. phaeochromocytoma, Cushing's disease, coarctation of aorta
6. Determine renal function (IVP rarely useful)

*B. Specific drug therapy.*
No patient is 'routine', each requires consideration of side-effects, contraindications etc., and the regime is fitted to the patient.
1. Hypertensive encephalopathy — see below.
2. Either  a.  β-blocker or thiazide diuretic.
   Then  b.  add β-blocker or thiazide to a. if inadequate response after 6 weeks.
   Then  c.  add vasodilator — hydralazine or nifedipine slow release or prazosin ('Triple Therapy').
3. For severe hypertension several approaches may need to be tried e.g.
   a. thiazide + β-blocker + hydralazine + prazosin ('Quadruple Therapy').
   b. thiazide + β-blocker + minoxidil.
   c. diuretic + captopril.
   d. substitute frusemide for thiazide in triple therapy (especially if creatinine clearance < 30 ml/min).
4. Other drugs such as methyldopa, clonidine may be useful in some cases but are regarded as second-line therapy.
5. Some patients fail to respond because of high salt intake; reduce to 100–150 mmol/day by avoiding added salt and salty food.

**Hypertension in pregnancy**
Raised diastolic BP associated with slower intra-uterine growth and increased stillbirth rate.
   Two different types of patient:
a. *Pregnant hypertensives* — higher the BP at mid-term the more likely is development of proteinuria and oedema (this may not be identical with pre-eclampsia).
b. *Pre-eclampsia* — hypertension in last trimester often accompanied by proteinuria and oedema which can progress to eclampsia (convulsions, CVA, renal failure, left ventricular failure and disseminated intravascular coagulation). Not clear whether eclampsia is type of malignant hypertension or a separate encephalopathy.

*Management*
1. Treat diastolic BP > 90–95 mmHg in pregnancy. Longest experience with methyldopa but oxprenolol may be as good. Avoid diuretics (ineffective in pregnancy; may decrease placental blood flow).

2. Bed rest if above insufficient — allows fetal monitoring. Hydralazine can be added to β-blocker treatment. Delivery necessary if control impossible.
3. In fulminating hypertension, hydralazine rapidly lowers BP; the baby should be delivered as soon as possible.

**Hypertension in elderly**
Treat if diastolic > 115 mmHg.
Below this, treatment controversial — the older the patient the less likely is treatment to be of benefit, the more likely it is to cause mischief. Several studies in progress to assess benefits and hazards of treatment but evidence of target organ damage suggests treatment should be given.
N.B. In the elderly:
 (i) malignant hypertension virtually unknown
 (ii) hypertension unusual cause of heart failure
(iii) systolic hypertension usually results from arterial rigidity and should be reduced cautiously since reduction may cause ischaemia.

*Treatment*
As for younger patients but should if possible be: simple (improves compliance); unlikely to cause postural hypotension/falls; without CNS effects.

DIURETICS AS ANTIHYPERTENSIVE AGENTS

**Differences from their use as diuretics**
1. Antihypertensive effects maximal at low doses, e.g. bendrofluazide 5 mg/day. N.B. Diuretics do not reduce BP in normotensives.
2. Loop diuretics not more effective than thiazides unless renal function impaired (when they are useful). Frusemide, bumetanide and metolazone (Metenix — a quinethazone derivative) are effective in patients with creatinine clearances down to 10 ml/min.
3. Spironolactone, a weak diuretic, has equal antihypertensive potency to thiazides.
4. In most patients $K^+$ loss is not a problem but important to ensure that plasma $K^+$ normal since hypokalaemia is adverse risk factor in myocardial infarction. Other side-effects (especially glucose intolerance and impotence) must be considered during chronic therapy.

**Types of hypertension particularly suitable for diuretic treatment**
1. Chronic renal failure.
2. Primary hyperaldosteronism — spironolactone treatment of choice.
3. Combined with other treatment specially β-blockers and vasodilators.

**Choice of diuretic**
No major differences between thiazides so choice made on cost, e.g. bendrofluazide presently cheapest in U.K.

Diuretics used almost exclusively for hypertension because long duration of action are:
Chlorthalidone (Hygroton)
— diuretic sulphonamide
— dose 25–50 mg/day.
Indapamide (Natrilix)
— ? vasodilator due to $Ca^{++}$ antagonism
— minimal $K^+$ loss and diuresis
— possibly no impairment glucose tolerance
— dose 2.5 mg/day

**Mechanism of action of thiazides in hypertension**
Two theories:
1. Natriuresis and volume depletion.
a. Dose-response curves for fall in BP and body weight similar.
b. Despite different structures, pharmacokinetics and pharmacology natriuretic diuretics are antihypertensive.
c. Onset of BP fall occurs with natriuresis and is accompanied by fall in blood volume, cardiac output but rise in TPR. Sodium infusion blocks BP fall.
d. Dietary sodium restriction (< 9 mmol/day) prevents BP rise when diuretics discontinued.
2. Vasodilator action.
a. Some diuretics, e.g. frusemide are vasodilators (cf. diazoxide a non-diuretic thiazide vasodilator)
b. TPR falls on continued treatment.
c. Early hypotensive action not reversed by salt-free dextran infusion or fludrocortisone.
d. Hypotheses:
  (i) diuretics reduce TPR by reducing $Na^+$ of blood vessel smooth muscle — no direct evidence.
  (ii) hydrolysis product of prostacyclin (6-oxo-$PGF_{1\alpha}$) found in blood after chronic therapy — vasodilator prostacyclin involved?

## β-ADRENERGIC BLOCKING DRUGS

Competitive inhibitors of catecholamine binding at β-adrenergic receptors.

Also have other pharmacological properties:

1. Membrane stabilising activity (quinidine-like or local anaesthetic activity)
— not responsible for anti-arrhythmic or negative-inotropic effects
— not related to β-blockade
— only occurs with high blood levels (may be relevant in overdose).

2. Intrinsic sympathomimetic (partial agonist) activity (ISA) — partially stimulate β-receptor but prevent effect of natural or exogenous catecholamines

Maximum effect of a partial agonist is less than maximum effect of full agonist like isoprenaline
— cause less slowing of resting heart rate but exercise rate is reduced similarly by drugs with or without ISA.
— no important influence on antihypertensive or anti-anginal efficacy
— may depress A-V conduction less
— controversial as to whether less dangerous in impending heart failure, peripheral vascular disease or asthma
— may produce less disadvantageous changes in plasma lipids.

3. Cardioselectivity: Some less-lipid soluble β-blockers have relatively higher affinity for $\beta_1$ (cardiac) adrenergic receptors. These have two *theoretical* advantages:
— may be safer in obstructive airways disease (but should *never* be used in such patients)
— do not block $\beta_2$ (vasodilator) receptors, may be relevant in peripheral vascular disease, hypoglycaemia and possibly hypertension.

### Effects of β-blockers

| | |
|---|---|
| C.V·S. | Reduction of exercise- and anxiety-induced tachycardia |
| | Reduced excitability of myocardium |
| | Negative inotropic action on heart and reduced cardiac output |
| | Reduction in blood pressure (often delayed) |
| | Reduced renin release from kidneys |
| | Reduced platelet aggregation (probably unimportant clinically) |
| R.S. | Bronchoconstriction in asthmatics |
| Metabolic | Hypoglycaemia due to block of gluconeogenesis |

| C.N.S. | Centrally mediated hypotension (controversial) Antipsychotic (controversial) |
| Peripheral nervous system | Reduction of tremor (e.g. due to anxiety thyrotoxicosis, hypoglycaemia) |

## Uses of β-blockers
1. Cardiovascular disease:
   Hypertension
   Angina
   Arrhythmias
   Post-myocardial infarction (cardioprotective agents) reducing incidence of sudden death
   Hypertrophic obstructive cardiomyopathy and Fallot's tetralogy
   Phaeochromocytoma (with α-blocker).
2. Nervous system:
   Migraine prophylaxis.
   Essential tremor.
3. Psychiatry:
   Anxiety (controls somatic symptoms)
   Schizophrenia (high dose therapy — controversial).
4. Opthamology:
   Open angle glaucoma (Timolol eye drops — probably decrease aqueous humour formation)
5. Endocrine:
   Hyperthyroidism (agents without ISA used to control tachycardia, tremor etc; no effect on thyroid hormones).

## Mechanism of antihypertensive action
Unknown: several theories, possibly more than one mechanism. Reason why action may take several days to manifest is unexplained.
1. Reduction of renin release: some studies show correlation between BP fall and reduced renin but others don't; Pindolol may raise renin but lower BP.
2. CNS action: intra-cerebral injection of β-blockers in animals causes BP fall but some don't enter CNS if given systemically.
3. Resetting baroreceptors to maintain BP at lower level due to attenuation of pressor responses to stimuli (similar to BP fall when patient put to bed). Some animal evidence but difficult to prove in man.
4. Effect on cardiac output: whilst lowering CO is hypotensive, this is not directly related to hypotensive effect of β-blockers (except when used with vasodilators). Possibly peripheral vascular adjustments to prolonged reduction of CO results in hypotensive effect.

5. Stimulation of vasodilator prostaglandins: action of propranolol antagonised by indomethacin (but latter also causes sodium retention).
6. Reduced plasma volume occurs with β-blocker treatment but is not correlated with antihypertensive effect.

**Adverse effects of β-blockers**

**A.  Cardiac**
 (i)  heart failure
 (ii)  bradycardia
(iii)  angina and infarction provoked by abrupt withdrawal during treatment of angina

*B. Peripheral vascular*
Cold extremities, Raynaud's phenomenon, gangrene.

*C. Pulmonary*
Bronchospasm (in unsuspected asthmatics).

*D. CNS*
 (i)  nightmares/vivid dreams (especially very lipid soluble drugs like pindolol, propranolol — use atenolol or timolol; avoid evening dose)
 (ii)  hallucinations — see (i)
(iii)  fatigue — try changing β-blocker
(iv)  migraine — avoid selective blocker
 (v)  impotence — rare

*E. Diabetes mellitus*
Alters control.

**Contraindications to β-blockers**

*A. Cardiac*
 (i)  Absolute
   a.  untreated heart failure except some cardiomyopathies (because cardiac output rate-dependent)
   b.  heart block/severe bradycardia (β-blockers slow heart further)
   c.  acute myocardial infarction unless monitored
 (ii)  Relative
   a.  treated heart failure (can use β-blockers with diuretics and digitalis)
   b.  atypical (Prinzmetal) angina (unopposed α-adrenergic stimulation encourages spasm)
   c.  high doses of verapamil (especially i.v.), nifedipine

B. *Peripheral vascular*
 (i) Absolute:  gangrene (unopposed $\alpha$-adrenergic effects cause vasoconstriction)
(ii) Relative:  Raynaud's phenomenon; cold extremities.

C. *Pulmonary*
 (i) Absolute:  asthma or bronchitis with spasm (unopposed $\alpha$-adrenergic bronchospasm)
(ii) Relative:  emphysema.

D. *CNS*
(i) Relative:  severe depression (use atenolol)

E. *Diabetes mellitus*
(i) Relative: insulin-dependent diabetes (non-selective agents decrease hypoglycaemic compensatory reactions by blocking $\beta_2$ receptors controlling glucose release mediated by catecholamines; $\beta$-blockers may increase blood glucose by 1–1.5 mmol/l — control requires adjustment).


## Labetalol (Trandate)

*Pharmacology*
Competitive $\alpha$ (mainly $\alpha_1$) and $\beta$-receptor blocker ($\alpha/\beta$ = 1 : 3 when given p.o.).
   Reduced BP, heart rate and peripheral resistance; postural hypotension occurs only with high doses.
   Less bronchoconstriction than propranolol (? $\alpha$-blocking effects protect).

*Pharmacokinetics*
Considerable first-pass metabolism interindividual oral dose variation wide.
$T_{\frac{1}{2}}$ 3–5 hrs.
Extensive hepatic metabolism (< 5% unchanged in urine).

*Dosage*
P.O. 100 mg 12–8-hourly after food — increase gradually up to 2.4 g/day max.
I.V. 50 mg over 1 min — repeat (× 1) in 5 mins if necessary.

*Uses*
Alternative to $\beta$-blocker
Phaeochromocytoma
Hypertensive encephalopathy
Controlled hypotensive anaesthesia with halothane.

**Table 20** Properties of some β-blockers

| | PROPRANOLOL | OXPRENOLOL | PINDOLOL | SOTALOL | ACEBUTOLOL | METOPROLOL | ATENOLOL | TIMOLOL | NADOLOL |
|---|---|---|---|---|---|---|---|---|---|
| Cardioselectivity | 0 | 0 | 0 | 0 | * | + | + | 0 | 0 |
| Intrinsic sympathomimetic activity | 0 | ++ | +++ | 0 | + | 0 | 0 | 0 | 0 |
| $T_{\frac{1}{2}}\beta$ (hours) | 2–4 | 1–3 | 3–4 | 12–16 | 6–8 | 3–4 | 6–9 | 3–4 | 12–24 |
| Interpatient variation in blood levels (n-fold) after single dose | 20 | 3 | 4 | 3 | * | 10 | 4 | 7 | 7 |
| Predominant route of excretion | Hepatic | Hepatic | Hepatic (60%) Renal (40%) | Renal (75%) Hepatic (25%) | Hepatic (60%) Renal (40%) | Hepatic | Hepatic (80%) Renal (20%) | Hepatic (80%) Renal (20%) | Biliary (75%) Renal (25%) |
| Significant CNS penetration | ++ | ++ | +++ | 0 | – | + | 0 | 0 | 0 |
| Daily dose (mg) (i) Hypertension | 120–1000 | 80–480 | 15–45 | 240–600 | 400–1200 | 200–400 | 50–200 | 15–45 | 80–240 |
| (ii) Angina | 120–480 | 40–160 | 7.5–30 | 240–480 | 400–1200 | 100–200 | 50–200 | 15–45 | 40–240 |

*Acebutolol metabolised to acetylated metabolite (not dependent upon fast/slow acetylator status) with non-selective β-blocking effects

*Adverse effects*
1. Postural hypotension, uncommon except with high doses or with excess diuretic treatment.
2. Expected adverse effects of β-blockers.

**Combined diuretic/β-blocker therapy**
Controls about 80% hypertensives.
Many combined tablets containing both drugs now on UK market
— examples:
Co-Betaloc   = Metoprolol (100 mg) + Hydrochlorothiazide
              (12.5 mg)
Inderetic    = Propranolol (100 mg) + Bendrofluazide (2.5 mg)
Tenoretic    = Atenolol (100 mg) + Chlorthalidone (25 mg)
Trasidrex    = Oxprenolol (160 mg) + Cyclopenthiazide
              (0.25 mg)
Advantage is reduced number of tablets to take and thus better compliance.
Disadvantages are:
Inability to manipulate dosage of separate components.
Danger of overlooking nature of components e.g. administration to patient with asthma or thiazide hypersensitivity.

**Autonomic neurone inhibiting drugs**
*Pharmacology*
Selectively concentrated (uptake$_1$) in terminals of postganglionic sympathetic nerves — lower BP by inhibiting noradrenaline release.
   Guanethidine (but not bethanidine or debrisoquine) depletes nerve NA stores (like reserpine).
   Hypotensive action mainly by ↓ peripheral resistance so postural hypotension occurs. BP low in morning and rises during day.

**Guanethidine**
— variable GI absorption (constant within patients)
— long $T_{\frac{1}{2}}$ so adjust dose at 3–4 day intervals and give only once daily
— 10–1000 mg
— mainly hepatic elimination.
**Debrisoquine**
— acts within hours
— metabolised by polymorphic hydroxylation (see Chapter 3) which is important determinant of dose
— 5–180 mg 12-hourly
**Bethanidine**
— acts in hours
— 5–350 mg 8 hourly
— mainly renal excretion (care in renal failure).

*Adverse effects*
1. Postural, exercise, post-prandial, Valsalva hypotension and/or faintness.
2. Abolish ejaculation (inhibit contraction internal urethral sphincter so ejaculation retrograde); occasionally impotence.
3. Guanethidine only — diarrhoea (60%); bethanidine occasionally — constipation.
4. Fluid retention and oedema.
5. Interaction with amphetamine, tricyclic antidepressants, chlorpramazine which inhibit action of these hypotensives.

**Centrally acting anti-hypertensive drugs**
$\alpha_2$ adrenoceptor agonism in brain stem inhibits sympathetic vasoconstrictor outflow to vessels and thus lowers BP. Associated effects of this $\alpha_2$-agonism are
 (i) sedation
(ii) dry mouth.
1. *Clonidine* Also peripheral site of action
    (i) modifies response of vascular smooth muscle to vasoconstrictors (hence use in migraine)
    (ii) $\alpha_2$-agonism reduces NA release in peripheral sympathetic nerves.
2. *Methyldopa* — metabolised like dopa to methylnoradrenaline an $\alpha_2$-agonist.

Methyldopa  $\rightarrow$  Methyldopamine  $\rightarrow$  Methylnoradrenaline

**Vasodilators in hypertension**
Adverse effects predictable from
 (i) vasodilator action:
    Headache
    Flushing
    Nasal congestion
    Tachycardia, palpitations, angina (not prazosin or indoramin)
    Hypotension — often postural
    Lethargy and weakness
(ii) secondary sodium and water retention with oedema resulting from increased renin and aldosterone secretion (not prazosin or indoramin).

*Specific $\alpha_1$ blockers*
  Prazosin
  Indoramin
  *Cause* Vasodilatation without tachycardia

*Mainly $\alpha_1$ agonists*
  Phenylephrine
  Methoxamine

  *Cause* Vasoconstriction

*Non-specific $\alpha_1$, $\alpha_2$ blockers*
  Phentolamine
  Phenoxybenzamine
  *Cause* Vasodilatation accompanied by tachycardia

*Mainly $\alpha_2$ agonist*
  Clonidine

  *Causes* Hypotension via central $\alpha_2$ effects

**Table 21** Centrally-acting antihypertensive agents — clinical aspects

| Drug | Dosage | Adverse effects |
|---|---|---|
| Methyldopa (Aldomet; Dopamet; Medomet). | 250 mg 8-hourly p.o. up to 3 g daily 250–500 mg i.v. 6-hourly (for hypertensive emergencies). | 1. CNS a. Lethargy; lack of concentration<br>b. Depression<br>c. Dry mouth; nasal congestion<br>d. Impotence<br>2. Blood a. Positive direct Coomb's test (20%), dose-related, interferes with cross-matching.<br>b. Haemolytic anaemia (0.2%) — not dose-related.<br>3. Fever<br>4. Hepatitis<br>5. CVS a. Bradycardia — usually asymptomatic<br>b. Postural and exercise hypotension<br>c. Salt and water retention<br>6. Others: Gynaecomastia; Parkinsonism (rare). |
| Clonidine (Catapres) | 0.05–0.1 mg 8-hourly increasing every 3rd day to maximum 1.2 mg/day. Sustained release preparation (Perlongets) available. | 1. Withdrawal hypertensive crisis (similar to phaeochromocytoma crisis with BP, plasma and urinary catecholamines) begins 18–72 hrs after stopping drug. Treat as phaeochromocytoma.<br>2. Sedation (60%)<br>3. Dry mouth (60%)<br>4. Constipation (? $\alpha_2$ agonist effect in GI tract) |

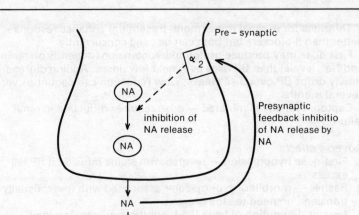

Pre – synaptic

NA

inhibition of
NA release

NA

Presynaptic
feedback inhibitio
of NA release by
NA

NA

Post – synaptic $\alpha_1$ receptor (mediates
vasoconstriction in arteries

N.B.  Mianserin is $\alpha_2$ blocker — ↟ NA in synaptic cleft and acts as
antidepressant.

**Captopril (Catapres)**
*Pharmacology*
Inhibitor of angiotensin converting enzyme (identical with kininase
II which breaks down the vasodilator bradykinin).
1. Renin and angiotensin II also occur in blood vessel walls and
   may be elevated in hypertension — they are also affected by
   captopril.
2. Effects on bradykinin of relatively minor importance.

*Uses*
Renal hypertension — renal artery stenosis; chronic renal failure.
Essential hypertension — reserved for severe cases not responding
to other agents because of possible long-term toxicity.
Malignant hypertension.
Severe congestive heart failure (as vasodilator therapy).

*Dose*
Initially 25 mg 8-hourly increased to 50 mg 8-hourly after 2 weeks.
Maximum dose 450 mg/day.

Thiazides (or in renal impairment, frusemide) enhance response better than β-blockers but both can be used concurrently.

First dose may produce profound hypotension (depends on renin and $Na^+$ levels) then BP rises over next few doses. Adding diuretic slowly drops BP over 3–4 weeks; slow reduction can continue over several months.

Captopril renally eliminated — dose requires reduction in renal failure.

*Adverse effects*
1. First-dose hypotension — reverse with saline infusion if BP fall excessive.
2. Rashes — morbiliform or macular associated with fever; usually transient, no need to stop drug.
3. Loss or diminution of taste (6%); aphthous ulcers; 'scalded' sensation in mouth.
4. Proteinuria and nephrotic syndrome — mainly with previous renal disease.
5. Neutropenia — especially in patients with SLE and other collagen diseases. Reversible if drug stopped.
6. Serum $K^+$ may rise during therapy so $K^+$ supplements or $K^+$ retaining diuretics are not used.

N.B. Test urine for protein at each visit.

w.b.c. counts every 2 weeks for first 3 months of therapy then periodically.

Patients told to report any signs of infection (sore throat, fever etc).

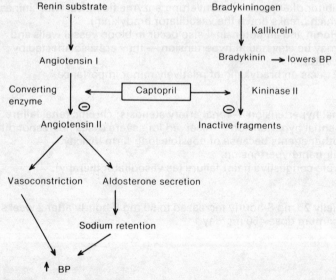

**Actions of captopril**

**Table 22** Vasodilators for chronic administration in hypertension

| Drug | Dosage | Pharmacology | Specific adverse effects |
|---|---|---|---|
| Hydralazine (Apresoline) | 25 mg 12-hourly up to 200 mg/day (slow acetylators) or 300 mg/day (fast acetylators) | Direct acting arterial vasodilator. Subject to polymorphic acetylation. Duration of effect $> T_{\frac{1}{2}}$. | S.L.E.-like syndrome (commoner slow acetylators) Peripheral neuropathy (pyridoxine antagonised by metabolite). Serum sickness-like syndrome early in therapy. |
| Prazosin (Hypovase) | Initially 0.5 mg 12-hourly beginning at night. Increase to max 20 mg/day. | $\alpha_1$ (post-synaptic) adrenergic blocker | First-dose dizziness or syncope (unusual with low starting dose). |
| Indoramin (Baratol) | 25 mg 12-hourly up to 200 mg/day | $\alpha_1$ (post-synaptic) adrenergic blocker. V-W Class I anti-arrhythmic properties (lignocaine-like). | Sedation (55% on 200 mg/day). Ejaculatory failure (may disappear on continued treatment). Caution in Parkinson's disease (weak anti-dopamine action). |
| Minoxidil (Loniten) | 2.5 mg-12 hourly up to 50 mg/day | Direct acting arterial vasodilator (? via metabolite). Duration of effect $> T_{\frac{1}{2}}$. | Excessive hair growth (hypertrichosis) of face, limbs and body. T wave inversion or flattening (80% but transient). |
| Nifedipine (Adalat Retard) | 20 mg 12-hourly — important to specify retard form | Calcium ion antagonist (No anti-arrhythmic effects). | Hyperglycaemia — rare (? interferes with $Ca^{++}$ entry associated with insulin release from $\beta$ cells in pancreas) |

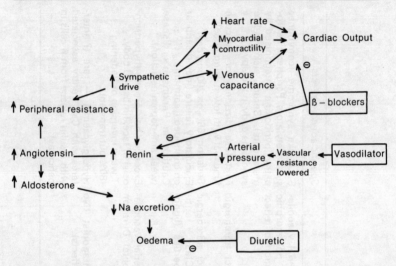

**Rationale of triple therapy**

**Table 23** Treatment of some hypertensive emergencies

| | Drugs | Comments |
|---|---|---|
| 1. Acute hypertensive encephalo-pathy | 1. Hydralazine 5 mg i.v. or 10–30 mg i.m. — effective 3–8 hrs and BP may fall over several hrs.<br>2. Sodium nitroprusside infusion 1 $\mu$g/kg/min up to 8 $\mu$g/kg/min.<br>3. Labetalol infusion 20–160 mg/hr. 300–400 mg p.o. effective within 30–60 minutes.<br>4. Diazoxide 100 mg i.v. as rapid bolus (not recommended). BP may fall over several hrs. | |
| 2. Dissecting aneurysm of aorta | Sodium nitroprusside infusion (as above) accompanied by oral propranolol so that nitroprusside can be gradually stopped. | BP lowered until pain disappears provided urinary output maintained. Anatomy defined by radiography and decision for surgery (mainly type 1 and 2) or medical (usually type 3) management made. |
| 3. Phaeochromocytoma | Phenoxybenzamine 10 mg p.o. 12-hourly increased to 40–100 mg 12-hourly as required plus propranolol p.o. in low doses if arrhythmia or tachycardia occur. | Definitive treatment is surgery. Drugs required pre-operatively. $\alpha$-blockade lowers BP, $\beta$-blockade protects heart (NB $\beta$-blockers never used alone as unopposed $\alpha$-effects increase BP) Acute BP crisis treated with phentolamine 5 mg i.v. or by infusion. |

# Drugs acting on the kidneys

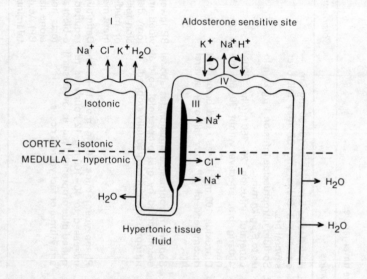

Tubular sites of ionic and water reabsorption
GFR = 180 1/day
Plasma $Na^+$ conc = 140 mmol/l
so Filtered load of $Na^+$ = 25 200 mmol/day. Fate of this $Na^+$:
Site I — removes 67% filtered load
          = 16 800 mmol/day
Site II — removes 25% filtered load
          = 6300 mmol/day
Site III — removes 5% filtered load
           = 1200 mmol/day
Site IV — removes 3% filtered load
          = 750 mmol/day
Urine contains about 0.6% filtered load
          = 150 mmol $Na^+$/day
Dietary intake of $Na^+$ = 150 mmol/day to maintain $Na^+$
homeostasis.

**Table 24** Summary of effects of diuretics on sodium reabsorption in the nephron

| Diuretic | Glomerular filtration | Zone I | Zone II | Zone III | Zone IV | % filtered sodium excreted |
|---|---|---|---|---|---|---|
| Benzothiadiazines* | Decreased | Minor inhibition | 0 | Inhibited | ↑ $Na^+$ delivery* increases $K^+$ and $H^+$ loss | 5–10 |
| Loop† | Possibly increased | Minor inhibition | Inhibited† | Inhibited | ↑ $Na^+$ delivery increases $K^+$ and $H^+$ loss | 15–40 |
| Spironolactone Triamterene Amiloride | 0 | 0 | 0 | 0 | Inhibited (spironolactone competitively blocks action of aldosterone; others are non-competitive inhibitors at this site). | 2–5 |
| Carbonic anhydrase inhibitors | 0 | Weak inhibition | 0 | 0 | Weak inhibition | 1–2 |
| Osmotic | Possibly increased | Inhibited | 0 | 0 | ↑ $Na^+$ delivery increases $K^+$ and $H^+$ loss | 5–10 |

* also reduce the permeability of tubules to water and hence relieve diabetes insipidus
† primary action is powerful inhibition of chloride reabsorption in Zone II

## BENZOTHIADIAZINES

| Approved name | Proprietary name | Usual daily dose range (mg) | Approximate duration of action (hours) |
|---|---|---|---|
| *Thiazides & hydrothiazides* | | | |
| chlorothiazide | Saluric | 500–2000 | 10 |
| hydrochlorothiazide | Esidrex | | |
| | HydroSaluric | 25–100 | 10 |
| bendrofluazide | Neo-Naclex | | |
| | Aprinox | 2.5–10 | 20 |
| | Berkozide | | |
| | Centyl | | |
| polythiazide | Nephril | 1–4 | 24–30 |
| cyclopenthiazide | Navidrex | 0.25–1.0 | 12–24 |
| methyclothiazide | Enduron | 5–10 | 24 |
| *Quinazolinones* | | | |
| quinethazone | Aquamox | 50–100 | 18–24 |
| metolazone | Metenix | 5–10 | 18–24 |
| *Phthalimides* | | | |
| chlorthalidone | Hygroton | 50–200 | 48 |
| clorexolone | Nefrolan | 10–100 | 72 |
| *Chlorbenzamide* | | | |
| clopamide | Brinaldix | 20–80 | 12–15 |
| *Benzene disulphonate* | | | |
| mefruside | Baycaron | 12.5–50 | 20–24 |

## Actions

The benzothiadiazines all have similar actions — but the more water-soluble ones are shorter-acting as they have a lower $V_d$ and more rapid elimination. High protein binding — correlates with increasing duration of action.

1. Diuresis mainly by action on Zone III (inhibit $Na^+$, $K^+$-ATPase and limit energy available for transport) reducing $Cl^-$ reabsorption
   Also inhibition of carbonic anhydrase
   Stimulation of $K^+/Na^+$ exchange at Zone IV (therefore $K^+$ loss)
2. Hypotension (see page 169)
3. Thiazides also produce antidiuresis in diabetus insipidus patients: possibly by reduction in GFR and/or reduction in thirst and/or increase permeability of tubules to water
4. Reduction in $Ca^{++}$ excretion useful in idiopathic hypercalciuria

## Interrelationships of thiazide adverse effects

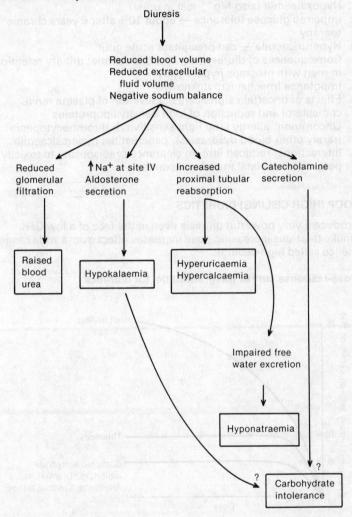

Diuresis

↓

Reduced blood volume
Reduced extracellular
fluid volume
Negative sodium balance

Reduced glomerular filtration

↑Na⁺ at site IV Aldosterone secretion

Increased proximal tubular reabsorption

Catecholamine secretion

Raised blood urea

Hypokalaemia

Hyperuricaemia Hypercalcaemia

Impaired free water excretion

Hyponatraemia

Carbohydrate intolerance

## Uses

1. generalised and localised oedema (e.g. heart failure, nephrotic syndrome, liver failure)
2. hypertension
3. diabetes insipidus
4. reduction of urinary stone formation in idiopathic hypercalciuria.

**Adverse effects**
1. Hypokalaemia (also $Mg^{++}$ lost in urine)
2. Impaired glucose tolerance — about 10% after 6 years chronic therapy
3. Hyperuricaemia — can precipitate acute gout
4. Consequences of diuresis, e.g. hyponatraemia; urinary retention in men with prostatic hypertrophy
5. Impotence (mechanism unknown)
6. Effects of uncertain significance: Elevation of plasma renin, cholesterol and reduction of high density lipoproteins
7. Uncommon: allergy (and light sensitivity); thrombocytopenia (rarely other blood dyscrasias); pancreatitis; hypercalcaemia
8. Interactions: reduced lithium clearance predisposing to toxicity; potentiates skeletal muscle relaxants.

## LOOP (HIGH CEILING) DIURETICS

Produce a very powerful diuresis even in the face of a low GFR. Unlike thiazides increasing dose increases effect over a wide range (hence called high-ceiling).

### Dose-response curves (diagrammatic) for diuretics

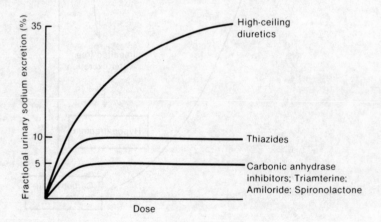

## Loop diuretics

| Approved name | Proprietary names | Usual dose | Start of action | Duration of action | Special properties |
|---|---|---|---|---|---|
| Frusemide | Lasix Dryptal Frusid | Orally 20–120 mg i.m. or<br>i.v. 20–80 mg (but up to 2 g are used in renal failure) | 30 mins<br>10 mins | 6 h<br>6 h | Can produce hypochloraemic alkalosis; $Ca^{++}$ loss |
| Ethacrynic acid | Edecrin | Orally 50–400 mg<br>i.v. 50 mg | 30 mins<br>10 mins | 6 h<br>6 h | Increased urinary $Ca^{++}$ loss |
| Bumetanide | Burinex | Orally 1–4 mg<br>i.v. 0.5–2 mg | 20 mins<br>5–10 mins | 4–6 h<br>4–6 h | Less $K^+$ loss than frusemide |

**Adverse effects**

| | Frusemide | Ethacrynic acid | Bumetanide |
|---|---|---|---|
| Acute hypovolaemia Hyponatraemia | +++ | +++ | +++ |
| $K^+$ deficiency | +++ | +++ | ++ |
| $Ca^{++}$ loss in urine | ++ | ++ | 0 |
| Uric acid retention and gout | ++ | ++ | + |
| Carbohydrate intolerance | ++ | ++ | ++ |
| Blood dyscrasias | rare | ? | ? |
| Ototoxicity | deafness with high peak levels (reversible) | deafness with high peak levels (reversible) | ? less than frusemide |
| Nephrotoxicity | especially with cephaloridine or gentamicin | | |
| Muscle pain | 0 | 0 | + |
| GI haemorrhage | 0 | 4.5% of patients | 0 |

```
  0  =  absent
  +  =  mild
 ++  =  moderate
+++  =  considerable
```

N.B.
1. All loop diuretics can produce hyponatraemia (without reduced total body $Na^+$) due to 'inappropriate' ADH secretion in response to stimulus of reduced ECF volume. Treat by water restriction.
2. Frusemide potentiates renal toxicity of cephaloridine. Frusemide potentiates ototoxicity of gentamicin.
3. Actions of frusemide antagonised by indomethacin, aspirin.

# K RETAINING DIURETICS

| Drug | Proprietary name | Dose | Duration of action | Special properties |
|---|---|---|---|---|
| Spironolactone (Canrenone is active metabolite of spironolactone) | Aldactone Spiroctan | Orally 25 – 50 mg 8-hourly | 10 h | Useful in hyperaldosteronism Can produce: hyperkalaemia nausea hirsutes gynaecomastia menstrual irregularity abolishes activity of carbenoxolone large doses: ataxia, confusion |
| Amiloride | Midamor | Orally 10 – 20 mg daily | 6 h | Weak diuretic. Can produce: hyperkalaemia fall in GFR can impair renal function rise in blood urea |
| Triamterine | Dytac | Orally 100 mg twice daily | 2 h | as amiloride |

**Uses**
1. Generalised/localised oedema.
2. Pulmonary oedema — frusemide has powerful vasodilator action which accounts in part for effectiveness.
3. Natriuresis in renal failure.
4. Hypercalcaemia (frusemide).

## CARBONIC ANHYDRASE INHIBITORS

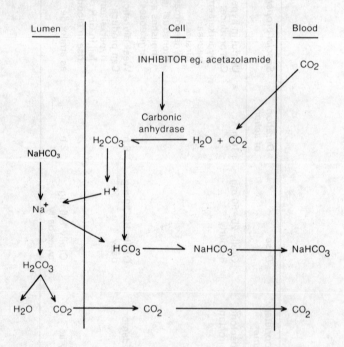

## ACETAZOLAMIDE (DIAMOX)

Inhibits carbonic anhydrase in eyes, brain and kidney; weak diuretic, action terminated by acidosis produced by the drug.

**Uses**
1. Narrow angle glaucoma: i.v. 250–500 mg in acute cases followed by 250 mg orally 6-hourly (sustained release tabs — Sustets — given twice daily)
2. Cysteine renal calculi.
3. Prophylaxis of mountain sickness.
4. Rarely for epilepsy in childhood.

5. Periodic paralysis (both hyperkalaemic and hypokalaemic varieties).
6. Reduction of intracranial hypertension (reduces CSF formation).

**Adverse effects**
1. Paraesthesia, fatigue, somnolence, malaise.
2. Dyspepsia, substernal burning
3. Hypersensitivity and blood dyscrasias

## OSMOTIC DIURETICS
MANNITOL

Administered i.v. as a 10 or 20% solution for:
1. Accelerating elimination of poisons
2. Impending renal failure
3. Reduction of intraocular pressure ⎫ i.v. urea or glycerol
4. Reduction of intracerebral pressure ⎬ alternative
⎭ osmotic diuretics

**Adverse effects**
1. Increase in plasma volume may precipitate heart failure.
2. Potassium loss.

## POTASSIUM AND DIURETICS

Serum $K^+$ is unreliable indicator of total body $K.^+$ (98% of body's 3500 mM is intracellular). Acid-base changes also disturb extra/intra cellular balance.

In practice if levels < 3 mmol/l a significant $K^+$ deficit (up to 400 mM) is assumed. This needs treatment to prevent cardiac arrhythmias, ileus, nephropathy, muscle weakness and potentiation of digitalis toxicity.

$K^+$ status of all patients on diuretics (± $K^+$ supplements) requires monitoring at least pre-treatment, after 3 months diuretics and then yearly.

**Hypokalaemia following diuretic therapy**
Diuretic therapy produces initial fall in serum $K^+$ within 1–2 weeks of starting treatment — but new steady-state then established and progressive deficit does not occur. Up to 50% of hypertensives on thiazides have serum $K^+$ between 3.0 and 3.5 mmol/l (represents 5–10% reduction in total body $K^+$). Less than 10% of patients have serum $K^+$ < 3.0 mmol/l. In patients with mild heart failure on frusemide corresponding figures are 5% < 3.5 mmol/l and 0.2% < 3.0 mmol/l. Average fall in serum $K^+$ is 0.6 mmol/l after thiazides; 0.3 mmol/l after 40–80 mg frusemide.

Patients with hypertension or mild heart failure exhibit similar falls in serum $K^+$ but in heart failure initial levels are higher and the incidence of hypokalaemia is decreased.

**Measures to reduce potassium loss**

Patients with heart failure — small doses of loop diuretics — waste less potassium than thiazides.

Patients with hypertension — doses of thiazides as low as 5 mg bendrofluazide produce near maximal effects.

Moderate salt restriction (to 70–80 mM daily) — no added salt and avoidance of salty foods — lowers diuretic requirements and reduces renal potassium losses.

Dietary measures — Additional meat and fish expensive but potassium rich foods also include milk, potatoes, carrots, parsnips, tomatoes, celery, leeks, dried fruits, nuts, bananas, rhubarb and soft fruits.

**Indications for potassium replacement**

Provided no contraindications (e.g. renal impairment) *prophylactic potassium* replacement needed in the following 'high risk' situations:

*High doses* of diuretics.

Concurrent digoxin, acute myocardial infarction or serious heart disease.

Concurrent drugs altering ventricular repolarisation (phenothiazines, tricyclic antidepressants).

Hyperaldosteronism

— severe congestive cardiac failure.

— severe liver disease, e.g. cirrhosis (hypokalaemia precipitates coma).

— nephrotic syndrome.

Concurrent potassium-losing therapy

— corticosteroids and ACTH.

— carbenoxolone.

— laxatives.

Poor $K^+$ intake — usually elderly (check renal function).

Pre-treatment potassium level < 3.5 mmol/l.

Serum potassium levels falling below 3.0 mmol/l require *correction*.

**Potassium replacement**

*Potassium supplements*

Limited effect in the prevention of diuretic-induced hypokalaemia. 24–48 mmol/day is needed and correction of hypokalaemia may require more. As most preparations contain 8–12 mmol, daily doses of at least 3–6 tablets can cause problems with compliance.

Combined diuretic/potassium tablets (contain only 7–8 mmol $K^+$) may be inadequate.

KCl preferred as corrects hypochloraemia and alkalosis associated with hypokalaemia.

| Proprietary name | Constituents | K$^+$ content | Presentation |
|---|---|---|---|
| Kay-Cee-L | KCl 10 ml–75 mg | 1 mmol K$^+$/ml | Liquid |
| Sando-K | KHCO$_3$ 400 mg<br>KCl 470 mg in<br>one tablet | 12 mmol K$^+$ | Effervescent<br>tablet |
| Kloref | KHCO$_3$ 455 mg<br>KCl 140 mg in<br>one tablet | 6.7 mmol K$^+$ | Effervescent<br>tablet |
| Slow K<br>Leo K | KCl 600 mg | 8 mmol K$^+$ | Slow release<br>tablet |

*Adverse effects*
Nausea, vomiting, diarrhoea, abdominal discomfort, bad taste.
Small risk of ulceration if GI transit delay.

**Potassium sparing diuretics**
Reduce urinary potassium loss, more effective in preventing
hypokalaemia and can replace depleted body stores. Expensive and
increase risk of adverse effects but of value if additional diuretic is
needed, e.g. where aldosterone levels are high as in hepatic
cirrhosis with ascites.

Hyperkalaemia especially in the elderly, in diabetics and patients
with impaired renal function is particular danger. Use with
potassium supplements should be avoided except with very close
monitoring.

**Drugs producing salt and water retention**
Result in oedema; hypertension; increased cardiac failure.
1. Corticosteroids and ACTH (occasionally anabolic steroids)
2. Oestrogens
3. Non-steroidal anti-inflammatory drugs, e.g. phenylbutazone
4. Carbenoxolone
5. Arterial vasodilators, e.g. hydralazine, minoxidil
6. Sometimes other antihypertensive agents in particular
   guanethidine, methyldopa
7. Lithium

**Drugs containing unexpectedly large amounts of sodium**
1. Antacids — some, e.g. Gaviscon, Aluminium hydroxide gel.
   — also over the counter preparations, e.g. Andrew's Liver Salts.
2. Penicillins — large doses given i.v., e.g. carbenicillin sodium.
3. X-ray contrast media, e.g. Conray.

**Treatment for ascites**
1. Salt and water restriction — mild cases Na intake <
   22 mmol/day (0.5 g); severe cases < 10 mmol/day. Diets
   unpalatable.

2. Diuretics — spironolactone (counteracts hyperaldosteronism) but slow and care needed if renal impairment. Add frusemide if no effect after few days on 100 mg 6-hourly. Thiazides also used with spironolactone.
3. Bed rest (but look out for DVTs!).
   Aim for loss of no more 1000 ml/day (best judged by body weight) since mobilisation of oedema fluid is slow and greater diuresis 'shrinks' plasma volume and is dangerous.
   Resistant cases try:
1. Infusion of salt-poor albumin (not more than 50 g) with large dose diuretic if severe hypoalbuminaemia present. Maintain albumin around 40 g/l if possible.
2. Corticosteroids may produce effect if given for up to a week (? mechanism)
3. Mannitol
4. Rarely haemodialysis

## Management of gravitational oedema
1. Diuretics — alone do not control postural oedema
2. Mobilise
3. Support legs with elastic stockings
4. Isometric exercises especially for chair-bound
5. Elevate foot of bed and feet when seated
6. Treat heart failure, hypoalbuminaemia, anaemia

## ALTERATION OF URINARY pH

### 1. To increase drug elimination in overdose.

*Principle*
Non-ionised drug equilibrates rapidly across membranes and can be reabsorbed from renal tubule into blood.
Ionised drug cannot be reabsorbed.
Thus adjusting urinary pH to promote drug ionisation increases urinary drug excretion.
Henderson-Hasselbalch equation:

$$pH = pK_a + \log \frac{[A^-]}{[HA]}$$

$$[A^-] = H^+ \text{ acceptor; } [HA] = H^+ \text{ donor}$$

so

$$\log \frac{[A^-]}{[HA]} = pH - pK_a$$

N.B.
a. If pH = $pK_a$ both acids and bases are 50 per cent ionised.

b. Acids are more ionised when pH > p$K_a$.
   Bases are more ionised when pH < p$K_a$.

*Example*
Phenobarbitone p$K_a$ 7.3.

| *Urine* | *Plasma* | *Urine* |
|---|---|---|
| pH 5.3 | pH 7.3 | pH 8.3 |

$$\log\frac{[A^-]}{[HA]} = 5.3 - 7.3 \qquad \log\frac{[A^-]}{[HA]} = 7.3 - 7.3 \qquad \log\frac{[A^-]}{[HA]} = 8.3 - 7.3$$

$$= -2 \qquad\qquad\qquad = 0 \qquad\qquad\qquad = 1$$

$$\frac{[A^-]}{[HA]} = 10^{-2} \qquad\quad \frac{[A^-]}{[HA]} = 1 \qquad\qquad \frac{[A^-]}{[HA]} = 10$$

$$= \frac{0.01}{1} \qquad\qquad\qquad = \frac{1}{1} \qquad\qquad\qquad = \frac{10}{1}$$

*Conclusion*: The proportion of ionised (and therefore non-reabsorbable) phenobarbitone increases 1000 fold by changing urinary pH from 5.3 to 8.3.

Drugs whose elimination is usefully promoted by manipulation of urinary pH:

| Alkaline diuresis | Acid diuresis |
|---|---|
| Barbitone | Amphetamine |
| Phenobarbitone | Pethidine |
| Salicylate | |

N.B. Most barbiturates are eliminated by metabolism and are not amenable to forced alkaline diuresis.

**2. To increase efficacy of antimicrobials in urine.**

| Acid | Alkali |
|---|---|
| Tetracycline | Streptomycin |
| Penicillin | Sulphonamides |

**3. To discourage growth of certain urinary pathogens, e.g. E. coli (alkaline).**

**4. Symptomatic relief of 'cystitis'.**

**5. To render drugs or metabolites more soluble to prevent crystalluria (e.g. sulphonamides-alkaline) or stone formation (e.g. urate-alkaline).**

**Drugs for alkalinisation**
1. i.v. or oral sodium bicarbonate.
2. i.v. sodium lactate (converted to bicarbonate in vivo).
3. Oral sodium or potassium citrate.

**Drugs for acidification**
1. Oral ammonium chloride (converted to ammonia (→ urea) and HCl).
2. Oral methionine (converted to equivalent of $H_2SO_4$).
3. Oral arginine hydrochloride (equivalent to HCl).
4. Oral or i.v. ascorbic acid.

# Drugs acting on the respiratory system

## ASTHMA

Asthma: a condition of airways obstruction which (in the earlier stages of the disease at least) is reversible.

Asthmatics may show several peculiarities:

 (i) Many cells (including leucocytes) contain reduced amounts of cAMP and show an attenuated rise of cAMP when exposed to $\beta$-agonists. Abnormal $\beta$-receptors may underlie this.
 (ii) High levels of circulating reaginic antibody (IgE) and increased proneness to types I and III and allergic reactions.
(iii) Bronchospasm readily provoked by $\beta$-blockers and by inhalation of $SO_2$ or histamine.
(iv) Degranulation of mast cells by trivial stimuli (e.g. exercise, laughing, cold).
 (v) Ready production of bronchospasm by physical stimuli (iv) may also involve vagal pathways.

Airways obstruction is due to:

 (i) plugging of small bronchi with viscid mucus
 (ii) mucosal swelling
(iii) bronchiolar constriction

Therapeutic agents have complex actions:

 (i) $\beta$-agonists and phosphodiesterase inhibitors raise intracellular cAMP. This causes bronchiolar relaxation and diminishes mediator release from mast cells.
 (ii) Corticosteroids: anti-inflammatory actions by inhibiting phospholipase thus inhibiting prostaglandin synthesis; reduction of capillary permeability and vasoconstriction thus reducing mucosal swelling; potentiation of catecholamine actions by blockade of $uptake_2$; stabilisation of mast cells.
(iii) Disodium cromoglycate and ketotifen may reduce mast cell degranulation, but they have other actions (e.g. phosphodiesterase inhibition).
(iv) Anticholinergic drugs block vagus-induced reflex airways obstruction.

## β-agonists

All can induce tremor ($\beta_2$ actions) and non-selective agonists also produce tachycardia and other arrhythmias ($\beta_1$ actions).

### Adrenaline

No longer used in routine or emergency treatment of asthma, apart from a life saving role in acute anaphyllaxis (0.6–0.8 ml of 1: 1000 adrenaline is given i.m. as soon as possible).

### Ephedrine

Becoming obsolete in adult asthma, but still used in paediatrics.
Kinetics: well absorbed from gut, $T_{\frac{1}{2}} = 6$ h.
Toxicity: excitement, anxiety, insomnia, hesitancy of micturition, tremor, tachycardia, tachyphyllaxis.
Dose: 15–60 mg/70 kg bodyweight.

### Selective $\beta_2$-agonists

Most useful (see Table 25).

## CORTICOSTEROIDS

Anti-inflammatory glucocorticoids are effective in chronic asthma which has not responded adequately to β-agonists and may be life saving in status asthmaticus.

## MAST CELL STABILISERS

Most useful in allergic and exercise provoked asthma.

### Disodium cromoglycate (DSCG; Intal)

#### Administration

1. As Spincaps (20 mg) inhaled as a powder using a Spinhaler. (Intal Compound: DSCG 20 mg with isoprenaline 0.1 mg. Not approved by experts, but very useful in prevention of exercise provoked asthma if taken 15 mins beforehand).
2. Nebuliser solution 10 mg/ml. 20 mg nebulised 4–6 times daily. Can be used in young children.
3. Metered aerosol 1 mg/puff. Probably dose is 3–4 puffs 5 hourly.

#### Pharmacokinetics

Not absorbed from gut. Only 10% of inhaled Spincap reaches alveoli. Most is swallowed.

#### Toxicity

Hoarseness and mild wheezing. Severe bronchospasm can be precipitated, but this is rare.

**Table 25(a)** β-agonist drugs in asthma

| Drug | Administration | Selectivity | Clinical properties |
|---|---|---|---|
| Isoprenaline (Aleudrin) (Medihaler 150) | Aerosol 0.08–0.4 mg/dose. Sublingual 10–20 mg (considerable 1st pass metabolism). | Not selective | Little use for asthma now because of powerful excitatory effect on heart. Fatal reactions also due to hydroxymethylisoprenaline (β-blocker) formed in lungs. |
| Orciprenaline (Alupent) | Aerosol 0.75 mg/dose. Oral 20 mg 6-hourly 5% solution for inhalation via nebuliser. I.M. 0.5 mg injection. | Not selective | Long duration of action, $T_{\frac{1}{2}}$ = 6 h. Excitatory effect on heart. |
| Salbutamol (Ventolin) | Aerosol 100 μg/dose. Rotacaps 400 μg 6-hourly. Oral 2–4 mg 6-hourly. i.v. 4 μg/kg by slow injection. s.c. & i.m. 8 μg/kg. 5 mg/ml solution for inhalation. | Selective β$_2$-agonist. (Equieffective β$_2$ action to isoprenaline with 1/10 of β$_1$ effect). | No hepatic or pulmonary 1st pass metabolism, $T_{\frac{1}{2}}$ = 2–4 h. Can produce tremor and mild tachycardia. Leg cramps at night are common. |
| Terbutaline (Bricanyl) | Aerosol (also spacer aerosol) 0.25 mg/dose. Oral 5 μg 8–12-hourly. 10 mg/ml solution for inhalation via nebuliser. | Selective β$_2$-agonist (twice bronchodilator action of isoprenaline with 1/4 of cardiostimulatory effect). | Small degree of 1st pass metabolism (sulphatation by gut wall) but effective orally. Not metabolised when given IV $T_{\frac{1}{2}}$ = 3–4 h. |
| Rimiterol (Pulmadil) | Aerosol 0.2 mg/dose. Can be given i.v. | Selective β$_2$-agonist (similar to salbutamol when given i.v. but similar to isoprenaline inhaled). | $T_{\frac{1}{2}}$ approx 2 h. |
| Fenoterol (Berotec) | Aerosol 0.2–0.4 mg/dose 2 or 3 times daily. | Selective β$_2$-agonist (similar to salbutamol). | Similar properties to salbutamol but longer acting $T_{\frac{1}{2}}$ = 7 h. |

**Table 25(b)** Glucocorticoids used in asthma

| Drug | Dose | Properties | Uses |
|---|---|---|---|
| Cortisol (Hydrocortisone) | Initial i.v. dose of 4 mg/kg of hemisuccinate, followed by 3-hourly doses of 3 mg/kg or continuous infusion of 3 mg/kg 6-hourly. | Subjective improvement in 1–4 hours, objective improvement from 6 h after first dose. (Plasma levels of cortisol of 100 $\mu$g/100 ml needed for optimum response.). | Emergency treatment in status asthmaticus |
| Tetracosactrin (Synacthen) | 1 mg i.m. | Similar time course of effects as cortisol. Cortisol plasma levels of 100 $\mu$g/100 ml by 8–24 h. | Emergency treatment of status asthmaticus. Can be used in chronic refractory asthma using twice weekly injections. |
| Corticotrophin (Acthar) | 40 i.u. i.m. | | |
| Prednisolone | 5–100 mg orally (see below). | Similar properties to cortisol (but 4–5 × anti-inflammatory with same mineralocorticoid effects). | Status asthmaticus (usually after initial improvement has been attained by cortisol). Also in chronic refractory asthma. |
| Beclomethasone dipropionate (Becotide) | 400 $\mu$g as daily dose (divided) from aerosol. 200–400 $\mu$g 6 hourly as Rotacaps. | Powerful anti-inflammatory actions — little is absorbed systemically from lungs. No evidence of prolonged supression of pituitary-adrenal axis Moniliasis of pharynx in 13% or of larynx in 5% of patients | Chronic asthma unresponsive to β-agonists |
| Betamethasone valerate (Bextesol) | 400 $\mu$g as daily dose (divided) from metered aerosol. | | |

### Ketotifen (Zaditen)

*Administration*
1 mg capsule oral twice daily.

*Pharmacokinetics and action*
Absorbed from gut. In addition to mast cell stabilisation, blocks histamine $H_1$ receptors (and has anticholinergic and sedative actions).

*Toxicity*
Sedation, dry mouth. Drying of bronchial secretions may aggravate asthma.

## PHOSPHODIESTERASE INHIBITORS

Only theophylline and its derivatives are widely used members of this group. Aminophylline is theophylline with ethylene diamine.

### Administration
*Oral*:  many forms, e.g. choline theophylline (Choledyl), sustained
  release aminophylline (e.g. Theodur, Phyllocontin) 225 mg.
*Rectal*:  aminophylline suppositories 50, 100, 150, 360 mg.
*i.v.*:  aminophylline given by *slow* injection of 250–500 mg over
  5–10 mins.

### Pharmacokinetics
Absorbed well from gut and rectum. $T_{\frac{1}{2}}$ = 3–10 h; elimination mainly by hepatic metabolism and 10% excreted unchanged in urine. Reduced clearance in infants under 6 months, acutely ill adults with cirrhosis, cardiac failure, cor pulmonale. Increased clearance in smokers.

### Effective plasma level
Mild asthma 4–5 $\mu$g/ml; severe asthma 10–20 $\mu$g/ml.

### Toxic effects
  nausea, vomiting, peptic ulceration
  tachycardia, cardiac arrhythmias
  hyperventilation
  insomnia, anxiety, headache, fits

## ANTICHOLINERGICS

| Drug | Dose/administration | Properties |
|---|---|---|
| Ipratropium (Atrovent) | Metered aerosol 20 $\mu$g/puff 1–2 puffs 6-hourly. | More bronchodilatation but less drying of secretions than atropine. Slow onset but prolonged effect $T_{\frac{1}{2}} = 3–4$ h. |
| Deptropine citrate (Brontina) (in Brontisol) | 1 mg tablets 12-hourly | Similar to atropine. |
| | metered aerosol each puff given 4–5-hourly hourly. { 0.1 mg deptropine 0.15 mg isoprenaline | |
| Atropine methonitrate (in Brovon, Eumydrin and Rybarvin). | Inhalation of a mixture of substances. | Bronchodilatation with drying of secretions. |

## DRUG TREATMENT OF ASTHMA

### A. Chronic
1. Bronchodilators to stop wheezing attacks. Preferably selective $\beta_2$-agonists (such as salbutamol) given by a metered aerosol. Metered aerosols can be used by children — but oral therapy may be required by very young children (e.g. salbutamol, terbutaline or ephedrine).
2. Disodium cromoglycate should be tried for 3 weeks in all patients, but particularly when attacks are provoked by allergies or exercise, and if other atopic phenomena are present. Improvement assessed by history, use of bronchodilator aerosol and PEFR before and after exercise.
3. Steroids used when
   (i) 1 and 2 (above) are not effective
   (ii) repeated attacks interupt work or school
   (iii) the growth of children is impaired (but systemic steroids can also stunt growth).
   Steroid aerosols or Rotahaler should be tried before giving oral prednisolone.
4. Nocturnal attacks or regular deterioration in the early hours of the morning ('dipping') may be prevented by an evening dose of theophylline (e.g. as 200–400 mg of slow release tablets or 360 mg aminophylline suppositories).

5. Antibacterials (e.g. cotrimoxazole; amoxycillin) are given if there is a respiratory infection — preferably at the first sign of a cold if this is usually followed by worsening of the asthma.
6. Anticholinergics are not successful in all patients but ipratropium aerosol may benefit some patients with a bronchitic component to their asthma and those with exercise induced spasm.

## B. Refractory severe asthma

1. Sedatives and narcotic analgesics are contraindicated.
2. If salbutamol aerosol is ineffective then arrange to admit to hospital. While waiting for the ambulance give: 375 mg aminophylline i.v. over 5–7 mins and 300 mg of cortisol i.v. (as succinate or hemisuccinate).
3. Because steroids take several hours to act, bronchodilator therapy is given:
   a  0.5% of salbutamol aerosol delivered by IPP ventilation in 40% oxygen from a Bird ventilator via a tightly fitting facemask. Given for 2–3 min every 1–2 h. OR
   b. i.v. aminophylline as a continuous infusion: 1.5 g in 5% glucose given over 24 h. If 4 h has elapsed since the initial bolus dose of 375 mg then the infusion is started by giving 375 mg over 20 mins. Ideally plasma levels are measured. OR
   c. i.v. salbutamol 4 $\mu$g/kg bodyweight given over 5–7 mins.
4. Hydrocortisone is given by continuous intravenous infusion (3 mg/kg/6 h).
*3 & 4 are initiated as soon as the patient is admitted and a 5% glucose drip set up.*
5. If $Pa_{O_2}$ < 8.5 kPa (< 65 mmHg)   } give 65% $O_2$ by
     $Pa_{CO_2}$ normal or low      } MC mask.

   if $Pa_{CO_2}$ raised                 give 28% $O_2$ by Ventimask.

   if $Pa_{CO_2}$ < 6.5 kPa (< 50 mmHg) }
     $Pa_{CO_2}$ rising                 }
     pulse > 130/min          } intubate IPP ventilation
     pulsus paradoxus        } for 24–48 h.
6. Antibacterial chemotherapy, e.g. amoxycillin, cotrimoxazole or oxytetracycline.
7. After 48 h of hydrocortisone treatment replace steroid with prednisolone 80 mg daily and then gradually reduce dose over 10 days.
8. Assess fluid balance and prevent dehydration.

## COMMON COLD

Very little can be done. 0.5–1 g of ascorbic acid may reduce the severity and possibly shorten the course of the disease. Proprietary mixtures containing antihistamines and various analgesics and vasoconstrictors may also alleviate some of the symptoms.

## ACUTE BRONCHITIS

No benefit (but possible harm) from antibiotics in otherwise fit persons, but serious deterioration can be prevented if they are used in patients with underlying lung disease.

## CHRONIC BRONCHITIS WITH EMPHYSEMA

1. Stop smoking; avoid cold and damp atmospheres; avoid irritating pollutants.
2. Treat acute exacerbations due to bacterial infections with chemotherapy: ampicillin penetrates into purulent sputum but 1 g 6 hourly required for H. influenzae; amoxycillin produces double the sputum concentration of same dose of ampicillin; tetracycline effective in bacterial and mycoplasmal infections and penetrate sputum adequately at a dose of 500 mg 6-hourly. Doxycycline (200 mg stat and 100 mg daily) also effective and can be used in renal insufficiency. Cotrimoxazole (2 tablets, 12 hourly) effective but sulphamethoxazole penetrates sputum poorly.
3. Improve sputum removal with exercise and postural drainage. Bromhexine and other mucolytics help some patients.
4. Prevent exacerbations, e.g. amantadine; influenza immunisation; antibacterials at first sign of a cold; avoid outdoor work in bad weather.
5. Airways resistance treated with bronchodilators (e.g. ventolin aerosol, ipratropium aerosol). Some patients respond to steroids (e.g. beclomethasone Rotacaps) and very severely affected patients should undergo a trial of steroids (e.g. 40 mg of prednisolone daily for 3 weeks) to assess the potential benefit.
6. Long-term oxygen therapy in severely disabled patients — 15 h daily for 6 months.

*Table of expectorants*

| Drug | Action |
|---|---|
| Mist sod chlor Co BP | Increases bronchial watery secretions, mainly by reflex action on stomach and duodenum. |
| Squill opiate linctus BPS | |
| Ammonium + Ipecacuanha mixture BPC | |
| Iodides e.g. isopropamide (in Escornade); iodinated glycerol (in Organidin) | |
| Guaiphenesin (Robitussin) | |

| Drug | Dose | Action |
|------|------|--------|
| Bromhexine (Bisolvon) | 8–16 mg 6–8-hourly (tablets, elixir, injection). | Fragments mucopolysaccharide fibres and thus reduces sputum viscosity. |
| Acetyl cysteine (Airbron) Methyl cysteine (Visclair) | Administered as an aerosol: acetylcysteine 2–5 ml of 20% solution 8-hourly. Also methyl cysteine 100 mg table (Visclair) 2, 6–8-hourly for 6 weeks then 2, 12-hourly. | Splits disulphide bonds in sputum proteins and thus reduces sputum viscosity. |
| Tyloxapol (Alevaire) | 0.125% solution for nebuliser. | Detergent |

## RESPIRATORY FAILURE

Defined as $Pa_{O_2} < 8$ kPa ($< 60$ mmHg) with or without $Pa_{CO_2} > 6.3$ kPa ($> 47$ mmHg)
1. Ventilation/perfusion inequality (pneumonia, LVF, pulmonary fibrosis, shock lung) gives a normal or lowered $Pa_{CO_2}$.
2. Ventilatory failure. (chronic airways obstruction, respiratory depression) gives increased $Pa_{CO_2}$.

*Treatment*
1. Ventilation perfusion inequality
   a. treat underlying disease.
   b. give oxygen at high rate (nasal cannula, MC or polymask).
2. Ventilatory failure
   a. encourage coughing and deep breathing; analeptics may be tried. Sedatives absolutely contraindicated.
   b. oxygen may depress respiration: try 24% $O_2$ via Venturi mask
      — if $CO_2$ does not rise and conciousness not impaired then increase $O_2$ to 28% then 35%
      — if respiratory depression with 24% $O_2$ then assisted ventilation urgently required.
   c. treat infection, pulmonary oedema, bronchospasm.

**Table 26** Analeptics

| Drug | Administration | Duration of action | Ratio of convulsive to stimulant dose | Toxicity |
|------|---------------|-------------------|--------------------------------------|----------|
| Nikethamide (Coramine) | i.v. injection 0.5–2 g every 15–30 mins | Short — single dose produces effects for 5–10 mins. | 95 : 1 | Repeated doses produce tachycardia, sneezing, itching, tremor, fever and convulsions. |
| Doxapram (Dopram) | i.v. infusion or bolus 0.5–1.5 mg/kg/h. | $T_{\frac{1}{2}} = 2.5$–$4$ h | 70 : 1 | Wider therapeutic ratio but similar effects as nikethamide contraindicated in epilepsy, hypertension, cerebral oedema and hyperthyroidism. |

# Drugs for gastro-intestinal disease

### ANTI-EMETICS

Different emetic mechanisms involved in different cases.
Anticholinergic drugs useful in motion sickness (probably mainly act on vomiting centre) and are useless in vomiting due to cancer chemotherapy. Phenothiazines and metoclopramide (act mainly on chemoreceptor trigger zone) have little effect on motion sickness.
Useful anti-emetics include:
  (i) Metoclopramide
 (ii) Anticholinergics
(iii) Antihistamines
 (iv) Phenothiazines
  (v) Butyrophenones
 (vi) Betahistine (for Meniere's disease only)
(vii) Experimental drugs based on cannabinoids, e.g. nabilone.
   Vomiting in pregnancy treated if possible by diet and reassurance regarding its self-limiting nature.
   Drugs may be held responsible for fetal malformation, ideally no drugs should be given in the first trimester. Evidence for anti-emetic teratogenicity is minimal. Meclozine as Ancoloxin (Meclozine HCl 25 mg; Pyridoxine HCl 50 mg) given as 2 tablets at bedtime has been used for many years. Prochlorperazine is used in severe vomiting in pregnancy.

### METOCLOPRAMIDE (Maxolon, Primperan)

**Pharmacology**
Derivative of procainamide.
1. Blocks central dopaminergic receptors and so
    (i) is anti-emetic via blockade in chemoreceptor trigger zone,
   (ii) induces extrapyramidal syndromes,
  (iii) stimulates prolactin secretion,
   but has virtually no antipsychotic actions (so maybe acts only on a subgroup of dopamine receptors).

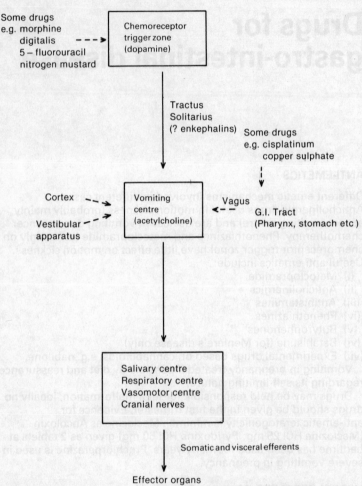

**Emetic pathways (putative transmitter shown in brackets)**

2. Sensitises gut muscle to acetylcholine so requires background cholinergic activity for effect; also releases acetylcholine from cholinergic nerves in gut; little effect on other cholinergic mechanisms.
   Actions on gut include:
   (i) increased tone of lower oesophageal sphincter,
   (ii) increased gastric tone,
   (iii) increased contraction of oesophagus, antrum and small intestine,
   (iv) increased co-ordination of mechanical activity of gut.
   (NB) Little effect on colon; no effect on gastric secretion.

## Pharmacokinetics
Rapidly absorbed from the gut. About 80% is excreted in urine as metabolites. $T_\frac{1}{2}$ = 4h. and is increased by renal failure.

## Uses
1. Anti-emetic, e.g. in anaesthesia, cancer chemotherapy, radiation sickness but *not* motion sickness.
2. Gastro-oesophageal reflux and oesophagitis.
3. Diagnostic radiography and intubation.
4. Gastric motor failure, e.g. post-vagotomy, diabetic autonomic neuropathy.
5. To improve analgesic absorption in migraine attacks, e.g. Migravess (aspirin + metoclopamide); Paramax (paracetamol + metoclopramide).

## Dosage
Orally: Up to 10 mg (5 mg in young adults up to 20 years) 8 hourly.
Lower doses in children: not greater than 0.1 mg/kg.
i.v. or i.m. doses similar.
Usual maximum dose (all ages, all routes) is 0.5 mg/kg/day.

## Adverse effects
CNS:  Drowsiness, dizziness and faintness.
       Extrapyramidal syndromes — akathisia, dystonia; oculogyric crises, torticollis, facial spasms. Commoner in young.
Endocrine:  Galactorrhoea, menstrual disorders.
GI:  Constipation.

## Drug interactions
1. Increased absorption of: aspirin, paracetamol, tetracycline, ethanol, levodopa. Decreased absorption of digoxin.
2. Antagonises anticholinergics, e.g. atropine, propantheline.
3. Potentiates extrapyramidal effects of phenothiazines and butyrophenones.

## OESOPHAGEAL DISORDERS

LESP (lower oesophageal sphincter pressure) most important factor in controlling gastro-oesophageal reflux).

### Drug effects on LESP

| Increased LESP | Decreased LESP |
| --- | --- |
| Antacids | Nicotine (smoking |
| | Caffeine (coffee, tea, chocolate) |
| Metoclopramide | Nitrates |
| Cholinergic drugs | Anticholinergic drugs (e.g. propantheline) |
| Protein meals | Fatty meals |

**Table 27** Some anti-emetic Drugs

| Drug | Dose | Mode of action | Toxicity | Uses |
|---|---|---|---|---|
| Anticholinergics: hyoscine | 0.3–0.6 mg 8-hourly | Antimuscarinic action on the gut and central inhibition of vomiting centre | Drowsiness Dry mouth Blurred vision Urinary retention | Preoperative medication, Motion sickness, Labyrinthitis, Meniere's disease |
| Antihistamines: cyclizine (Marzine) dimenhydrinate (Dramamine) | 50 mg, 8-hourly  50–100 mg 4–6-hourly. Suppositories (100) available. | Have an anticholinergic hyoscine-like action | Drowsiness Dry mouth Blurred vision | Motion sickness and other forms of labyrinthin vomiting |
| promethazine (Phenergan) cinnarizine (Stugeron) | 25–50 mg daily in divided doses 15–30 mg 8-hourly | | | |
| Neuroleptics: Phenothiazines, e.g. chlorpromazine (Largactil) prochlorperazine (Stemetil) | 25–50 mg 8-hourly  10 mg 8-hourly or 12.5 mg i.m. stat | Block dopamine receptors in chemoreceptor zone | Postural hypotension Extrapyramidal effects Ataractic states | Postoperative, post radiation, drug induced vomiting |
| Butyrophenones, e.g. haloperidol (Serenace) | 0.5–5 mg 8–12-hourly | | | |

| Betahistine (Serc) | 8–16 mg 8-hourly | Partial agonist of histamine — exerts vasodilatation like histamine, but can relieve histamine headache. | Aggravation of asthma and peptic ulcer. Can produce nausea. Contraindicated in phaeochromocytoma. | Reduced vertigo and nausea in Meniere's disease. No value in other types of vomiting. |

## 1. Reflux oesophagitis

May occur in absence of anatomical hiatus hernia.

a  General advice: reduce weight; raise head of bed (but not to
   sleep with more pillows which raises intra-abdominal pressure);
   avoid stooping and abdominal constriction; eat prudently; stop
   smoking.
b.  Antacids ± polymethylsiloxane preparations to relieve
    flatulence and pain. Used after meals and at bed-time.
c.  Metoclopramide 30 mins before meals aids gastric emptying
    and increases LESP.
d.  Alginate-antacid preparations (e.g. Gaviscon) produces viscous
    raft of antacid floating on surface of gastric contents.
e.  Cimetidine: reduces acidity; no effect on LESP.
N.B.  Anticholinergic drugs contraindicated.

## 2. Diffuse oesophageal spasm

a.  Nitrates, e.g. nitroglycerine, or long-acting erythritol tetranitrate
    sometimes used for pain and dysphagia.
b.  Avoid anticholinergic agents
c.  Anxiety and reflux oesophagitis should be treated on their
    merits.

## MANAGEMENT OF PEPTIC ULCER

### A. General

1. Bed rest — heals G.U., may symptomatically improve D.U.
2. Stop smoking.
3. Diet — food acts as antacid so frequent small meals help
   symptoms.
4. Avoid 'irritants', e.g. caffeine, alcohol, drugs (e.g. aspirin,
   indomethacin, phenylbutazone).

### B. Drugs

Remember disappearance of symptoms does not prove ulcer
healed. Endoscopy ensures accurate diagnosis and excludes
carcinoma.

1. G.U.: Carbenoxolone or chelated bismuth or $H_2$-blockers for
   initial therapy. Antacids are used symptomatically.
   Carbenoxolone unsuitable for elderly, in renal or cardiorespiratory disease. Colloidal bismuth relatively
   unpalatable. $H_2$-blockers safe and effective but may need
   maintenance treatment. If none of these tolerated try
   deglycyrrhizinated liquorice. Replases and slow healing with
   disruption of social life and work are indications for surgery.
2. D.U.: $H_2$-blockers (+ antacids for symptoms) treatment of choice.
   Maintenance treatment for relapses should not be continued for
   more than a year or so because long-term safety uncertain.
   Duogastrone may be tried if $H_2$-blockers not tolerated.

CIMETIDINE (Tagamet)

**Actions**
Prevents gastrin, vagal stimulation and histamine from enhancing gastric acid secretion by competitive antagonism of histamine at $H_2$-receptor. Volume of acid secreted is reduced and pepsin secretion secondarily decreased. No effect on intrinsic factor secretion or gut motility. No rebound increase in gastric acid secretion when treatment stopped.

**Pharmacokinetics**
80–90% absorbed p.o. Absorption delayed by food: recommended to sustain blood levels and prolong effect. Plasma $T_{\frac{1}{2}}$ = 2h (increased up to 5h in renal failure). Elimination mainly renal as unchanged drug but some metabolism mainly to sulphoxide. Biliary secretion may become important in renal failure. 20–25% protein bound. Removed by haemodialysis.

**Clinical uses**
1. Duodenal ulcers.
2. Gastric ulcers — evidence for efficacy in lesser curve and proximal ulcers less convincing than for pyloric and prepyloric ulcers.
3. Postoperative stomal ulcers.
4. Peptic oesophagitis.
5. Zollinger-Ellison syndrome.
6. Prevention of upper GI bleeding after burns, trauma, acute renal failure etc.
7. Prevention of acid inactivation of pancreatic extracts (enzymes) in pancreatic insufficiency.
8. No good evidence of efficacy in established GI bleeding or in acute gastritis.
9. Reduces liver blood flow in portal hypertension and bleeding oesophageal varices.
N.B. Malignant gastric ulcers may symptomatically respond: exclusion of malignancy is mandatory before cimetidine treatment.

**Dose**
400 mg at breakfast and bedtime for at least 4 weeks then 400 mg once nightly to prevent relapse for 6 months. Reflux oesophagitis requires higher doses: 400 mg 6–8-hourly with meals and at bedtime.
    In patients with very high gastric acid secretion (e.g. Zollinger-Ellison syndrome) up to 2 g/day used.

    Cimetidine may not give immediate symptomatic relief and antacids should be available until symptoms disappear.
    Intravenous infusion is at a rate of 100 mg/hour for 2 hours every 4–6 hours.

## Adverse effects
Usually well tolerated — minor effects include diarrhoea, dizziness, myalgia and rashes.

GI — No convincing evidence of carcinogenesis in man.

CVS — Cardiac arrhythmias (bradycardia, A–V dissociation) are very rare. Rapid i.v. injection rarely causes hypotension.

CNS — Reversible confusional states, hallucinations, drowsiness tremor and dizziness can occur usually but not necessarily in elderly or in renal failure.

Endocrine — Breast tenderness, gynaecomastia and galactorrhoea (? direct action on breast tissue, ?? hyperprolactinaemia). Anti-androgenic: loss of libido, erectile impotence, reduced sperm count (? raised gonadotrophin secretion) — reverses when treatment ceases.

Blood — marrow suppression rarely occurs.

## Drug interactions
Cimetidine inhibits cytochrome $P_{450}$ microsomal enzymes — interactions, possibly of clinical importance, with increased levels and effects of chlordiazepoxide, diazepam, theophylline, propranolol, phenytoin.

## RANITIDINE (Zantac)

A substituted furan not an imidazole (like cimetidine and histamine), more specific competition with histamine on gastric $H_2$-receptors, 4–9 times more active than cimetidine. Without effects on CNS, androgen receptors and cytochrome $P_{450}$ enzymes (c.f. cimetidine).

## Pharmacokinetics
Rapid oral absorption, unaffected by food or antacid administration. Plasma $T_{\frac{1}{2}} = 2$ h but probably increased by renal impairment (and ? biliary obstruction but not hepatic disease). Excreted mainly unchanged in urine and also in bile.

## Clinical uses
As for cimetidine: has been used successfully in cimetidine resistant cases.

## Dose
Oral: 150 mg 12-hourly has similar effects to cimetidine 1 g daily. For maintenance treatment 150 mg at night.
Injection: 50 mg 6–8-hourly (oral bioavailability about 50%).

## Adverse effects and interactions
Too new to be certain.
No evidence of effects on CNS, or endocrines. Very rarely causes bradycardia. No interaction with warfarin, diazepam or antipyrine.

## ANTACIDS

Neutralise HCl and raise gastric pH so reducing irritation and inactivating pepsin but several proteolytic enzymes in gastric juice with activity at high pH. Less effective than cimetidine in suppression of nocturnal acid secretion but similar effect on daytime secretion.

Mainly for symptomatic treatment but given frequently in large doses (enough to neutralise 1000 mmol $H^+$/day) may heal ulcers. Usual doses: between meals and at bedtime but may be taken at hourly or more frequent intervals. GI bleeding associated with severe acute illness may be prevented by antacids.

Up to 18-fold differences in acid neutralising power in vitro. Some antacids in common use shown in Table 28. Others include aluminium phosphate and glycate, magnesium oxide and bismuth aluminate (latter not recommended as weak antacid and can cause encephalopathy). *Sodium bicarbonate* acts rapidly but produces systemic alkalosis and is not recommended. *Calcium carbonate* can cause hypercalcaemia and acid rebound and should be used sparingly. Antacid mixtures frequently used to avoid undesirable effects of each component, especially on colonic function. Remember presence of $Na^+$ in some mixtures, e.g. mist. mag. trisil if patient requires $Na^+$ restriction.

Choice of liquid or solid preparations — former may be preferred because act rapidly and less unpalatable for chronic use.

Some mixtures, e.g. Andursil, Asilone, contain *dimethacone* — causes gas bubbles to coalesce by reducing surface tension. May reduce functional and postoperative gaseous distension. Not absorbed, has no known adverse effects.

Antacid mixtures containing barbiturates and anticholinergics should be avoided.

Antacids used for:
1. Peptic ulcer
   — symptom control
   — adjunct to $H_2$-blockade.
2. Non-ulcer dyspepsia.
3. Reflux oesophagitis.
4. Prevention of acute gastric erosions in shocked, burned or seriously ill patients on ventilators etc.

### LIQUORICE DERIVATIVES

#### 1. CARBENOXOLONE

Synthetic triterpenoid derived from liquorice root has a steroid-like molecule.

**Table 28** Antacids in common use

| Drug | Pharmacology | Adverse effects | Drug interactions |
|------|--------------|-----------------|-------------------|
| Aluminium hydroxide | Inhibits smooth muscle contraction so delays gastric emptying, decreases gut mobility. Binds bile acids, pepsin, phosphate — latter used to reduce hyperphosphataemia in renal disease. | Constipation, nausea, bloating ? Aluminium toxicity in renal failure | Reduced absorption of tetracyclines isoniazid, digoxin, vitamin A. Increased blood levels of pseudoephedrine. |
| Calcium carbonate | Produces $CO_2$ on reaction with HCl. Acid rebound secretion occurs due to local gastrin release + systemic hypercalcaemia. 40% $Ca^{++}$ absorbed. | Belching. Constipation. Hypercalcaemia. Milk-alkali syndrome (hypercalcaemia, calcinosis renal failure). | Reduced blood levels of tetracyclines and iron. Increased blood levels of some sulphonamides, amphetamine, naproxen. |
| Magnesium hydroxide | Most potent $H^+$ neutralising effect/g of all nonsystemic antacids. Acid rebound is minimal. Stimulates gut mobility. | Diarrhoea, hypermagnesaemia (CNS depression hypotension, muscle weakness) in renal failure. | Reduced blood levels of tetracyclines, digoxin. Increased blood levels of dicoumarol, some sulphonamides. |
| Magnesium trisilicate | Slowly reacts with HCl. Stimulates gut mobility. | Diarrhoea, hypermagnesaemia in renal failure. | Reduce absorption of tetracyclines. |

## Pharmacology

No effects on acid secretion or gut motility.
Increases mucosal resistance by:
  (i)  increases (up to 50%) gastric epithelial cell life-span.
 (ii)  enhances secretion and changed composition of mucus so
       reducing back-diffusion of $H^+$ into mucosa.
(iii)  reduced activity of pepsin and chymotrypsin.
       Carbenoxolone is potent mineralocorticoid causing:
  (i)  hypokalaemia — increases colonic $K^+$ loss, minor increase in
       renal $K^+$ excretion.
 (ii)  sodium and water retention.
(iii)  hypertension.
       Also has mild glucocorticoid and anti-inflammatory properties.

## Pharmacokinetics

Well absorbed orally but absorption reduced by food so given
before meals.
  Rapid absorption (peak 1–2 h) by gastric mucosa, excreted in bile
and reabsorbed in small intestine (little carbenoxolone reaches
proximal duodenum). Biliary excretion main elimination route so
contra-indicated by biliary obstruction.
  99% bound to plasma protein. $T_{\frac{1}{2}}$ 13–24 h (longer in old ? cause
of higher incidence of toxicity). Effects not correlated with plasma
levels — ? related to local gastric effects.

## Clinical uses

Shown to heal gastric ulcers effectively, less evidence for efficacy in
duodenal ulceration, ? because of difficulty in getting drug to ulcer.
Used as:
  (i)  Biogastrone for G.U.: 100 mg 8 hourly for 1 week then 50 mg 8
       hourly until ulcer healed (4–6 weeks).
 (ii)  Duogastrone (positioned release capsules to liberate drug in
       duodenum): 50 mg 6 hourly with fluid for 6–12 weeks.
  Also used for oesophagitis as combination preparation with
aluminium hydroxide, magnesium trisilicate and sodium
bicarbonate (Pyrogastrone).

## Adverse effects

Common (up to 50% with 100 mg 8-hourly) — most at risk are old and
patients with cardiac, renal and hepatic disease.
1. *Sodium retention*: Hypertension, oedema, heart-failure. May
   counter effects of digitalis and antihypertensive drugs.
   Spironolactone blocks effect of carbenoxolone on ulcers so
   triamterene or amiloride preferred (thiazides aggravate
   hypokalaemia).
2. *Hypokalaemia* (muscle weakness, myasthenia, myoglobinuria,
   peripheral neuropathy) occurs in up to 40%. Give $K^+$
   supplements.

**Drug interactions**
Potentiation of digitalis toxicity.
Thiazide and loop diuretics potentiate carbenoxolone toxicity.
Antacids do not affect carbenoxolone absorption.

## 2. DEGLYCYRRHIZINATED LIQUORICE

Residue after extraction of glycyrrhizinic acid (precursor of
carbenoxolone) contains substances with less ulcer healing efficacy
than carbenoxolone but which lack its mineralocorticoid action.
Incorporated with antacids in Caved-S.
  Virtually without side effects.

## BISMUTH CHELATE

Bismuth compounds are weak antacids. Tripotassium dicitrato
bismuthate an alkaline colloidal solution (De-Nol) has been shown
to heal D.U. Mechanism of action unknown. Suggested that in
presence of acid it combines with proteins of ulcer base forming a
protective coat. Also may stimulate mucus production, combine
with mucoproteins and complex with pepsin producing inactive
chelate.
  Dose is 5 ml as elixir taken with water 30 minutes before meals
and two hours before last meal of the day.
  No serious acute adverse effects — can turn stools black
(confusion with melaena!) and has rather unpleasant taste. Chronic
treatment can cause encephalopathy, especially in renal failure.

## ANTICHOLINERGIC DRUGS

Reduce gastric acid secretion ('medical vagotomy') and motility
and possibly spasm ('antispasmodics'). Antimuscarinic
anticholinergics may be:
 (i) tertiary amines, e.g. dicyclomine — well absorbed; enter CNS.
(ii) quaternary amines, e.g. propantheline — less well absorbed; do
     not enter CNS; more effects at autonomic ganglia and
     neuromuscular junction (large doses).

**Pharmacology on GIT**
1. Decrease salivary secretion
2. Inhibit cholinergic component of gastric acid secretion by 40%
   (less than cimetidine) and reduce pepsin, mucus and volume
   output so $H^+$ concentration (as reflected by gastric pH) is little
   affected.
3. Potentiate effect of cimetidine on acid secretion and reduce
   pepsin secretion more than cimetidine.
4. Inhibit GI motility: delayed gastric emptying may prolong phase
   of acid secretion; cause constipation.

5. Mild relaxation of gallbladder and bile ducts insufficient to reverse spasm produced by narcotics. Minimal effects on biliary or pancreatic secretion.

**Clinical use**
Efficacy questionable — may be useful symptomatically in a few patients. Effective dose to suppress acid secretion may be close to or exceed toxic dose. Can be used at night since side-effects less troublesome. Dosage gradually increased to maximum tolerated given in divided (usually 6-hourly) doses:

| | | |
|---|---|---|
| Atropine sulphate | Daily dose | 0.25–2 mg |
| Dicyclomine hydrochloride (Merbentyl) | Daily dose | 30–60 mg |
| Poldine methylsulphate (Nacton) | Daily dose | 8–16 mg |
| Propantheline bromide (Pro-Banthine) | Daily dose | 150 mg |

Avoid in pyloric stenosis and oesophageal reflux because of reduced gastric emptying.

**Adverse effects**
Dry mouth and skin, thirst
Pupil dilatation, paralysis of accommodation, glaucoma, blurred vision.
Tachycardia
Constipation
Urinary retention
Excitement, confusion and delirium — rarely convulsions.
Postural hypotension and impotence (quaternary salts only due to effects on ganglia).

**Drug interactions**
Delayed absorption of some drugs, e.g. mexiletine, paracetamol, ketoconazole; occasionally enhanced absorption of slowly absorbed drugs, e.g. digoxin.
 Antagonism of effects of metoclopramide on GI motility.
 Potentiation of anticholinergic effects of other drugs, e.g. tricyclic antidepressants, antihistamines.
 Absorption of propantheline markedly reduced by food.

**SUCRALFATE (Antepsin)**
Basic aluminium salt of sucrose octasulphate.
 Forms chemical complex with protein in ulcer crater by electrostatic interaction to form a protective antacid barrier in ulcer so blocking diffusion of acid and pepsin. Directly inhibits action of pepsin and bile and acts as local antacid (i.e. overall stomach pH unchanged).

**Dose**
1 g 6-hourly before meals and at night for 6 weeks heals D.U. and
G.U. (70–80%). Role in ulcer treatment not yet established.
  No systemic absorption but may cause constipation.
  Could interfere with absorption of other drugs, e.g. tetracycline.

## ACUTE PANCREATITIS

1. *Supportive treatment*: Fluid replacement — usually plasma or
   albumin required as well as electrolytes.
     Nasogastric suction optional — prevents gastric contents
   entering duodenum to release secretin and
   cholecystokinin-pancreozymin which increase pancreatic
   secretion.
2. *Analgesia*: Pethidine or pentazocine.
3. *Antibiotics*: No value in alcoholics; may be useful in pancreatitis
   associated with ascending cholangitis; perforated peptic ulcer;
   necrotising or haemorrhagic pancreatitis or with septic
   complications.
4. *Peritoneal lavage*: Removes toxic products released into
   peritoneum by necrotic pancreas.
5. *Other measures*: Proteolytic enzyme inhibitor (Trasylol) does not
   alter mortality — unknown if it alters complication rate. Similar
   comments apply to glucagon.
*Anticholinergic drugs*: useless and cause tachycardia, ileus and
confusion thereby masking clinical signs of deterioration.

**Drug-induced pancreatitis**
  Azathioprine
  Corticosteroids
  Diuretics: frusemide, thiazides
  Methyldopa
  Oestrogens
  Pentamidine
  Sulindac
  Sulphonamides
  Tetracycline

## PURGATIVES (LAXATIVES; CATHARTICS)

Avoid unless:
 (i) straining at stool will cause damage, e.g. postoperatively, in
     haemorrhoids, post-myocardial infarction.
(ii) in hepatocellular failure (page 233).
(iii) occasionally in drug-induced constipation.
  Divided into
a. Bulk

b. Osmotic
c. Stimulant
d. Lubricant
but some may have more than one type of activity.

Diagnosis of the cause of constipation is important: faecal impaction, obstruction and carcinoma must be excluded. Constipation best treated by increasing fibre and fluid content of diet. Purgatives should be used in lowest dose possible and only for short periods.

## BULK PURGATIVES

Contain non-digestible, unabsorbed polysaccharides.

*Wheat bran* contains 30% fibre. This consists of: cellulose, hemicelluloses, pectins, lignins. These take up water and so increase the bulk of stools. Stretching the colonic wall stimulates peristalsis, thus reducing transit time. Wheat fibre binds bile salts and increases their excretion. However, blood cholesterol is not reduced on a bran-supplemented diet, although this does occur with guar gum or fruit pectin.

Bran either native or as tablets (Fybranta, Proctofibe) is given in divided doses 12–24 g/day with fluid. Acts within 24–72 hours.

Bran is of value in treating:
    constipation
    diverticulosis
    spastic colon
    ulcerative colitis.
It probably could play a role in preventing:
    haemorrhoids
    anal fissure
    appendicitis
    diverticulitis.
It has been suggested that it may reduce the likelihood of:
varicose veins
cholecystitis
carcinoma of the colon
coronary artery disease
obesity.

**Adverse effects**
Flatulence
Reduced absorption of calcium and iron
Avoid in coeliac disease and gluten enteropathy
If taken with insufficient fluid may form masses in gut and produce obstruction.

Other bulk purgatives with similar effects (used if bran not tolerated) are Ispaghula busk (Fybogel; Isogel); Methylcellulose (Celerac); Sterculia (Normacol).

**Table 29:** Purgatives

| Drug | Pharmacological properties | Approximate dose effect interval | Toxicity | Special uses |
|---|---|---|---|---|
| *Osmotic purgatives:* | | | | |
| Sodium sulphate | Largely unabsorbed from gut and so osmotically active. Increased bulk of water in lumen stimulates peristalsis | 2 h | Sodium absorption | |
| Magnesium sulphate | Acts like sodium sulphate, in addition Mg stimulates peristalsis by liberating cholecystokinin | 2 h | Magnesium can be absorbed and be of clinical significance in renal failure | Hepatocellular failure |
| Lactulose (Duphalac) | Disaccharide split by bacteria in colon to organic acids which are unabsorbed and act osmotically to increase bulk of stools. Gas formation is increased. | 46 h | Contraindicated in galactosaemia | Hepatocellular failure |
| *Chemical stimulants of colonic action:* | | | | |
| Castor oil | Inhibit Na and water absorption, increase K secretion (? by inhibiting Na$^+$, K$^+$-ATPase). Digested in small intestine to ricinoleic acid. Can stimulate uterine contractions at full term. | 2 h | Excessive loss of water and electrolytes (including potassium) | Initiation of labour (obsolete) |

| Drug | Action | Time | Side effects | Notes |
|---|---|---|---|---|
| Senna (e.g. Senokot, Agiolax) | Contains glycosides which are hydrolysed by colonic bacteria to sennosides A and B. These are absorbed and then stimulate colonic peristalsis by acting on mural nerve plexuses. Enters milk. | 8 h | Griping and diarrhoea. Diarrhoea in suckling child. Melanosis coli. Red or yellow colouration of urine. | |
| Danthron (Dorbanex; Normax) | Partly absorbed from small intestine and detoxified by liver — otherwise similar to senna but 100 mg equivalent to 15 mg sennoside because of hepatic destruction | 8 h | As for senna. Avoid prolonged skin contact (e.g. in incontinence) since irritation can occur | |
| Bisacodyl (Dulcolax) | Deacetylated in gut, absorbed, glucuronidated in liver and enters enterohepatic circulation. Has a direct action on gut wall to stimulate peristalsis. Also absorbed into circulation and reaches gut wall in arterial blood. | 10 h | Abdominal cramps | Can be given by suppository |

**Table 29** (continued)

| Drug | Pharmacological properties | Approximate dose effect interval | Toxicity | Special uses |
|---|---|---|---|---|
| Phenolphthalein | 15% absorbed from gut, excreted in bile and undergoes an enterohepatic circulation — resulting in a prolonged effect. Active fraction produced in liver and undergoes further modification in colon. | 8–10 h | 4% develop a fixed drug eruption. Other rashes. SLE-like syndrome. Alkaline urine coloured pink. | Use has greatly declined over last 25 years. Use is not recommended. |
| *Lubricants and stool softeners:* | | | | |
| Dioctyl sodium sulphosuccinate (DSS: dioctyl) | Surface agent allows water into inspissated colonic contents | 1 day | Detergent action alters intestinal mucosa permeability. | Faecal impaction |
| Liquid paraffin | Lubricates contents of colonic Not digested. | 1 day | Interferes with absorption of fat soluble vitamins. Aspiration lipid pneumonia. Anal leakage. Absorption into tissues (e.g. after intestinal operations) Can cause granuloma formation. Possible carcinogenicity. | (Should be not used) |

## TREATMENT OF ACUTE DIARRHOEAL SYNDROMES

Replace lost fluid and electrolytes
Most attacks are self-limiting.
  Consider use of symptomatic treatment with codeine,
diphenoxylate etc, or with an absorbent mixture such as:
a. Kaolin
b. Chalk
c. Methylcellulose — useful in control of ileostomy and colostomy
d. Sterculia — useful in control of ileostomy and colostomy
  Infective diarrhoeas should *not* be treated with antibodies or
sulphanamides which may prolong the diarrhoea or carrier state;
encourage resistance; produce pseudomembranous colitis (page
324). Chemotherapy is indicated for:
a. *Shigellosis* — only severe, invasive cases with systemic
   manifestations require chemotherapy: ampicillin 2–4 g/day;
   cotrimoxazole tablets 2, 12-hourly;
b. *Enteric fever* — chloramphenicol 500 mg, 4 hourly until
   defervesence then 6 hourly for total period of 14 days;
   cotrimoxazole 2 or 3 tablets 12-hourly for 14 days is equally
   effective for chloramphenicol-resistant *Salmonella typhi*
   infections and does not suppress bone marrow.
c. *Salmonella food poisoning* — only when septicaemia occurs
   then chloramphenicol, cotrimoxazole or amoxycillin used.
d. *Cholera* — toxin increases adenyl cyclase activity raising cyclic
   AMP which reduces $Na^+$ absorption and increases $Cl^-$ and $HCO_3$
   secretion by gut. $Na^+$ absorption encouraged by giving oral
   glucose/saline: glucose and $Na^+$ absorption are coupled
   together in mucosal cells. Give mixture of 4 g NaCl, 4 g $NaHCO_3$,
   1 g KCl, 20 g glucose in 1 litre water — may need 10–15 litres in
   24 hours. Oral tetracycline eliminates vibrio and reduces toxin
   formation but tetracycline resistant strains have appeared in
   Bangladesh.

### Travellers' Diarrhoea
Various causes: toxigenic *E. coli*, Shigella, *Giardia lamblia*,
Salmonella, *Entamoeba histolytica*, Campylobacter.
  Acute onset of watery diarrhoea and abdominal cramps
occurring a few days after arrival, usually self-limiting.

*Prophylaxis*
Doxycycline 100 mg/day.

*Treatment*
Replace fluid and electrolytes orally.
Absorbent mixtures may help. Possibly salicylates
  (inhibit intestinal secretion by anti-prostaglandin action).
Avoid drugs inhibiting intestinal mobility which prevents
elimination of pathogens.

**Table 30:** Symptomatic drug treatment of diarrhoea

| Drug | Proprietary name | Dose | Special features | Adverse effects | Mechanism of action |
|---|---|---|---|---|---|
| Codeine phosphate | | 45–120 mg daily in 4–8-hourly doses | Opiate (p. 128) — tolerance and dependence can occur rarely. Contraindicated by hepatic or diverticular disease. | Nausea, dizziness and sedation. Constipation | Opiates decrease propulsive and increase tonic gut contractions allowing prolonged contact of gut contents with mucosa and greater water absorption |
| Diphenoxylate HCl | | 10 mg start then 5 mg 6-hourly | Pethidine derivative — dependence can occur. Contraindicated by hepatic or diverticular disease. Also with small doses of atropine (0.025 mg) as Lomotil and Reasec dose 4 tablets stat then 2 tablets 6 hourly — dangerous in overdose especially in children. | Euphoria, nausea, dizziness and sedation. Rarely ileus. | As codeine |
| Loperamide HCl | Imodium | 4 mg stat then 2 mg after each loose stool up to total 16 daily | No CNS effects — so no synergism with tranquillizers, sedatives or alcohol. No major anticholinergic actions. | Occasionally dry-mouth, headache, dizziness, vomiting, abdominal colic. | Interacts with cholinergic and non-cholinergic mechanisms in gut wall to inhibit motility |

| Cholestyramine | Questran | 12–24 g daily in 4–8 hourly | Used only for diarrhoea after ileal resection, vagotomy, bile acid malabsorption. | See page 241 | Basic anion-exchange resin to bind bile salts preventing reabsorption. So used for bile acid diarrhoea. |
|---|---|---|---|---|---|

## SULPHASALAZINE (Salazopyrin)

### Possible mechanisms of action
1. Prostaglandins ($PGE_2$) cause diarrhoea and colonic inflammation experimentally and increased production occurs in ulcerative colitis. 5-aminosalicylate inhibits prostaglandin synthesis and is anti-inflammatory.
2. Sulphapyridine's antibacterial effect changes colonic bacterial flora (reduces *E. coli* and Clostridia).

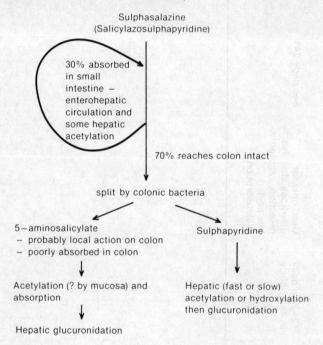

Sulphasalazine
(Salicylazosulphapyridine)

30% absorbed in small intestine — enterohepatic circulation and some hepatic acetylation

70% reaches colon intact

split by colonic bacteria

5–aminosalicylate
— probably local action on colon
— poorly absorbed in colon

Sulphapyridine

Acetylation (? by mucosa) and absorption

Hepatic (fast or slow) acetylation or hydroxylation then glucuronidation

Hepatic glucuronidation

### Pharmacokinetics
Very little sulphasalazine or acetylsulphasalazine excreted — all eliminated as metabolites of 5-aminosalicylate or sulphapyridine.

Toxic effects associated with high plasma levels ($> 50 \mu g/ml$) of sulphapyridine — commoner in slow acetylators.

Therapeutic plasma sulphapyridine concentration approximately $20-50 \mu g/ml$.

**Dose**
1 g 6-hourly p.o. in acute exacerbations of colitis and 1 g 8–12 hourly p.o. during quiescent periods. Given after meals or as enteric coated drug. Also as enema (3 g) or suppositories (500 mg).

**Uses**
Ulcerative colitis
Crohn's disease
Radiation enteritis

**Adverse effects**
Cross allergy with sulphanamides.
   Dose-dependent effects: nausea, vomiting, headaches, fever, arthralgia, transient leucocytosis, bluish colour of skin, reversible male sterility. Haemolytic anaemia in G6PD deficiency (see page 36)
   Sensitivity reactions: rash, blood dycrasia, bronchospasm, hepatotoxicity, peripheral neuropathy, toxic epidermal neurolysis
   Folate malabsorption.

**Interaction**
Concomitant use of ferrous sulphate lowers plasma sulphasalazine and sulphapyridine concentrations due to chelation.
   Can displace bilirubin, warfarin and oral hypoglycaemics from plasma protein binding.

**Treatment of ulcerative colitis**
A. *Mild attacks* without systemic features, usually confined to rectum and sigmoid colon. Can often be managed as out-patients.
1. Sulphasalazine 0.5 mg 12-hourly increasing to 1 g 6–8-hourly.
2. Topical corticosteroid — Prednisolone disodium phosphate (Predsol) suppositories 2, once or twice daily or as enema.
3. If 1 and 2 ineffective, prednisolone 40 mg/day p.o.
4. Disodium cromoglycate (Nalcrom) 200 mg 6-hourly p.o. — efficacy under investigation.
B. *Moderately severe attacks* — some systemic upset usually involving at least the left side and sigmoid colon and rectum and requiring hospital admission.
1. Prednisolone 40 mg/day p.o.
2. Replacement of fluid, electrolytes, iron and blood as required. Possibly parenteral feeding.
3. If no response, intravenous hydrocortisone or ACTH.
   As patient improves prednisolone dose slowly reduced, topical corticosteroids and sulphasalazine begun.
C. *Severe attacks* with major systemic effects and bowel involvement.
1. Prednisolone-21-phosphate 60 mg i.v./day, hydrocortisone hemisuccinate 300–400 mg i.v./day or ACTH gel 80 units i.m./day.

2. Replacement of fluid, electrolytes and blood (fresh if possible)
3. Parenteral feeding.
4. Collaborative management with surgeons.
D. *Maintenance of remission.*
1. Sulphasalazine is the only drug clearly shown as effective prophylactic but it is ineffective in significant relapse: the converse applies to steroids. Maintenance sulphasalazine dose is 1 g 8–12-hourly.
2. Azathioprine (2–2.5 mg/kg) may prevent recurrent relapse but ineffective during exacerbation.
3. Avoid precipitating factors: intestinal infections, stress, 20% have milk intolerance.
4. Prompt treatment of impending relapse.
E. *Systemic manifestations*
Arthritis; sacroiliitis; ankylosing spondylitis; erythema nodosum; pyoderma gangrenosum; iritis; urethritis; chronic active hepatitis.
   These are all indications for corticosteroid treatment.

**Treatment of Crohn's disease**
A. *Acute attack*
1. Bed rest
2. Codeine phosphate or diphenoxylate (see page 228).
3. If severe or no response, hydrocortisone hemisuccinate 100 mg 6-hourly i.v. or ACTH gel 80 units i.m./day or if oral drugs appropriate prednisolone 60 mg daily in limited doses. Then doese carefully reduced.
B. *Prevention of relapse and treatment in remission*
1. Sulphasalazine 1 g 12- or 8-hourly p.o. is less effective than in ulcerative colitis.
2. Azathioprine 2–2.5 mg/kg p.o. or cyclophosphamide 1.5–2 mg/kg p.o. have been used but carry greater hazard.
3. Others of unproven efficacy: dapsone 100 mg/day; Metronidazole 400 mg 8 hourly.
4. Diarrhoea may result from fat malabsorption and may respond to a low fat or medium chain triglyceride diet. Alternatively it may result from bile salt colitis due to terminal ileitis or a blind loop syndrome: these may respond to cholestyramine (see page 241). Otherwise symptomatic treatment with codeine phosphate, Lomotil or methylcellulose.
5. Pain, if not due to obstruction, is treated with a mild analgesic; sometimes mebeverine helps. Exclusion of milk from the diet may help.

**Treatment of irritable bowel syndrome**
1. Dietary
   — High fibre diets using bran (12–24 g/day).
   — Reduced sugar diets
   — Eliminate lactose in lactase-deficient patients.

2. Avoid stress; simple psychotherapy.
3. Anticholinergic drugs if above fail. No evidence that any is better than atropine but commonly used are propantheline bromide (Pro Banthine) 15–30 mg 8-hourly; dicyclomine (Merbentyl) 10–20 mg 8-hourly.
4. Smooth muscle relaxants without anticholinergic properties, e.g. Mebeverine 135 mg 8-hourly before meals.
5. Psychotropic agents, e.g. amitriptyline, imipramine which also have anticholinergic activity have been used as adjunctive treatments.

## HEPATIC ENCEPHALOPATHY

### A. Precipitating factors of encephalopathy (in approximate order of frequency) in patients with chronic liver disease

| Factor | Presumed mechanism |
|---|---|
| Uraemia | Ureases in gut split urea to $NH_3$. |
| Sedatives, analgesics | Direct CNS depression. Impaired hepatic drug metabolism. |
| GI haemorrhage | Blood is substrate for $NH_3$ production in gut. Shock, hypoxia and hypovolaemia impair CNS and hepatic function. |
| Hypokalaemia/Diuretics | Hypokalaemia and alkalosis decrease renal $NH_3$ loss. Alkalosis increases $NH_3$ entry into CNS. Vigorous diuresis produces hypovolaemia and impaired cardiac, CNS, hepatic and renal function. |
| Excess dietary protein | Substrate for $NH_3$ production — especially in patients with porto-caval shunt. |
| Infection | Tissue catabolism increases $NH_3$ Dehydration, hypotension, hypoxia. |

N.B. Drugs to be avoided in patients with liver disease:
1. Narcotics, e.g. morphine, pethidine, codeine.
2. Sedatives, e.g. pentobarbitone, amylobarbitone (barbitone may be used with care), glutethimide, chloral.
3. Benzodiazepines: diazepam should be used in reduced dosage; better use oxazepam (mainly renal excretion; no active metabolites; short $T_{\frac{1}{2}}$).
4. Tranquillizers, e.g. chlorpromazine.
5. Ethanol: acute alcoholism precipitates encephalopathy by reducing hepatic and cerebral function.
6. Diuretics: Thiazides and loop diuretics (but amiloride and spironolactone can be used with care).

**B. Treatment of acute hepatic failure and encephalopathy (in ICU)**
1. Remove or treat precipitating causes.
2. Reduce $NH_3$ production.
   a. No protein, high carbohydrate diet prevents protein catabolism and $NH_3$ production — 1500 ml fluid, 1000 cals, 200 g carbohydrate in 24 hours given i.v. or p.o.
   b  Mg $SO_4$ purge.
   c. Empty colon with enemas (acid or neutral to reduce $NH_3$ absorption).
   d. Alter colonic flora and reduce toxin absorption:
      Lactulose 50–200 ml/day p.o. — acidifies stools and reduces $NH_3$ absorption.
      Neomycin 4–6 g/day p.o.
3. Correct metabolic/respiratory disturbances
   a. Electrolytes:
      hyponatraemia (partly dilutional, partly shift into cells)
      hypokalaemia
      hypomagnesaemia and hypophosphataemia occasionally require correction.
   b. Acid-base disturbances — respiratory alkalosis common but does not require correction.
   c. Hypoxia — give oxygen by mask or intermittent positive-pressure ventilation with PEEP.
   d. Hypoglycaemia can develop rapidly.
   e. Watch for acute tubular necrosis or pre-renal failure.
4. Control haematological disturbances.
   a. Fresh frozen plasma partially repairs deficit in levels of fibrinogen and clotting factors synthesised in liver (II, VII, IX, X). Vitamin K, (Menadiol sodium phosphate, Synkavit) 10 mg i.m. may help.
   b. Platelet transfusions if count $< 30 \times 10^9$/l.
5. Be wary of infection.
6. Experimental procedures
   a. Levodopa ($\pm$ decarboxylase inhibitor) may replenish depleted neurotransmitters — 1–2 g/day but GI side effects limit dose. Bromocriptine may be an alternative.
   b. Charcoal haemoperfusion.

**C. Treatment of chronic hepatic failure and encephalopathy**
1. Avoid precipitating factors.
2. Diet: re-introduce protein (vegetable rather than animal) 20 g alternate days to limit of tolerance (usually 20–40 g/day).
3. Lactulose begun at 30–45 ml 6–8-hourly, increased if necessary to give 2–3 bowel movements of pH 5.5–6. Better than neomycin chronically because of danger of aminoglycoside toxicity from minimal absorption.
4. Consider levodopa or bromocriptine.

**D.  Treatment of cirrhotic oedema and ascites**
1. General
    a. Bed rest with daily measurement of weight, girth, electrolytes (urinary and plasma) and fluid balance.
    b. Salt restriction (no added salt = 50 mmol/day; low salt diet = 20 mmol/day).
    c. Fluid restriction < 1500 ml/day..
2. Diuretics
    — if trial of general measures fails.
    — avoid weight loss > 1.5 kg/day.
    — avoid hypokalaemia and hyperkalaemia
    — remember ascites may not need aggressive treatment, that diuretics can cause complications and do not increase life expectancy.
    a. Spironolactone (begin with 50–100 mg/day but can increase slowly to 500 mg/day); triamterine (150–300 mg/day) or amiloride (5–20 mg/day) counter secondary hyperaldosteronism,
    b. If these fail add frusemide (up to 150 mg/day) cautiously.
3. Infuse salt-free albumin if hypoalbuminaemia a major factor but effect usually transient.
4. Paracentesis for symptomatic relief, e.g. nausea, respiratory distress, abdominal pain.
5. Ascites ultrafiltration and re-infusion.
6. Le Veen peritoneal-jugular shunt.

**E.  Management of bleeding oesophageal varices**
1. Resuscitation with fresh blood if possible, CVP line and naso-gastric tube.
2. Early diagnosis — usually endoscopic.
3. Control of bleeding in order of preference:
    a. Vasopressin 20 units in 100 ml 5% destrose given i.v. over 15 mins. Causes intense splanchnic vascoconstriction and reduces hepatic portal blood flow. Also gives colic, facial pallor, and rarely hypertension and angina.
    b. Sengstaken-Blakemore tube to compress varices.
    c. Surgical and endoscopic procedures.
4. Treatment for acute encephalopathy usually required.


## MEDICAL TREATMENT OF GALLSTONES

Cholesterol stones comprise 75% of all gall stones: these alone are amenable to dissolution by medical treatment. Result from secretion of cholesterol-saturated bile by the liver but cause of this super-saturation is uncertain. Cholesterol stones may be dissolved by making bile unsaturated with respect to cholesterol so that cholesterol in the stones redissolves in bile acid and phospholipid micelles.

CHENODEOXYCHOLIC ACID (Chendol)

**Pharmacology**
Reduces biliary cholesterol saturation by reducing hepatic
cholesterol synthesis — inhibits hydroxymethylglutaryl
coenzyme-A reductase (HMGCoAR), the rate-limiting enzyme for
cholesterol synthesis from acetate. May act directly or via its
metabolite ursodeoxycholic acid. Also increases the bile acid pool
(reduced in patients with gall stones) and becomes major
component of pool. Output of phospholipids is also increased thus
allowing micelles to hold more cholesterol in solution.

Well absorbed orally, undergoes reabsorption after biliary
excretion in terminal ileum so completing enterohepatic circulation.
Some metabolised by bacterial gut flora to secondary bile acids
(Lithocholic and 7-keto-lithocholic acid). Later undergoes hepatic
metabolism to ursodeoxycholic acid (a tertiary bile acid).

**Patient selection**
1. Cholesterol stones: calcified stones do not dissolve. Radiolucent
   stones with regular outlines on oral cholecystography are likely
   to be cholesterol. Can be used for non-obstructing stones in
   common bile duct.
2. Normal functioning gallbladder giving good opacification and
   contraction after fats is necessary so that stones come into
   contact with desaturated bile.
3. The smaller the stone, the faster it dissolves.
4. Should not be given to fertile women unless they are on low
   dose oestrogen contraceptive pill because risk to fetus unknown.
5. Indicated for frail, elderly patients, those fearful of surgery or in
   whom operation is contraindicated.
6. Patients with frequent symptoms should have surgery not drugs
   since dissolution therapy can take many months.

**Dose**
13–15 mg/kg/day in divided doses. Obese (25%+ over ideal body
weight) are relatively resistant and require 18–20 mg/kg/day. Small
stones (<5 mm diameter begin dissolving after 6 months, but
stones >10 mm diameter only begin after 2 years treatment).
Treatment checked by 6 monthly oral cholecystograms.

Drug continued for 3 months after complete dissolution. Bile
reverts to supersaturated state 3 weeks after stopping treatment:
some patients develop further stones (30% in first year) —
maintenance regimes presently under investigation. Medical
treatment of gallstones is expensive.

**Adverse effects**
1. Diarrhoea (about 30–40%)
2. Transiently raised serum transaminase levels without evidence
   of liver damage.

## URSODEOXYCHOLIC ACID (Destolit)

Similar mode of action to chenodeoxycholic acid of which it is a metabolite. May be more active injibitor of HMGCoAR.

Patients selected as for chenodeoxycholic acid.

### Dose
10 mg/kg/day gives similar efficacy to chenodeoxycholic acid. May act more quickly than chenodeoxycholic acid but dissolution still takes many months.

### Adverse effects
Diarrhoea unusual and no reported effects on liver failure.

## ROWACHOL

Proprietary mixture of terpenes (menthol, menthane, pinene, borneol, camphene, cineol) which lowers hepatic HMGCoAR activity. Induces hepatic enzymes, e.g. glucuronyl transferase, and enhances cholesterol solubility of bile. Active component(s) unknown.

### Dose
1 capsule/10 kg body weight/day for 6 months or more. Presently under evaluation.

# Obesity, vitamins, hyperlipoproteinaemias and nutrition

## TREATMENT OF OBESITY

### 1. Dieting
  (i) assess calorie needs and what patient consumes.
 (ii) put on a *balanced* diet with a deficit of 500 cal/day (should lose 0.5 kg/week). Total starvation not recommended because long term success is low and risks are high; unbalanced diets (e.g. grapefruits only; low carbohydrate) lead to nutritional and intestinal problems.
(iii) teach patient to count calories; particular care to include sweet drinks; alcohol; sugar in tea and coffee; fat used in cooking.
 (iv) change patterns of eating:
      *Antecedent events* (e.g. attractive adverts, visits to food shops) must be recognised.
      *Behaviour of eating* — learn only to eat at mealtimes and sitting at a table. No standing in kitchen or by 'fridge. Have breakfast but no snack after evening meal. Making a complete list of what is eaten can alone improve eating pattern. Also keeping a record of hunger helps to space meals.
      *Consequences of eating* — understanding the depressive effect of guilt about breaking diet. Rewards include improved appearance, interpersonal relationships.

### 2. Exercise
Not only increases calorie consumption, but may readjust appetite to match energy needs. Strenous physical exercise hazardous for grossly obese, but a planned progressive programme used. Exercise *daily* for at least 30 mins.

### 3. Drugs
Controversial (but patients lose 0.25 kg/week more than those receiving placebo).
  (i) Thyroid hormones — only large doses are effective and produce no dependence. However, lean bodyweight also decreased and cardiac toxicity likely. Not recommended.
 (ii) Amphetamines, diethylpropion, phentermine, phenbutrazate

diethylpropion, mazindol: effective but produce excitement, tolerance, risk of dependence. Cannot be used with MAOI, in CVS disorder (including hypertension).
(iii) Fenfluramine (Ponderax) (40–120 mg daily in divided doses) is anorectic but sedative. Can precipitate depression.
(iv) Bulk agents (cellulose, guar gum, sterculia, bran) not shown to be effective.

## 4. Surgery
 (i) Intestinal bypass: lose 5–70 kg in first year.
disadvantages: haemorrhoids; fluid and electrolyte imbalance; protein malnutrition; liver failure; renal stones; metabolic bone disease; polyarthritis. Mortality is 3%.
 (ii) Gastric bypass: slightly less hazardous than intestinal bypass.
(iii) Vagotomy: patients lose hunger and lose weight.
(iv) Jaw wiring: lose 20 kg in first 5 months.
disadvantages: dental damage; risk of aspiration; gain weight when wires removed.

# VITAMINS

## Vitamin A
A number of forms of vitamin A exist, e.g.:
    retinol (vitamin $A_1$)
    3-dehydroretinol (vitamin $A_2$)
    retinoic acid (vitamin A acid)

*Deficiency*
1. Earliest signs: follicular hyperkeratosis and infections of skin.
2. Reduced visual dark adaptation is a feature of severe lack.
   Permanent blindness follows prolonged deficiency.
3. Blindness may also be the result of keratomalacia, xerophthalmia and corneal scarring.
4. Bronchorespiratory keratinisation, mucus plugging and infections.
5. Urinary calculi; impaired spermatogenesis.
6. Metaplasia of pancreatic duct epithelium; diarrhoea.
7. Skin: atrophy of sweat glands; papular rashes.
8. Bone: increased formation of cancellous bone.
9. Sense organs: decreased hearing, taste, smell, + 2 & 3.

*Hypervitaminosis*
Usually due to excess intake of retinol with a relative lack of vitamin E.
Chronic:
1. Irritability, headache, fatigue.
2. Anorexia, vomiting.

3. Dry itching skin, skin desquamation, erythema.
4. Loss of body hair, deposition of carotenoids.
5. Myalgia, pain in feet and legs.
6. Gingivitis, mouth fissures.
7. Nystagmus, papilloedema.
8. Enlargement of liver, spleen and lymph nodes.

Acute:
1. Drowsiness.
2. Headache, vomiting, papilloedema (bulging fontanelle in infants).
3. Desquamation of skin.

Uses:
1. Prevention of deficiency: normal daily requirement 800 r.e. for women; 100 r.e. for men (r.e. = 1 retinol equivalent = 1 μg retinol = 1 unit of vitamin A, assuming that 50% of dietary vitamin A is from retinol and 50% from β-carotene).
   Infants: 400–700 r.e./day.
   Pregnancy & lactation: 1000–1200 r.e./day.
2. In severe deficiency (e.g. Kwashiorkor): a single i.m. injection of 30 mg retinol (as palmitate), then 60–120 mg retinol every 3–6 months.
3. Desquamation of skin, e.g. in Darier's disease; ichthyoses and severe psoriasis: retinoic acid (tretinoin) or etretinate (Tigason) orally 0.75–1 mg/kg/day in divided doses for 2–4 weeks. Oral 13-cis-retinoic acid (2 mg/kg/day) for severe cystic acne.
4. Topical tretinoin for acne vulgaris (Retin A lotion and gel is 0.025% tretinoin).

## Ascorbic acid (vitamin C)

*Ascorbic acid deficiency*
Dietary lack in elderly, alcoholics, drug addicts, infants on poor diets.
1. Perifollicular hyperkeratosis in skin.
2. Petechiae and ecchymoses in skin.
3. Slowed healing of wounds.
4. Loose teeth, gingivitis, bleeding gums.
5. Anaemia.
6. In babies: irritability, painful sub-periosteal haemorrhages.

*Toxicity*
Excessive doses may produce dysuria, oxalate kidney stones and interfere with anticoagulant action — but such toxic effects are uncommon.

*Uses*
1. Prevention of scurvy: 60 mg ascorbic acid daily (increased needs: smokers, oral contraceptive use, infections, wound healing). Usual route is oral.
2. Malabsorption and during parenteral nutrition i.m. or i.v. 200 mg sodium ascorbate/day.
3. Idiopathic methaemoglobinaemia: 150 mg ascorbic acid/day.
4. Prevention and/or cure respiratory viral infections: large dose used — results are inconclusive (high doses in pregnancy can produce rebound scurvy in offspring).

## HYPERLIPOPROTEINAEMIAS (HYPERLIPIDAEMIAS)

### Steps in management
1. Confirm raised blood lipid(s) and look for treatable underlying cause.
2. Family history and investigation for raised lipids, early CVS disease and pancreatitis.
3. Treat to prevent atherosclerosis and pancreatitis.
4. If decide to treat try diet first.
5. If 4 fails try 4 plus drugs.
Decide to treat:
1. Young patients with hypercholesterolaemia or hypertriglyceridaemia with family history of early atherosclerotic disease.
2. All patients with serum triglycerides above 15–20 mmol/l.

### Diet
1. Primary lipoprotein lipase deficiency: very low fat diet.
2. All other types:
   (i)   treat obesity with calorie restriction and exercise.
   (ii)  reduce dietary saturated fats.
   (iii) partially replace (ii) with unsaturated fats.
   (iv)  increase complex (starchy) carbohydrate content of diet to 55–60% of total calories.

### Drugs
*Hypercholesterolaemia*
1. Cholestyramine (Questran) 12–32 g/day in divided doses before meals.
   Toxicity:
   anorexia, nausea
   constipation (responds to bran)
   paradoxical rise in triglycerides
   vitamin deficiency (give supplements at night).
2. Colestipol (Colestiol) 15–40 g/day in divided doses before meals. Like cholestyramine is a bile acid binding resin and has the same toxic effects.

3. Nicotinic acid 2 – 9 g/day in divided doses (but start with 250 mg/day and gradually increase dose). Lowers both cholesterol and triglycerides. Useful in resistant familial hypercholesterolaemia (with resins) and in combined lipid disease (with resins if necessary).
   Toxicity:
   flushing
   GI toxicity
   impaired glucose tolerance
   hyperuricaemia
   abnormalities in liver function tests.
   hyperlipoproteinaemias

*Hypertriglyceridaemia*
1. Clofibrate (Atromid-S) 1 g twice daily. Can prevent pancreatitis in massive hypertriglyceridaemia.
   Toxicity:
   gallbladder disease
   GI disturbances
   thrombophlebitis and pulmonary emboli
   cardiac arrhythmias (possibly raised incidence of sudden death).
   myopathy
   abnormal liver function tests
   Because of toxicity, clofibrate has limited uses.
2. Nicotinic acid (see above).

## ENTERAL NUTRITION

Used to provide calories and nitrogen if a negative balance has occurred due to starvation, trauma, infection, burns or surgery. Also used in malabsorption, post-gastrectomy and dysphagia. Cheaper and safer than parenteral nutrition.
Usual daily adult need: 8 – 20 g nitrogen in 1500 – 4000 cals (6270 – 16720 kJ). Administration best via small (1 mm) bore tube with continuous gravity feed.

**Some proprietary enteral feeds**

| Name | Energy content | Additional features |
| --- | --- | --- |
| Clinifeed 400 | 1674 kJ/375 ml tin<br>593 kJ/gN = 142 cals/gN | Complete nutrition.<br>Casein is protein source.<br>Gluten free. |
| Ensure | 450 kJ/100 ml<br>643 kJ/gN = 154 cals/gN | Complete nutrition.<br>Casein and soya protein.<br>Gluten and lactose free. |
| Flexical | 1850 kJ/100 ml<br>1070 kJ/gN = 256 cals/gN | Complete nutrition.<br>Casein amino acids.<br>Gluten and lactose free. |

| Forceval | 1540 kJ/100 g | Low fat. Gluten and lactose free. |
| Isocal | 445 kJ/100 ml | Complete nutrition. Casein and soya protein. Gluten and lactose free. |

## Toxicity

Lactose intolerance (Asians and Africans esp.) can cause diarrhoea — if likely choose lactose-free solution.

Abdominal distension, colic, diarrhoea (usually when full strength feeds introduced too rapidly).

Tube problems (e.g. irritation, ulceration of oesophagus, accidental insertion into lung)

Hyperglycaemia (give insulin to keep blood glucose normal)

Low blood levels of K, Ca, Mg, Zn, $PO_4$ (measure these $\times$ 2 weekly)

Abnormal liver function tests.

## Chronic renal failure and hepatic failure

Require high energy, low fluid and low electrolyte diet, e.g:

Caloreen (polyglucose polymer, low in electrolytes, low protein, lactose and fructose free) 1.67 mJ/100 g.

Hycal (carbohydrate as corn syrup, lactose, fructose, sucrose, protein free. Low in electrolytes) 1.03 mJ/100 ml.

## PARENTERAL NUTRITION

Only used when the enteral route cannot be used in malnourished patients.

## Requirements

*1. Nitrogen*

As crystalline L-amino acid mixtures (not partial hydrolysates of whole protein).

Essential amino acids should be approx 40% (w/w) of total.

Higher proportion of branched amino acids (valine, leucine and isoleucine) lower proportion of phenylalanine and tyrosine in liver failure, sepsis and severe injuries. Several formulations are available, including:

| | |
|---|---|
| Synthamin 9 (9.3 gN/l) | also contain Na, K, Cl, Mg, $PO_4$, acetate |
| Synthamin 14 (14.4 gN/l) | (but also electrolyte free) |
| Synthamin 17 (17.9 gN/l) | |

Vamin N (9.4 gN/l also contains Na, K, Cl, Mg, Ca (with or without glucose and fructose)

## 2. Energy

As glucose *or* glucose plus lipid. Basal requirement is 25 cal/kg/day and the usual need is 150–250 cals (627–1045 kJ) of non-protein energy/k nitrogen supplied.

In severely negative nitrogen balance, only glucose is used, but in other types of patient the combination is given because less water retention results. i.v. lipid preparations:

Intralipid 10% (soya bean oil + egg phospholipid) emulsion 4620 kJ/l

Intralipid 20% (soya bean oil + egg phospholipid) emulsion 8400 kJ/l.

## 3. Vitamins

Recommended daily intake:

| | |
|---|---|
| retinol | 700 IU |
| thiamine | 1.4 mg |
| riboflavin | 2.1 mg |
| nicotinamide | 14 mg |
| pyridoxine | 2.1 mg |
| folic acid | 2 mg |
| cyanocobalamin | 2.0 $\mu$g |
| biotin | 350 $\mu$g |
| pantothenic acid | 14 mg |
| ascorbic acid | 35 mg |
| calciferol | 100 IU |
| tocopheryl acetate | 30 IU |
| phytomenaquinone | 140 $\mu$g |

Preparations include:

Multibionta
Parentrovite
Solivito

none are ideal, e.g. care not to give excess retinol. Supplements of vitamins and ascorbic acid for alcoholic and catabolic patients.

## Problems in patients needing parenteral nutrition:

A. Catheter — sepsis, etc.
B. Metabolic changes
  1. Hyperglycaemia
  2. Intracellular ion deficiency, e.g. $PO_4$, Zn, Mg, Cu. Check $K^+$ if glucose and insulin used.
  3. Vitamin deficiencies, e.g. folate.
  4. Essential fatty acid deficiency
  5. Abnormal liver function tests and intrahepatic cholestasis with jaundice.
  6. Hyperosmolality due to excess glucose and relative insulin deficiency.

## PANCREATIC ENZYME REPLACEMENT

Used in pancreatic insufficiency due to cystic fibrosis, chronic pancreatitis etc to reduce diarrhoea, steatorrhoea and weight loss. Pancreatin B.P. contains proteases, lipases and amylase — available as enteric and sugar-coated (e.g. Pancrex V) capsules, enteric-coated granules to be taken dry or with liquid (e.g. Protopan) or capsules to be opened and sprinkled on food (e.g. Cotazym). Usual dose is 2–8 g in divided dose. Concurrent use of cimetidine to reduce gastric acidity improves delivery of intact enzyme to the duodenum. Adverse effects include irritation of skin surrounding mouth and anus; hyperuricosuria and uric acid stones (in children with cystic fibrosis ingesting excessive amounts of purine-containing pancreatic extract).

Patients also require supplemental water and fat-soluble vitamins.

# Drugs affecting the blood

## COAGULATION PATHWAYS

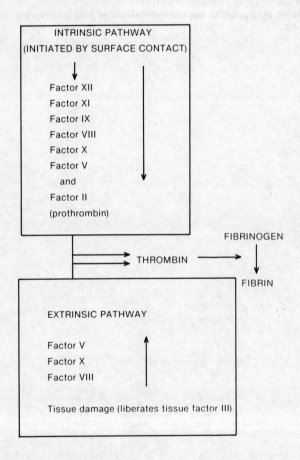

**Nomenclature of clotting factors**
  I  fibrinogen
 II  prothrombin
III  thromboplastin (tissue factor III)
 IV  calcium
  V  pro-accelerin
(VI) not used)
VII  proconvertin
VIII antihaemophilic factor (AHF)
 IX  Christmas factor (Plasma thromboplastin component (PTC))
  X  Stuart-Prower factor
 XI  plasma thromboplastin antecedent (PTA)
XII  Hageman factor (contact factor)
XIII fibrin stabilising factor.

Antithrombin III is a naturally occuring inhibitor of coagulation
enzymes:
XIIa
XIa
IXa
Xa
thrombin.
Heparin greatly accelerates the action of antithrombin III.

## ANTICOAGULANTS

### A.  Drugs affecting the clotting process

#### 1. Heparin
A mixture of sulphated polysaccharides (MW 6000–20 000) 120 U
= 1 mg. Active in vitro and invivo. Acts immediately.

*Actions*
In the presence of heparin cofactor (antithrombin III) in plasma acts
as an antithrombin (i.e. inhibits fibrinogen → fibrin); and as an
inhibitor of factor Xa. Heparin also inhibits:
    factor IXa (even low doses do this);
    activation of factor IX by factor XIa;
    activation of lipoprotein lipase;
    platelet aggregation due to fibrin.

*Pharmacokinetics*
Precipitated by gastric acid, but can be absorbed from s.c., i.m. or
i.v. injection (but i.m. commonly causes haematomas and (rarely)
s.c. may produce skin necrosis). $T_{\frac{1}{2}} = 60$–90 mins. 20% excreted in
urine unchanged; 80% metabolised in liver (to sulphates,

oligosaccharides and uroheparin). Metabolism reduced in shock. Does not cross placental barrier or enter milk.

*Indications*
When oral anticoagulants are used, heparin may be given during the first 36 h of treatment (i.e. until the oral agent has produced its effect) (see warfarin);
    haemodialysis and other mechanical circulation techniques;
    acute arterial obstruction of a limb;
    disseminated intravascular coagulation;
    prophylaxis of deep vein thrombosis;
    anticoagulation in pregnancy.

*Dose and control of dose*
Heparin prolongs: whole blood clotting time (WBCT), activated partial thromboplastin time (APTT or Kaolin-cephalin time) and thrombin time. (The latter is normally 10–12s and may be prolonged to 60s with therapeutic doses). Therapeutic range is 1.5–2.5 × normal for APTT and 2–3 × normal for WBCT). Therapeutic range for Xa inhibition has not yet been defined. Control tests only done if treatment prolonged beyond 48 h. Continuous infusion: loading dose 5000 U then 1500 U hourly for 7–10 days (control tests at 0, 6 and 24 h then 12-hourly). Intermittent i.v.: 10 000 U 6-hourly (control tests before each dose). Low dose s.c.: 5000 U s.c. or 5000 U 4 hourly every 12 h (lab control not necessary). Never given i.m.

*Toxicity*
1. Spontaneous haemorrhage (very important and occurs in up to 5% of patients) — reverse effect with 1 mg protamine sulphate per 100 U heparin.
2. Allergy (uncommon).
3. Osteoporosis (chronic administration of 10 000 U daily).
4. Alopecia (rare).
5. Thrombocytopenia (rare).

## 2.  Oral anticoagulants (vitamin K antagonists)
*4-hydroxycoumarins*: warfarin; bishydroxycoumarin

*Indan 1:3 diones*: phenindione

*Actions*
Prevent synthesis of factors II, VII, IX and X by inhibiting regeneration of vitamin K oxide.

*Pharmacokinetics*
Complete absorption from gut. All oral anticoagulants enter the fetus. Warfarin is 97% bound to plasma albumin. Warfarin: mean $T_{\frac{1}{2}}$ = 44 h (but 12-fold variation). Eliminated by hepatic microsomal metabolism. Phenindiones (but very little warfarin) enter breast milk.

*Warfarin is racemic* — S and R forms: S isomer 3–4 × more potent but rapidly metabolised. Main metabolite of S isomer is 7-hydroxywarfarin. Main metabolite of R isomer is warfarin alcohol. Phenylbutazone reduces metabolism of S warfarin and increases metabolism of R warfarin — net effect is same amount of racemic warfarin but more anticoagulation (because S more active).

*Indications*
Much difference of opinion.
Limited administration:
prophylaxis of thromboembolic disease, e.g. myocardial infarction
    (some give warfarin up to 1 year in young patients), repair of
    fractured femur, caesarean section;
deep vein thrombosis — 2 weeks treatment;
pulmonary embolism — 6 weeks to 6 months treatment;
cerebrovascular disease (if CSF free from blood).
Long term or permanent administration:
atrial fibrillation or a large left atrium;
artificial heart valves;
pulmonary hypertension (subacute thromboembolic).

*Contraindications*
Absolute
    active bleeding, e.g. ulcerative colitis, peptic ulcer, haematuria;
    haemorrhagic diathesis;
    dissecting aneurysm;
    surgery of CNS or eye.
Relative
    potential bleeding lesion, e.g. papilloma of bladder, history of
    peptic ulcer;
    severe hypertension;
    severe diabetes;
    chronic alcoholism;
    pregnancy;
    hepatic or renal insufficiency;
    poor patient complicance.
Increased susceptibility in old age.

*Dose and control of dose*
Prothrombin time increases with reduced activity of factors II, VII, X; thrombotest sensitive to factor IX. Initial daily dose of warfarin is 10–15 mg and; phenindione 200–300 mg. After 48 h prothrombin

time used to modify dose (prothrombin time also measured before start of treatment). Maintenance daily dose usually in range 2–20 mg warfarin and 25–200 mg phenindione. At first daily tests carried out — but when anticoagulation established, every 4–12 weeks. Therapeutic range of prothrombin time corresponds to 20–30% prothrombin activity; for thrombotest, range is 5–15%.

*Toxicity*
1. Haemorrhage (very important and common: 5% per treatment year). Effect terminated by oral or i.v. vitamin K (5–25 mg) or water soluble analogue (e.g. phytomenadione 10–20 mg; menadiol diphosphate 10–100 mg). Check prothrombin time at 3h and repeat if very prolonged. Prothrombin time returns to normal in 12–36 h.
2. Coumarins: skin necrosis; alopecia; abortion; congenital abnormalities (nasal hypoplasia).
3. Phenindiones: block $I_2$ uptake by thyroid; uricosuria; congenital nasal abnormalities; renal tubular damage; hepatitis; dermatitis; agranulocytosis; pink urine (fades with acetic acid); up to 3% of patients on phenindione develop sensitivity reactions.

## Oral anticoagulants — interactions
1. *Enhanced effect*

| Drug | Mechanism |
|---|---|
| 1. phenylbutazone<br>alcohol<br>anabolic steroids<br>chloramphenicol<br>colchicine<br>reserpine | Inhibition of hepatic metabolism anticoagulant |
| 2. oral antibiotics | Less vitamin K made by micro-organisms in the gut |
| 3. chloral<br>sulphonamides<br>phenytoin<br>phenylbutazone &<br>oxyphenbutazone<br>mefenamic acid<br>indomethacin<br>feprazone & azapropazone<br>ketoprofen<br>aspirin<br>amiodarone<br>danazol<br>metronidazole | Displacement of anticoagulant from protein binding sites |

   4. thyroxine                    Unknown
      triiodothyronine
      chloroquine

   5. liquid paraffin              Reduces vitamin K absorption

   6. clofibrate                   Lowers plasma triglycerides
                                   which carry vitamin K

II. *Reduced effect*

   1. barbiturates                 Enzyme induction
      glutethimide
      phenytoin
      primidone
      carbamazepine
      glucocorticoids
      rifampicin

   2. contraceptive pill           Increased synthesis of clotting
                                   factors
      vitamins K$_1$ & K$_2$       Allows activation of clotting
      antacids                     factors
      cholestyramine               Impair absorption

Drugs potentiated by oral anticoagulants:
   chlorpropamide, tolbutamide
   phenytoin
Oral anticoagulants more active in:
   alcoholism
   hepatic failure, cholestasis
   renal failure
   cardiac failure
   diarrhoea
   malnutrition
   thyrotoxicosis
   fever
   hypoalbuminaemia

**Ancrod (Arvin)**
Snake venom glycoprotein.

*Actions*
Converts fibrinogen to imperfect fibrin polymer that is readily
degraded.
No effect on platelets or clotting factors.

*Uses*
Treatment of established deep vein thrombosis.
Prevention of deep vein thrombosis.

*Dose and control of dose*
Induction dose (2 units/kg over 6-12 h) given slowly so that
  physiological mechanisms for fibrin disposal not overloaded.
Maintenance dose (2 units/kg every 12 h by slow i.v. infusion or
injection).
Also given s.c.
Monitor plasma fibrinogen concentration or clot quality.

*Toxicity*
Similar to heparin — especially haemorrhage, anaphylaxis.
Effects can be reversed by specific antiserum or fibrinogen.
Some patients become resistant.

## THROMBOLYTIC AGENTS

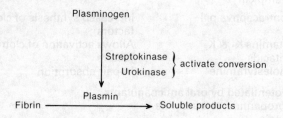

### Streptokinase
Used in:
  pulmonary embolism
  life-threatening venous thrombosis
Must be given within 1 hour of event. May cause allergy.

### Urokinase
Used for thrombolysis in eye and A-V shunts.
Not antigenic.
Experimental use in myocardial infarction, arterial thrombosis.
Both
 (i)  cause haemorrhage reversed by epsilon-aminocaproic acid
 (ii)  monitored with thrombin time (aim for 2-5 × control)
(iii)  are expensive.

## INHIBITORS OF FIBRINOLYSIS

Inhibitors of plasminogen activation and encourage clot
stabilisation.

## Uses

Menorrhagia especially associated with IUD.
Haemorrhage, e.g. prostatectomy, post-dental extraction, peptic ulcer.
Sub-arachnoid haemorrhage — prevention of re-bleeding in acute phase.
Reversal of action of fibrinolytic drugs.

## Drugs

Epsilon aminocaproic acid
— dose 3 g 4–6 times daily p.o.
Tranexamic acid
— dose 1 g 3–4 times daily p.o.
  or 1–2 g 3 times daily i.v. slowly.

## DEXTRANS

Glucose polymers impair platelet function and produce an altered fibrin which is susceptible to fibrinolysis.

Dextran 40 (avge MW 40 000) $T_{\frac{1}{2}}$ = 3 h. ⎫ 500–1000 ml infused
Dextran 70 (avge MW 70 000) $T_{\frac{1}{2}}$ = 24–48 h. ⎬ in 4–6 h during and
⎭ after surgery.

Used to prevent postoperative pulmonary embolism.

## Toxicity

Volume expansion (dextran 70); oliguria and renal failure (dextran 40); allergy; interference with cross matching.

## ANTIPLATELET DRUGS

Reduce platelet aggregation. May prevent thromboembolism in atheroma and prosthetic heart valves.

| Drug and dose | Action | Uses |
|---|---|---|
| Aspirin 300–600 mg daily | Prevents platelet prostaglandin generation; irreversible inhibition of prostaglandin synthetase. | Possible reduction in post MI mortality. Reduction in of stroke in men with transient ischaemic attacks (TIA). Reduces incidence of emboli with prosthetic valves (but risk of haemorrhage). Possible reduction in venous thrombosis after hip operations. |

| Sulphinpyrazone (Anturan) 200 mg 6-hourly | Reversible inhibition of prostaglandin synthetase. Metabolites more active than sulphinpyrazone. | Possible reduction in post MI mortality in first year. Probably ineffective in stroke prevention in TIA. |
|---|---|---|
| Dipyridamole (Persantin) 100 mg 6-hourly (or 100 mg daily with aspirin). | Inhibition of platelet phosphodiesterase, raises platelet AMP levels. | Used with anticoagulants in patients with prosthetic heart valves. |

## DISSEMINATED INTRAVASCULAR COAGULATION (DIC)

Many diseases can produce DIC.

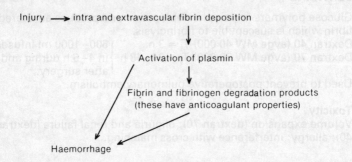

1. Correct primary condition if possible.
2. Treat shock, blood loss, pH disturbances, hypoxia.
3. Give i.v. heparin if thrombosis in limb, pulmonary embolus or peripheral gangrene.
4. If bleeding replace coagulation factors: e.g. platelets; fresh whole blood: fresh frozen plasma.
5. Inhibition of excessive fibrinolysis if lab tests show this with Epsilon — aminocaproic acid (Episcapron) or Aprotinin (Trasylol).
   Overall mortality is 50% — mainly due to underlying disease.

## HAEMOLYTIC URAEMIC SYNDROME

Usually a child under the age of 3 years, over a week after an upper respiratory or intestinal infection presents with anuria, anaemia and purpura. Untreated mortality is 30%. Treat with heparin plus peritoneal dialysis. Possible benefit with streptokinase and antiplatelet drugs.

## THROMBOTIC THROMBOCYTOPENIC PURPURA

Often follows an infection in adults but may be caused by contraceptive pill. Usually fatal if untreated. Syndrome is due to immune complex damage to the vessel wall plus a lack of a plasma inhibitor of platelet aggregation (which can be replaced by plasma transfusion).

Most effective treatment is exchange transfusion or plasmapheresis. Infusion of fresh frozen plasma may also be effective.

In the past some benefit has been observed by giving heparin with steroids, antiplatelet drugs (including dipyridamole) and by splenectomy.

## BLEEDING IN LIVER DISEASE DUE TO LACK OF CLOTTING FACTORS

The following are synthesized in the liver:
  fibrinogen (factor I)
  factors V, XI, XII, XIII
  factors II, VII, IX, X (vitamin K dependent)
  plasminogen
  fibrinolytic inhibitors
  coagulation inhibitors

### Obstructive jaundice
Coagulation defect corrected by parenteral vitamin K.

### Acute liver failure
Bleeding because of DIC plus lack of clotting factors.

### Chronic liver disease
Can result in DIC, thrombocytopenia, lack of fibrinogen and a readily lysed clot. If haemorrhage occurs or surgery is to be performed vitamin K is given parenterally plus fresh frozen plasma (up to 1 litre). Platelet infusions may be given in addition.

## HAEMOPHILIA

Haemophilia A — congenital bleeding disorder inherited as sex-linked recessive producing factor VIII activity deficiency in plasma.

Haemophilia B (Christmas disease) — similar inheritance and clinical features to haemophilia B but due to lack of factor IX.

Von Willebrand's disease — congenital bleeding disorder inherited as autosomal dominant. Patients have prolonged bleeding time, abnormal platelet function and reduced level of factor VIII activity.

Factor VIII: not stable at room temperature; in vivo $T_{\frac{1}{2}} = 6-8$ h.
Factor IX: not stable at room temperature; in vivo $T_{\frac{1}{2}} = 12-15$ h.

*The treatment of a bleeding episode* is intravenous replacement of clotting factors. For a haemarthrosis, infusion is for 4–6 h and clotting factor levels raised to 20–30% of normal. However visceral or intra-abdominal haemorrhage requires bed rest and clotting factors to be raised to 50%. For surgical operation infusions are continued until 10 days afterwards and during the procedure the deficient clotting factor is raised to normal levels. The concentrates used are:

*Cryoprecipitate* — stored frozen. Rapidly thawed at 37° in 200–300 ml batches and used immediately infusion over a 30 minute period.

*Factor VIII and IX concentrates* — stored in lyophilised form and diluted with water and then immediately injected (usually volumes of 50–100 ml).

Toxicity of concentrates

flushing, rash
bronchospasm, collapse (rare).

## IRON

Average Western diet contains 10–20 mg iron.

## ABSORPTION

Daily intestinal absorption 1 mg (males), 2 mg (females). Ferrous iron absorbed more readily than ferric iron. Enhancement of absorption by: low pH of intestinal contents; high protein diet; ascorbic acid; potentiated mucosal transport (as in iron deficiency and increased erythropoiesis).

## ADMINISTRATION

**Oral iron**
Iron deficiency — first exclude blood loss. Replace with: ferrous sulphate 400–600 mg orally daily (in divided doses) continuing for 2 months after Hb has risen to normal (i.e. 4 months in all).

Others: ferrous fumarate, gluconate and succinate absorbed as well as sulphate. Sustained-release preparations and those containing vitamin C are more expensive, have no greater bioavailability and are not more effective than simpler preparations.

*Toxicity*
GI upset (20–30%) — ferrous iron irritates mucosa causing nausea, discomfort and bowel disturbance, psychological factors may also be involved. Try changing preparation; reducing dose; giving with food (but may reduce absorption).

Hypersensitivity reactions, intestinal ulceration very rare.

**Parenteral iron**
Only justified if
  (i)  Genuine intolerance to oral iron
 (ii)  Failed oral iron therapy and causes below are excluded
(iii)  Poor compliance with oral therapy likely
N.B.  Bone marrow response to parenteral iron no faster than to oral iron.
i.v. route preferred as i.m. absorption erratic.

*Preparations available*
Iron dextran (Imferon; Imferon D) i.v. or i.m.
Iron sorbitol citric acid complex (Jectofer) only i.m.

   Both contain 50 mg/ml: total deficiency can be replaced by one i.v. injection to replace calculated deficit (see package insert for dose calculation). There is a greater risk of iron overload than with oral iron.

*Toxicity*
  (i)  Acute hypersensitivity (collapse, hypotension, respiratory arrest, urticaria)
 (ii)  Arthralgia and exacerbation of rheumatoid arthritis (? mechanism)
(iii)  Painful lymphadenopathy, fever, raised ESR and high serum and globulin concentration — probably immunological mechanism.

**Contraindications to iron**
Risk of iron overload and siderosis if iron given unnecessarily in:
haemolytic
hypoplastic    } anaemia
sideroblastic
renal failure
anaemia of chronic inflammation
thalassaemia

**Failed response to iron**
In patient with definite iron deficiency may be due to:
  (i)  compliance failure
 (ii)  combined $B_{12}$/folate deficiency
(iii)  continuing blood loss
(iv)  chronic infection
 (v)  malabsorption (usually clinically obvious)

## FOLIC ACID

= pteroylglutamic acid. Activated in the body to 5-methyltetrahydrolate, which acts as a 1C donor for several metabolic reactions including synthesis of purine and pyrimidine bases and interconversions of aminoacids. Folate deficiency results in megaloblastic anaemia.

### Pharmacokinetics

Daily requirement (100 $\mu$g) usually exceeded in normal diet (400 $\mu$g) absorbed in duodenum and jejunum, with no limitation on rate of transmucosal absorption. An enterohepatic circulation is present. Loose binding to plasma albumin. Body stores (10–15 mg) last for 4 months. Normal serum folate 3.0–15.0 $\mu$g/1.

### Administration

Care to exclude vitamin $B_{12}$ deficiency before starting. Oral folic acid 5 mg daily is initial treatment for folate deficiency and is continued for 4 months. Parenteral folic acid only needed for patients who cannot swallow.
Prophylactic folate given to:
pregnant women (4 mg daily)
babies under 1500 g (1 mg weekly)
patients on dialysis (5 mg daily)
chronic haemolytic anaemia (5 mg daily).

### Problems arising during treatment

Heart failure — diuretics.
Poor haematological response due to concomittant Fe deficiency — ferrous sulphate 400 mg–600 mg daily for 3–6 months.
Acute gout — treatment for acute then chronic gout.

## VITAMIN $B_{12}$

(= a group of cobalamins, including methyl cobalamin and deoxyadenosyl cobalamin. Hydroxycobalamin is used in treatment).
   Vitamin $B_{12}$ deficiency causes an arrest in folate metabolism by:
a. blocking demethylation of methyltetrahydrofolate,
b. failure of entry of folate into cells.

### Pharmacokinetics

Maximum daily absorption capacity (2 $\mu$g) is daily requirement. Absorption in ileum in presence of intrinsic factor. Bound in plasma to transcobalamin I. Enterohepatic circulation is present. Body stores (2–4 mg) last 3–4 yrs. Normal serum levels 160–925 $\mu$g/l.

## Administration
Initial treatment of megaloblastic anaemia due to vitamin B$_{12}$ deficiency:
1. 1000 $\mu$g hydroxycobalamin (Neo-Cytamen) i.m., two injections weekly for first 3 weeks. This replenishes stores.
2. Maintenance: 500–1000 $\mu$g i.m. every 3 months.
3. Prophylactic (after total gastrectomy) 1000 $\mu$g 3 monthly.

## Problems during treatment
Attempt to exclude gastric neoplasm
Iron deficiency
Hypothroidism
Cardiac failure
Gout
Vitamin B$_{12}$ allergy

## Response to treatment (Vitamin B$_{12}$ or folate)
Subjective improvement 24–48 h
Normoblastic marrow 48 h
Start of reticulocyte response 3 d
Peak of reticulocyte response 6 d
Hb normal 6 weeks

## ADVERSE HAEMATOLOGICAL RESPONSE TO DRUGS

### 1. Cytotoxic agents
— produce dose-dependent depression of all marrow elements (i.e. aplastic anaemia) e.g.:

6-mercaptopurine
azathioprine — toxicity potentiated by allopurinol
cyclophosphamide — possibly potentiated by allopurinol
methotrexate — recovery more rapid with folinic acid

### 2. Idiosyncratic agranulocytosis
phenylbutazone and oxyphenylbutazone
chloramphenicol
amidopyrines
sulphonamides and dapsone
phenothiazines
antithyroid drugs
captopril (particularly in patients with autoimmune disease on immuno-suppressants)

### 3. Idiosyncratic aplastic anaemia
phenylbutazone and oxyphenylbutazone
chloramphenicol
phenothiazines
phenytoin and troxidone
sodium aurothiomalate

*4. Idiosyncractic thrombocytopenia*
quinidine and quinine
phenylbutazone and oxyphenylbutazone
thiazides
heparin

*5. Anaemia*
dyshaemopoietic, e.g. folate deficiency due to methotrexate
haemolytic, e.g.  methyldopa
                 G6PD deficiency plus primaquine
haemorrhagic, e.g. NSAID
aplasia, e.g. chloramphenicol

## Management of aplastic anaemia
Transfusion to replace lacking components of blood.
Protect from and treat infection.
Attempt to promote marrow recovery.
1. Isolation, scrupulous cleaning of skin and mouth.
2. At presentation prevent infection from gut organisms with
   non-absorbable antibiotics.
3. Anabolic steroids,  e.g. oxymetholone (Anapolon) 2.5–5.0
                       mg/kg/day
                       or methandienone (Dianabol) 1 mg/kg/day.
   possible benefit in some patients after 2–3 months but
   cholestatic jaundice and hepatocellular carcinoma may occur.
4. Glucocorticoids may reduce bleeding due to thrombocytopenia
   if given in small doses (10 mg/day).
5. Neutrophil release (in moderate neutropenia): Li CO$_3$;
   etiocholanolone.
6. Bone marrow transplantation after irradiation followed by
   antilymphocyte globulin or cyclosporin. Especially < 30 years
   (older patients more prone to graft v host disease).

# Hormones and drugs acting on the endocrine system

## ANTERIOR PITUITARY HORMONES

Growth hormone (GH)
Prolactin
Gonadotrophins (FSH & LH)
Corticotrophin (ACTH)

## POSTERIOR PITUITARY HORMONES

Vasopressin
Oxytocin

## ANTERIOR PITUITARY

### Growth hormone (GH)

*Actions*
1. Potentiates protein synthesis.
2. Synergistic effect with insulin in increasing flow of amino acids into cells.
3. Stimulates somatomedin secretion by liver which mediates skeletal growth.

*Use of GH*
Only indication is growth failure in children due to GH lack.
However growth hormone releasing factor (GHRF) may become the treatment of choice for this.

### Prolactin
Hyperprolactinaemia
→ infertility, amenorrhoea, galactorrhoea in women.
→ hypogonadism, impotence, gynaecomastia in men.
Increased secretion: dopamine antagonists (neuroleptics; metoclopramine)
Decreased secretion: dopamine agonists (dopamine; bromocriptine)

261

**Bromocriptine (Parlodel)**
dopamine receptor agonist which reduces prolactin secretion.

*Uses*
1. Suppression of puerperal lactation: 2.5 mg initially followed by 2.5 mg twice daily for 2 weeks. Residual breast tenderness: given 2.5 mg daily for a further week.
2. Hyperprolactinaemia associated with infertility and hypergonadism: 2.5–7.5 mg twice daily for 2–6 months. Stop treatment (in females) if pregnancy occurs. Pituitary tumours may expand, thus measure visual fields.
3. Hyperprolactinaemic syndromes — e.g. galactorrhoea during drug therapy. (Exclude a pituitary tumour).
4. Acromegaly — probably suppresses GH, prolactin and somatomedin secretion. Give 5 mg 6-hourly.
5. Parkinsonism — up to 100 mg daily (in divided doses) may be required.

*Toxicity*
Constipation
Nausea, vomiting
Giddyness, hypotension and fainting
Cramps
Dystonia
Hallucinations

**Gonadotrophins**
FSH
— Controls development of primary ovarian follicle; stimulates granulosa cell proliferation; increases oestrogen secretion } females
— increases spermatogenesis     — males
LH
— Produces ovulation; stimulates thecal oestrogen secretion; initiates and maintains copus luteum } females

— stimulates androgen secretion from Leydig cells.   — males
Human menopausal urinary gonadotrophin (HMG, Pergonal) and human chorionic gonadotrophin (HCG) used for:
a. Primary or secondary amenorrhoea due to lack of gonadotrophins: HMG given for 8 days followed by a large dose of HCG on the 10th day.
b. Polycystic ovary syndrome: sequential treatment with HMG and HCG.
c. Diagnosis and treatment of secondary testicular failure.
d. Undescended testes: 1500 units of HCG thrice weekly for 6 weeks.

**Danazol (Danol)**
Inhibits gonadotrophin secretion. Used in:
a. Gynaecomastia in male; premature puberty in female
b. Endometriosis
c. Fibrocystic mastitis

**Corticosteroids**
Suppress hypothalamic and pituitary secretion. Used for this property in idiopathic hirsutes and in hirsutes in the polycystic ovary syndrome.


POSTERIOR PITUITARY

**Oxytocin and Vasopressin**
Synthesised in anterior hypothalamic nuclei and travel in nerve fibres to posterior lobe of pituitary.

**Oxytocin**
Octapeptide.
Produces contraction of uterus and mammary glands ducts.

*Kinetics*
Destroyed by trypsin.
Absorbed from buccal and nasal mucosae and from injection sites.
$T_{\frac{1}{2}} = 5 - 10$ mins (but action more prolonged).
Eliminated by tissue inactivation (small amount in urine)

*Uses*
1. Initiation of labour:
   Oxytocin injection (Syntocinon) 1 – 10 U/ml: i.v. or i.m. infusion 5 – 20 milli U/min.
   OR nasal spray (40 U/ml)      irregular absorption — less
   OR buccal tablets (200 U each)   effective or more effective
   (uterine rupture, fetal
   asphyxia) than injection.
2. Post partum haemorrhage: oxytocin or synthetic oxytocin (Syntocinon) 2 – 5 U i.m. or i.v. or Syntometrine (5 U synthetic oxytocin plus 0.5 mg ergometrine maleate/ml).

*Toxicity*
1. Excessive action (uterine rupture; fetal asphyxia)
2. Water retention and intoxication, hypertension with large doses.
3. Increased incidence of neonatal jaundice.

**Vasopressin (antidiuretic hormone; ADH)**
Similar octapeptide structure to oxytocin.

*Secretion*
Increased by:
raised plasma osmotic pressure
decreased blood volume
emotional and physical stress
morphine, nicotine

*Actions*
1. Increases water reabsorption by distal renal tubules and collecting ducts.
2. Vasoconstriction.

*Kinetics*
Similar to oxytocin — can be administered by injection or nasal insufflation.

*Uses*
In cranial diabetes insipidus:
1. Pig or beef vasopressin injections effective for 3–5 hours. Vasopressin snuff effective but allergenic causing rhinitis, bronchospasm and pulmonary fibrosis. Obsolescent.
2. Synthetic lysine vasopressin — Lypressin — nasal spray for mild diabetes insipidus but short lasting. No local or pulmonary complications: Plasma $T_{\frac{1}{2}}$ = 15 mins. Metered dose (each 5 U): 10 U 12-hourly or more frequently.
3. 1-desamino-8-D-arginine vasopressin — Desmopressin (DDAVP) — Synthetic long-acting analogue or vasopressin. $T_{\frac{1}{2}}$ = 75 mins. Administered i.v. (10–20 $\mu$g) or i.m. (1–2 $\mu$g) or intranasally once or twice daily. No local or pulmonary toxicity. At present drug of choice for diabetes insipidus.
4. In mild diabetes insipidus: chlorpropamide (increases renal sensitivity to vasopressin); carbamazepine (increases vasopressin secretion); demeclocycline also used.
5. Thiazide diuretics used in nephrogenic diabetes insipidus.

## ADRENAL CORTICOSTEROIDS

Secretions of adrenal cortex:
1. Glucocorticoids: cortisol and corticosterone
2. Mineralocorticoids: aldosterone and small amounts of desoxycorticosterone.
3. Small amounts of testosterone, androsterone, oestrogens, progesterone.

**Table 31:** Actions of cortisol and consequences of under- and over-secretion

| | Actions | Deficiency | Excess |
|---|---|---|---|
| Carbohydrate, protein & fat metabolism | Enhances gluconeogenesis; antagonises insulin hyperglycaemia ± diabetes mellitus; centripetal fat disposition; hypertriglyceridaemia; hypercholesterolaemia; decreased protein synthesis, e.g. diminished skin collagen. | Hypoglycaemia Loss of weight | Cushing's syndrome. Weight gain; increase in trunk fat; moon face; skin striae; bruising; trophy; wasting of limb muscles. |
| Water & salt metabolism | Inhibits fluid shift from extracellular into intra cellular compartment; antagonises vasopressin action on kidney; increases vasopressin destruction and decreases its production. Sodium and water retention, potassium loss. | Loss of weight Hypovolaemia Hyponatraemia | Oedema; thirst; polyuria. Hypertension. Muscular weakness. |
| Haematological | Lowers lymphocyte and eosinophil counts; increases RBC, platelets and clotting tendency. | | Florid complexion and polycythaemia |
| Alimentary | Increased production of gastric acid and pepsin. | Anorexia & nausea | Dyspepsia |
| CVS | Sensitises arterioles to catecholamines enhances production of angiotensinogen Fall in high density lipoprotein with increased total cholesterol. | Hypotension Fainting | Hypertension Atherosclerosis |

**Table 31** (continued)

| | Actions | Deficiency | Excess |
|---|---|---|---|
| Skeletal | Decreased production of cartilage and bone; osteoporosis; anti-vitamin D; increased renal loss of calcium; renal calculi formation. | | Backache due to osteoporosis Renal calculi Dwarfing in children (also anti-GH effect) |
| Nervous system | Altered neuronal excitability. Inhibition of uptake$_2$ of catecholamines. | | Depression and other psychiatric changes |
| Anti-inflammatory | Reduces formation of fluid and cellular exudate; reduces fibrous tissue repair. | | Increased spread of and proneness to infections |
| Immunological | Large doses lyse lymphocytes and plasma cells (transient release of immunoglobulin). | | Reduced lymphocyte mass Diminished immunoglobulin production |
| Feedback | Inhibits release of ACTH and MSH. | Pigmentation of skin and mucosa | |

**Table 32:** Relative activities of glucocorticoids and mineralocorticoids

| Drug | Compared with cortisol (w/w) Mineralocorticoid activity | Glucocorticoid & anti-inflammatory activity | Special features | Equivalent dose for anti-inflammatory effect (mg) |
|---|---|---|---|---|
| Cortisol (hydrocortisone) (Solu-Cortef, Efcortelan, Hydrocortone) | 1 | 1 | $T_{\frac{1}{2}}$ = 2 h (but biological effects $T_{\frac{1}{2}}$ = 12 h) | 80 |
| Cortisone | Inactive but converted to cortisol in liver | | | |
| Prednisolone (Deltastab, Deltacortyl) | × 0.8 | × 4 | $T_{\frac{1}{2}}$ = 2.5–3 h (but biological effects $T_{\frac{1}{2}}$ = 12 h). Mainly used for antiinflammatory actions | 20 |
| Prednisone | Inactive but converted to prednisolone in liver | | | |
| 6-α-methylprednisolone (Depo-Medrone, Solu-Medrone) | × 0.5 | × 5 | | 16 |
| Triamcinolone (9-α-fluoro-16-α-hydroxy prednisolone) (Adcortyl, Kenalog, Ledercort) | 0 | × 5 | Can produce flushes, sweating and muscular weakness. Arthritis on withdrawal. Plus glucocorticoid side-effects. Used for an anti-inflammatory. | 20 |
| Betamethasone (Betnelan, Betnesol) | 0 | × 25 | Used for anti-inflammatory actions. | 2 |
| Dexamethasone (Decadron, Dexacortisyl) | 0 | × 25 | Used for anti-inflammatory actions. | 2 |
| Fludrocortisol (9-α-fluoro-hydrocortisone) | × 125 | × 10 | Used for its mineralocorticoid activity in hypoadrenal states. | — |
| Aldosterone | × 1000 | 0 | Has to be injected. Not often used clinically. | |

**Uses of systemic steroids**

*Replacement*
Addison's disease and other forms of adrenal cortical insufficiency.
Hypopituitarism

*Anti-inflammatory*
Rheumatic disorders
Allergic reactions
Immunosuppression (e.g. organ transplantation, collagen diseases)
Specific clinical problems (e.g. status asthmaticus, eczema, shock)

*Suppression of ACTH*
Congenital adrenal hyperplasia.

**Chronic hypoadrenalism**
1. Oral cortisol — 20 mg morning+ 10 mg evening (prednisolone is an alternative)
2. More severely affected: add fludrocortisone 0.05–0.2 mg/day.
3. Intercurrent illness
   — mild: double cortisol dose
   moderate: i.m. or i.v. cortisol 100 mg 6-hourly
4. Surgery: i.m. or i.v. cortisol 100 mg 6-hourly, from 2 hours before operation till oral feeding resumed.

**Acute hypoadrenalism**
1. i.v. water + NaCl + glucose (enough to maintain fluid and salt balance and blood glucose)
2. i.v. cortisol (hydrocortisone hemisuccinate) 100 mg 6-hourly or more frequently (enough to maintain BP)
3. When electrolyte balance restored and vomiting stopped, give oral cortisol 20 mg 6-hourly initially then reduce.
   Mineralocorticoid may have to be introduced with lower doses of cortisol.

**Some important examples of anti-inflammatory uses of glucocorticoids**
temporal arteritis (giant cell arteritis) & polymyalgia rheumatica
myasthenia gravis (esp. failed thymectomy; patients unsuitable for thymectomy)
dermatomyositis & polymyositis
infantile salaam attacks with hypsarrhythmia
reduction of oedema around tumours (esp. mediastinum; intracranial)

severe bronchial asthma and bronchitis
pulmonary sarcoidosis
pulmonary alveolitis (allergic and fibrosing)
minimal change nephrotic syndrome
SLE
prevention of neonatal respiratory distress syndrome
septic shock
chronic active hepatitis
ulcerative colitis
Crohn's disease

## TESTIS

Main hormone is testosterone, secreted by interstitial (Leydig) cells.

**Actions of testosterone**
development of secondary male characteristics
anabolic effects (e.g. nitrogen retention, bone growth and
  maturation, muscle development)
temporal recession of hairline
sebum secretion
spermatogenesis and seminal fluid formation
psychological effects (e.g. libido, aggression)

**FSH**
Promotes spermatogenesis

**LH**
Stimulates testosterone production

**Testosterone kinetics:**
1. Absorbed orally but considerable first-pass metabolism
2. Satisfactory absorption sublingually and from injection
3. Esters are less polar and have a more prolonged effect than
   testosterone itself
4. Chief metabolites: androsterone, etiocholanolone

## Androgens used in therapeutics

| Androgen | Proprietary name | Administration |
|---|---|---|
| Testosterone propionate in waxy base | Testoral | 10–30 mg/day sublingually in divided doses |
| Testosterone propionate | Virormone | 100 mg i.m. 3 times/week |
| Testosterone oenanthate in oil | Primotestone Depot | 250 mg i.m. every 2–4 weeks |
| Testosterone esters in oil (propionate 30 mg; phenylpropionate 60 mg; isocaproate 60 mg; decanoate 100 mg) | Sustanon 250 | 250 mg 1 or 2 times monthly |
| Fluoxymesterone | Ultandren | 5–15 mg/day orally in divided doses |

## Less virilising preparations (anabolic steroids)

| Androgen | Proprietary name | Administration |
|---|---|---|
| Nandrolone phenylpropionate BP inj. | Durabolin | 25–50 mg weekly by i.m. injection |
| Nandrolone decanoate | Deca-Durabolin | 25–50 mg i.m. every 3 weeks |
| Methandienone | Dianabol | 5–10 mg daily orally for men 2.5 mg daily for women |

Use as tonics or for body-building unjustified.

*Uses*
1. Replacement therapy for primary or secondary hypogonadism (4.6 × 100 mg subcutaneous implants last up to 6 months).
2. Delayed puberty due to gonadal deficiency (125 mg i.m. testosterone esters in oil 2–3 weekly).
3. Anabolic effects used in renal failure, burns, injuries, osteoporosis (not obviously beneficial).
4. Hypoplastic anaemia and anaemia due to neoplasia and uraemia (not very effective in most cases).
5. 25–30% oestrogen-dependent metastases of breast cancer in premenopausal patients regress with androgen (? action via peripheral conversion to oestrogen).
6. Relief from itch in jaundice (not methyl-testosterone).

*Toxicity*
1. Virilisation in women, acne, facial hair, clitoral hypertrophy, baldness and deep voice.
2. Increased libido in men. Also aggressive behaviour, priapism.
3. Premature fusion of epiphyses.
4. Cholestatic jaundice from methyltestosterone.
5. Impotence and azoospermia (on prolonged use).
6. Hypercalcaemia (when used in malignant disease).
7. Salt and water retention (unusual).

**Cyproterone (Androcur)**
An anti-androgen with progestogenic properties. Used to suppress sexual activity in men with unacceptable sexual behaviour.

*Daily dose*
100–200 mg oral

*Toxicity*
reversible inhibition of spermatogenesis
gynaecomastia
drowsiness

## OESTROGENS

**Oral**
Ethinyloestradiol (Lynoral)
Oestradiol valerate (Progynova)
Stilboestrol
Quinestrol
Piperazine oestrone sulphate (Harmogen)
Dienoestrol
Oestriol
Oestrone

**Topical**
Dienoestrol (Hormofemin)
Premarin (oestrone, equilin and $17\alpha$-dihydroequilin)

**Also**
Conjugated oestrogens (equine) are used.

**Uses**
1. In combined contraceptive pill.
2. Replacement in hypofunctioning ovary (e.g. menopause).
3. Carcinoma of prostate (and some breast carcinomas).
4. Suppression of lactation (actually just reduce congestion, no primary effect on lactation).
5. Functional uterine haemorrhage.

**Specific indications in climacteric**
vasomotor instability
lower genital tract atrophy
prevention of osteoporosis (only during therapy)
— esp. with strong family history.

**Toxicity**
nausea
breast tenderness
vaginal discharge
leg cramps
weight gain
raised blood pressure
endometrial hyperplasia & carcinoma (incidence reduced by adding
progestogens to regime)
thromboembolism

**Contraindications to oestrogen treatment**
Absolute contraindications — breast carcinoma
                                              — endometrial hyperplasia or
                                                  carcinoma
myocardial infarction
stroke or other thromboembolic disease
porphyria
hyperlipoproteinaemia
pregnancy
obesity
heavy smoker
hypertension
active liver disease
breast dysplasia

## PROGESTOGENS

Act principally on reproductive organs.
   Unlike oestrogens and androgens, have few systemic effects but
synthetic progestogens variably metabolised to oestrogens and
androgens.
   Act mainly on tissues sensitised by oestrogens but effects
inhibited by oestrogens.

**Naturally occurring**:
Progesterone — 5–10 mg daily i.m. — Gestone
Cyclogest — 200–400 mg rectally or vaginally

**Testosterone-derived progestogens**
Noresthisterone — 10–20 mg p.o. daily
(Primolut N)

**Uses**
1. Contraception.
2. Climacteric symptoms — often combined with oestrogens e.g. Mixogen, Cyclo-Progynova.
3. Dysmenorrhoea — given on days 20–25 of cycle (oral contraceptives to suppress ovulation are effective).
4. Endometriosis — prolonged doses of progestogens or oral contraceptives with high progestogen content.
5. Functional uterine haemorrhage — induce regular bleeding with oral contraceptives or give progestogen on 20–25 days of cycle.
6. Threatened abortion — relatively ineffective, may cause virilisation of fetus.

## ORAL CONTRACEPTIVES

Despite their important social consequences and convenience these are potent drugs and because they are used in well women safety must be paramount.

**Three main types**
a. *Combination*:  one oestrogen/progestogen tablet daily for 21 days starting on day 7 of menstrual cycle, repeated after 7 pill-free days. Maximum oestrogen dose now 50 $\mu$g/day.
b. *Triphasic formulations* which more closely mimic endogenous cyclic hormonal activity, e.g. Logynon, Trinordiol. Beginning on first day of period daily regime is:

| Days | Content of each pill ($\mu$g) | |
| --- | --- | --- |
| | Ethinyloestradiol | Levonorgestrel |
| 1–6 | 30 | 50 |
| 7–11 | 40 | 75 |
| 12–21 | 30 | 125 |
| 22–28 | No pill taken | |

Efficacy and use of this formulation not established.
c. *Progestogen only* — continuous administration of progestogen one tablet daily starting on day 1 of period.

**Pharmacology**
a. Oestrogen-progestogen combined pill acts at several levels:
  (i) oestrogen inhibits FSH release and progestogen inhibits midcycle LH surge required for ovulation.
  (ii) ovarian steroidogenesis (especially progestogen) inhibited
  (iii) endometrial changes make implantation less likely
  (iv) cervical mucus remains thick and impermeable to sperm at ovulation.
  (v) ? interferes with coordinated contractions of cervix and fallopian tubes important for sperm transport.

Abrupt withdrawal of progestogen at the end of each dose interval (21 days) results in withdrawal uterine bleeding like a period.
b.  Progestogen only pill — main actions on cervical mucus and endometrium to prevent fertilisation and implantation. Inhibits ovulation (in 40% women). Success rate lower than combined pill.
Menstruation occurs despite continuous progestogen administration but bleeding less predictable and duration variable.

## Other important pharmacological effects
1. Enhanced blood clotting due to:
    (i)  increased platelet aggregation
    (ii)  decreased antithrombin III
    (iii)  increased clotting factors
    (iv)  decreased plasminogen activator in vessel walls.
2. Hypertension (? due to increased renin substrate synthesis) — usually resolved 6 months after discontinuation.
3. Decreased glucose tolerance.
4. Cholestatic jaundice (especially if history of pregnancy jaundice).
5. Secondary amenorrhoea and infertility after stopping pill.

## Pharmacokinetics
Natural oestrogens and progestogens undergo extensive first-pass metabolism and are ineffective orally so synthetic oestrogens (ethinyloestradiol or its methoxy analogue mestranol used) and progestogens (19-nortestosterone derivatives — levonorgestrel, norethisterone and ethynodiol) used. 19-nortestosterone derivatives can have some androgenic action and also metabolised to oestrogens (may account for anti-ovulatory effect in some women).
Undergo hepatic metabolism and enterohepatic recirculation — broad spectrum antibiotics inhibit gut flora which release hormone from glucuronide for reabsorption.

## Drug interactions
Contraceptive failure possible if inducing agents given, e.g. phenytoin, carbamazepine, phenobarbitone, rifampicin, or gut flora altered by antibiotic, e.g. ampicillin.

## Absolute contraindications
1. Thrombophlebitis, thromboembolic disorders, CVS disease, coronary artery disease (and past history of these).
2. Significantly impaired liver function.
3. Known or suspected breast cancer.
4. Known or suspected oestrogen-dependent neoplasm.
5. Undiagnosed cause of vaginal bleeding.
6. Known or suspected pregnancy.

## Increased risk of CVS disease if pill used in patients with
1. Hyperlipidaemia (especially type IIa)
2. Diabetes mellitus
3. Hypertension; previous hypertension of pregnancy
4. Obesity
5. Tobacco smoking
6. Progressive rise in risk over age 30 — especially with high oestrogen use for prolonged period.
7. Family history of MI, cerebrovascular disease or pulmonary embolism before age of 50.

N.B.: Risk may persist after stopping Pill (? how long).

## Increased risk of thrombophlebitis
1. Varicose veins
2. Obesity

## Diseases which may worsen or improve on pill
1. Fibrocystic breast disease
2. Asthma
3. Epilepsy
4. Migraine; other headaches
5. Depression
6. Leiomyoma of uterus
7. Ulcerative colitis

N.B. Most serious toxicity of pill related to oestrogen dose — apart from hypertension, diabetes and depression. Hypertension related to total hormone dose.

## Other contraindications to pill
Cholelithiasis (increased frequency of gall stones on pill)
Multiple sclerosis
Porphyria (precipitates acute attack)

## Initial choice of pill

| Clinical background | Type of pill indicated and other considerations | Examples |
|---|---|---|
| Regular, light periods 2–4 days flow. No dysmenorrhoea. | Low progestogen | Brevinor |
| Regular, moderate periods 4–6 days flow. Moderate dysmenorrhoea | Intermediate progestogen | Loestrin 20 Orlest 21 Norinyl |
| Regular, heavy periods, 6+ days flow. Severe dysmenorrhoea. | High progestogen | Norlestrin |

| | | |
|---|---|---|
| Irregular, heavy and infrequent periods. Acne, oily skin hirsutes. Possible polycystic ovarian syndrome hirsutes. | Pill: low androgen and 50 $\mu$g oestrogen. | Norinyl |
| Irregular, scanty periods. No androgenic features | Oral contraceptives not recommended. Possible hypothalamic insufficiency X-ray skull if galactorrhoea | |
| Patient over 35 years | Low oestrogen or progestogen only | Low oestogen: Loestrin 20 No oestrogen: Neogest |
| Weight over 75 kg | High progestogen | Norlestrin |
| History of toxaemia; family history of hypertension; tiredness, varicose veins, weight gain during pregnancy; excessive premenstrual oedema. | Measure BP 3-monthly Low progestogen pill (toxaemia and hypertension also indicates low oestrogen pill). | Brevinor |
| Excessive nausea, oedema in pregnancy. Hypertrophy of cervix or uterus. Uterine leiomyomas. Fibrocystic disease of breasts. | Low oestrogen | Loestrin 20 |
| Surgery within 4 weeks | No pill or progestogen-only pill | Neogest |
| Lactation | No oral contraceptives until weaning | |

## Toxicity of pill

| A. *Symptoms and signs* | *Pill must be stopped because possible cause is:* |
|---|---|
| Blindness, proptosis, diplopia, papilloedema | Retinal artery thrombosis |
| Unilateral or central chest pain or tingling. Pains or weakness in arms. Haemoptysis. Dyspnoea | Myocardial infarction; pulmonary embolism |

| Leg pains, tenderness or swelling | Thrombophlebitis |
| Slurring of speech | Stroke |
| Hepatic mass or tenderness | Liver neoplasm |
| B. | *Pill may be continued only if the following are excluded:* |
| Amenorrhoea | Pregnancy |
| Breakthrough bleeding | Genital cancer |
| Breast lumps, pain, swelling | Breast carcinoma |
| Right upper abdominal pain | Cholecystitis, cholelithiasis, liver cancer |
| Mid epigastric pain | Abdominal artery or vein thrombosis, pulmonary embolism, myocardial infarction |
| Migraine | Vascular spasm preceding a cerebral thrombosis |
| Non-migraine headache | Hypertension |
| Jaundice; itching | Cholestatic jaundice |
| Increase in uterine size | Uterine tumour; adenomyosis; pregnancy |

*C. Toxicity due to oestrogen excess:*
*Increased serum proteins* (including clotting factors, steroid and thyroid binding proteins, renin substrate, caeruloplasmin)
*Hypertriglyceridaemia*
*Vascular*: thromboembolic disease, migraine, myocardial infarction, stroke (increased 6–8 times)
*Skin*: cloasma, telangiectasia, capillary fragility.
*Gynaecological*: vaginal mucous discharge, uterine enlargement and leiomyomas, excessive uterine blood loss.
*Breasts*: cystic breast hypertrophy.

*D. Toxicity due to progestogen excess:*
*CNS*: tiredness, depression, decreased libido, increased appetite and weight gain.
*CVS*: dilated leg veins; decreased high density lipoprotein cholesterol (therefore possible increase in atheroma)
*Skin*: oily skin and scalp, acne, neurodermatitis.
*Gynaecological*: pelvic convestion, cervicitis, moniliasis, scanty periods.
*Breasts*: tenderness, increased alveolar mass.
*Liver*: jaundice

*C plus D*
Hypertension

### F.  Fluid retention effects
Due to oestrogen excess if occur on pill days and progestogen excess if occur on pill-free days: nausea and vomiting; dizziness and syncope; oedema; leg cramps; irritability; bloating cyclic weight gain; headaches or visual disturbances.

### F.  Relative oestrogen deficiency
Breakthrough bleeding days 1–7
Continuous breakthrough bleeding
Scanty or absent menstruation
Nervousness
Vasomotor symptoms
Dysparunia due to dry vagina

### G.  Relative progestogen deficiency
Breakthrough bleeding days 8–21
Heavy menstruation and/or delayed menstruation
Dysmenorrhoea
Weight loss

## Mortality

*Mortality per 100 000 women aged 35–49*
Oral contraceptive users — 3.9
Non pill users — 0.5
Risk of dying during pregnancy — 58
Risk of dying due to thromboembolism during pregnancy — 2.3
Mortality in pill users mainly consequences of thromboembolism
(blood group O pill users have $\frac{1}{3}$ this risk.)

## Morbidity versus Efficacy

| Method of contraception | Excess of admissions to hospital (per 100 women years) | | Pregnancies (per 100 women years) |
|---|---|---|---|
| Pill | Stroke | 0.035 | 0.36 |
| | Thromboembolic disease | 0.07 | |
| | MI | 0.01 | |
| IUD | Uterine perforation | 0.05 | 2.0 |
| | Pelvic inflammatory disease | 0.2 | |
| Occlusive devices | NIL | | 5.0 |

**Table 33: Stimulation of ovulation**

| Drug | Action | Use |
|------|--------|-----|
| Clomiphene (Clomid) | A mixed oestrogen/anti-oestrogen which blocks oestrogen receptors in hypothalamus and thus causes release of FSH and LH, which in turn stimulates ovulation and formation of corpus luteum | Main indication is infertile female, esp. with secondary amenorrhoea. Start drug on 2nd–3rd day after spontaneous or induced menstruation. Give 50 mg/day for 5 days for 5 cycles. |
| Human chorionic gonadotrophin (HCG) | Additional gonadotrophin (when LH is lacking) | Infertility when higher doses of clomiphene have not produced ovulation. HCG 5000 IU i.m. given 7 days after the last clomiphene tablet. *Toxicity*: flushing, abdominal distension or pain. Rarely nausea, breast discomfort, visual changes. |
| Gonadotrophins — human menopausal urine (HMG) and HCG | Stimulate ovulation and corpus luteum formation | Indications: infertility associated with (a) primary or secondary amenorrhoea with low gonadotrophins; (b) anovulation, menstrual abnormalities and normal gonadotrophins. *Administration*: variable dose according to oestradiol levels *or* fixed dose of HMG given on days 1, 3 & 5 followed by HCG 3 days later if oestradiol response satisfactory. *Toxicity*: multiple pregnancy, raised abortion rate, ovarian enlargement. |
| Bromocriptine (Parlodel) | Dopamine agonist. Dopamine inhibits prolactin secretion. Thus bromocriptine will correct hyperprolactinaemia. | Infertility associated with hyperprolactinaemia (when thyroid and pituitary diseases have been excluded). *Dose*: 7.6–30 mg daily usually restores ovulatory cycles. Drug is stopped as soon as pregnancy occurs. |

## Some contraceptive pills available in the UK

| Oestrogen | Progestogen | Proprietary name |
|---|---|---|
| a. *Combined pills* | | |
| Ethinyloestradiol 20 $\mu$g | Norethisterone 1 mg | Loestrin 20 |
| Ethinyloestradiol 30 $\mu$g | Levonorgestrel 250 $\mu$g | Eugynon 30 |
| Ethinyloestradiol 35 $\mu$g | Norethisterone 500 $\mu$g | Brevinor |
| Ethinyloestradiol 50 $\mu$g | Norethisterone 1 mg | Orlest 21 |
| Mestranol 50 $\mu$g | Norethisterone 1 mg | Norinyl-1 |
| b. *Progestogen only pills* | | |
| — | Norgestrel 75 $\mu$g | Neogest |
| — | Norethisterone 350 $\mu$g | Noriday |

# INSULIN

INSULIN

Proinsulin synthesized in $\beta$-cells of islets; C-peptide cleaved off in storage granules to form insulin. At secretion equivalent amounts of insulin and C-peptide released into blood.

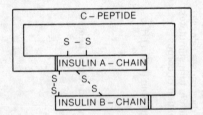

Blood insulin and C-peptide high when glucose is given. Endogenous insulin and C-peptide low when insulin is administered.

*Diabetic state* (diabetus mellitus; DM) is a sustained and abnormal elevation of blood glucose concentration which is due to a relative or absolute deficiency of insulin action

Most insulin used in treatment is beef or pig. Antigenicity mainly due to C-peptide and other non insulin peptides. Thus antigenicity is low in highly purified (monocomponent) insulins in which these have been removed.

## Actions of insulin

1. Increased glucose uptake by muscle and fat.
2. Inhibition of gluconeogenesis.
3. Conversion of glucose to glycogen and fatty acids promoted.
4. Conversion of fatty acids to triglycerides promoted and reverse reactions inhibited.
5. Conversion of aminoacids to proteins promoted and reverse reactions inhibited.

## Pharmacokinetics

Insulin polypeptide destroyed by gut enzymes and so given parenterally. $T_\frac{1}{2}$ is 6– 10 mins but various pharmaceutical processes can produce products with different absorption characteristics and therefore different durations of action.

HUMAN INSULIN

Recently available from two sources:
a. Semi-synthetic — chemical substitution of the alanine at B30 of porcine insulin by threonine
   — Human Actrapid
   — Human Monotard
b. Total synthesis of A and B chains separately by recombinant DNA techniques using *E. coli* which are then combined into biosynthetic human insulin.
   — Humulin S (like soluble insulin)
   — Humulin I (like isophane insulin)
   Effects similar to animal insulins but action may be faster and should not be allergenic. In future may replace animal insulins.

## Indications for insulin

1. DM with ketosis or polyuria and weight loss. Usually but not always present under 30.
2. DM not adequately controlled with diet and oral agent.
3. Hyperglycaemic ketoacidosis.
4. Critical episodes in DM, e.g. operations, infections, ischaemia, trauma and pregnancy.

## Clinical use

1. Take care with different strengths: 20, 40, 80, 320 IU/ml. Soon 100 IU/ml will replace all of these.
2. New patients started on highly purified MC insulins.
3. Most satisfactory regime is multiple dosing (single dosing with long acting insulins in elderly, visually disabled and those needing < 30 IU/day).
   a. Start with 2 injections of soluble insulin before breakfast and supper.

**Table 34:** Insulin preparations

| Type of insulin | Proprietary preparation | Type of insulin | Onset of activity (h) | Peak activity (h) | Duration of activity (h) |
|---|---|---|---|---|---|
| *1. Rapidly acting, short duration* | | | | | |
| Insulin BP (Soluble insulin) | Soluble | Solution. Beef | 1 | 3–5 | 6–8 |
| Neutral insulin BP | Hypurin Neutral | Highly purified.  Beef | ½ | 2–6 | 6–8 |
| | Actapid MC | Monocomponent.  Pork | 1 | 3–5 | 7 |
| | Velosulin (Leo Neutral) | Highly purified.  Pork | 1 | 1½–3½ | 7–8 |
| | Nuso (neutral soluble) | Solution.  Beef | 1 | 3–5 | 6–8 |
| *2. Intermediate duration of action* | | | | | |
| Isophane insulin BP (Isophane protamine insulin) | Insulatard (Leo Retard) | Highly purified crystalline suspension.  Pork | 2 | 4–12 | 24 |
| | Isophane NPH | Crystalline suspension.  Beef | 2½ | 5–14 | 18–27 |
| Insulin zinc suspension (amorphous) BP | Semitard MC | Monocomponent amorphous suspension.  Pork | 1½ | 4–10 | 16 |
| | Semilente | Amorphous suspension.  Beef | 1 | 4–8 | 12–16 |
| Globin zinc insulin BP | Globin | Crystalline suspension.  Pork | 2 | 6–12 | 18–24 |
| *3. Long duration of action* | | | | | |
| Insulin zinc suspension (crystalline) BP | Ultratard MC | Monocomponent crystalline suspension.  Beef | 4 | 10–30 | 35 |
| | Ultralente | Crystalline suspension | 4–8 | 10–30 | 30–35 |

| | | | | | |
|---|---|---|---|---|---|
| Protamine zinc insulin BP | Hypurin protamine zinc | Highly purified suspension. Beef. Contains excess protamine and zinc. | 4-6 | 10-20 | 24-35 |
| | Protamine Zinc Insulin (PZI) | Amorphous suspension. Beef. Contains an excess of protamine and zinc. | 4-8 | 10-20 | 24-34 |
| **4. Mixed preparations** Biphasic insulin BP | Rapitard MC | Monocomponent. Mixed beef and pork. Suspension of 25% Actrapid MC and 75% crystalline. | 1½ | 4-12 | 22 |
| | Mixtard 30/70 (Leo Mixtard) | Highly purified. Pork. 30% Velosulin and 70% of Insulatard. | ½ | 2-8 | 24 |
| | Monotard MC | Monocomponentms Pork Suspension of 30% amorphous and 70% crystalline | 3 | 6½-14 | 22 |
| Insulin zinc suspension BP (insulin zinc suspension (mixed)) | Lentard MC | Monocomponent. Mixed beef and pork. Suspension of 30% amorphous and 70% crystalline. | 3 | 6½-14 | 24 |
| | Lente | Beef suspension of 30% amorphous and 70% crystalline. | 2½ | 6-14 | 22-29 |

    b. If saw-tooth pattern of glycaemia then replace part or whole of one or both doses with intermediate acting insulin.

    c. If further smoothing needed, then a long acting insulin given before supper plus 2 or more injections of short acting insulin during the day.

    d. During childbirth, crises and in brittle diabetes closed or open loop systems (artificial pancreas) may be used.

4. Reduce insulin dose if unusual activity undertaken or if food consumption is reduced.

**Toxicity of insulin**

1. Hypoglycaemia
2. Post-hypoglycaemic hyperglycaemia (Somogyi effect)
3. Local and systemic allergy
4. Insulin resistance due to insulin antibodies (uncommon)
5. Acquired increased susceptibility to insulin
6. Lipodystrophy (becoming less common with use of purified insulins)

**Comas in diabetics**

| Type | Management |
| --- | --- |
| Hyperglycaemic with ketoacidosis | See Table 35 |
| Hyperglycaemic without ketosis | See Table 35 |
| Hypoglycaemic | *Prevent*: Care with different insulin strengths; patient takes meal or glucose tablets when early symptoms appear. 20 ml of 10% glucose i.v. usually successful *or* 1 mg of glucagon i.m. I.V. injection of 50% glucose not usually required. |
| Lactic acidosis | i.v. fluids containing bicarbonate. Dialyse. |
| Renal failure | Renal failure regime including dialysis, treatment of encephalopathy, correction of electrolyte disturbances. |

**Diet in diabetes**

1. Patient education — including spacing of meals, relationship of food and hypoglycaemic agents, lipids and atheroma, recognition of hyper and hypoglycaemia.
2. Initial dietary trial for 4 weeks in order to assess whether symptoms, 2 h post prandial hyperglycaemia (< 13–14 mmol/l) and ketonuria can be readily controlled by diet alone.
3. If patient is obese restrict calories and increase exercise to attain ideal weight. Fat must be restricted more than carbohydrate. Calorie needs:
   inactive — ideal body weight (lbs) × 10
   sedentary — ideal body weight (lbs) × 15
   active — ideal body weight (lbs) × 20
   growing child — ideal body weight (lbs) × 20
4. Distribute calories during day to match insulin effects e.g.: 2/7 at each of 3 meals plus 1/7 at bedtime.
5. Reduce proportion of fat to 20% of calories; increase carbohydrate to 60% of calories.
6. Fat should have a reduced proportion from animal sources and more from fish and vegetable sources (i.e. lowered amount of saturated lipids and cholesterol). Measure plasma lipids before and after initial 4 weeks.
7. Carbohydrates should be complex starches (as in bread, rice, potato, pasta and other cereal products). Rapidly absorbed simple sugars and oligosaccharides are reserved for hypoglycaemic episodes only and have no place in the usual diet.
8. Some fibres (non-absorbable carbohydrates) such as guar gum, pectins and those in pulses (peas and beans) reduce insulin requirements when mixed with other foods — probably by slowing and lowering glucose absorption curve. A high fibre diet should be encouraged, but fibre in the form of leguminous seeds (e.g. soya beans) not as cereals is beneficial in diabetic control.

## ORAL HYPOGLYCAEMIC AGENTS

Oral agents are used — particularly in adult onset diabetes without ketosis — when an initial 4 week trial on diet alone has failed to control symptoms and hyperglycaemia.

### A. Sulphonylureas

1. Stimulate insulin release from pancreatic β-cells. Also hepatic and peripheral hypoglycaemic actions. Possibly increase insulin receptor density. Functioning pancreatic tissue necessary for action.
2. Increase appetite.

**Table 35:** Management of hyperglycaemic coma (Guy's Hospital — from H Keen & J Jarrett)

1. History and examination — previous severity and treatment of diabetes and complications. Look for infection infarction, trauma. Monitor ECG, temperature, pulse, respiration, blood pressure hourly.
2. Set up IV line and CVP line; take blood initially for glucose, electrolytes, arterial pH, $PO_2$ $PCO_2$, FBP and culture. Repeat blood glucose hourly. $Na^+$ and $K^+$ hourly for 2 hours then 4 hourly.
3. Nasogastric tube and aspirate stomach contents.
4. Catheterise bladder — test urine hourly: volume output, glucose, ketones.
5. Give the following:

| Time (hrs) | Fluid (saline) | Potassium | Insulin | | Bicarbonate | |
|---|---|---|---|---|---|---|
| | | | i.m. or Continuous i.v. infusion (by pump or i.v. drip) | | Only give if considerable acidosis: | |
| | | | I.M. | I.V. | Arterial pH | I.V. |
| 0–1 | 1 l in first 30 mins then 0.5 l in second 30 mins. | 13 mmol/h initially | 5 U | 5 U/h | < 7 | 100 mmol $HCO_3$ with 26 mmol $K^+$ |
| 1–2 | 1 l/h | Change rate of administration of K according to plasma K: | 5 U | 5 U/h | 7.0–7.1 | 50 mmol $HCO_3$ with 13 mmol $K^+$ |
| 2–3 | 0.5 l/h | | | | | |

Fluid (saline) note: (NaCl 154 mM; but change to 5% glucose when blood glucose < 14 mmol/l; if blood $Na^+$ > 155 mmol/l then give NaCl 77 mM)

Bicarbonate note: ∴ give over 30–40 mins.

0.5 l/h
0.25 l/h
0.25 l/h

3–4
4–5
5–6

| Plasma K (mmol/l) | ∴ Give K (mmol/h) |
|---|---|
| > 6 | 0 |
| 6–4.5 | 13 |
| 4.5–3 | 26 |
| < 3 | 39 |

If no fall in blood glucose then switch to i.v. regime.

When blood glucose < 14 mmol/l switch to 4-hourly s.c. injections according to urine glucose:

| Urine glucose | |
|---|---|
| 2% | |
| 1% | |
| < 1% | |

If no fall in blood glucose then double rate.

∴ give insulin s.c. 4-hourly
32 U
16 U
8 U

Measure pH 30 mins after and repeat schedule until pH < 7.1.

**Table 36:** Oral hypoglycaemic agents — A. sulphonylureas

| Drug | Metabolism & Elimination | $T_\frac{1}{2}$ (h) | Dose | Duration of action (h) | Special features |
|---|---|---|---|---|---|
| Tolbutamide (Rastinon) | Oxidised in liver, excreted in urine | 4–5 | 0.5–3 g in divided doses | 6–12 | Action prolonged by phenylbutazone sulphaphenazole and coumarins. Alcohol enhances action and may produce mild disulfiram type reaction. Less active in chronic alcoholics. |
| Chlorpropamide (Diabinese) | Little metabolised, mainly excreted unchanged in urine | 36 | 0.1–0.5 g single daily dose | 60 | Responsible for half cases of sulphonylurea hypoglycaemia. Aspirin inhibits excretion of chlorpropamide. Antidiuretic and can cause hyponatraemia and water intoxication. Some individuals develop severe disulfiram effect with alcohol; reaction inherited as dominant; ?retinopathy more severe in non reactors. |
| Acetoheximide (Dimelor) | 60% activated in liver to hydroxyhexamide which is secreted by renal tubules | 6–8 | 0.25–1.5 g as one or two doses daily | 12–24 | |

| Drug | Pharmacokinetics | | Dose | Duration of action | Special features |
|---|---|---|---|---|---|
| Glibenclamide (Daonil; Euglucon) | 95% metabolised to inactive hydroxylated derivatives Excreted in bile and urine | 1.5–2.5 | 2.5–20 mg as one or two daily doses | 12 | Mildly diuretic |
| Glibornuride (Glutril) | 95% metabolised to inactive products | 5–12 | 12.5–75 mg one or two daily doses | 16 | |
| Glipizide (Glibenese) | 85% metabolised to inactive hydroxyl derivative | 2.5–4 | 2.5–30 mg; doses below 10 mg given as single daily dose | 6–10 | |
| Gliquidone (Glurenorm) | 95% metabolised 95% excreted in bile | 2.5–4 1.5 (α-phase) | 45–180 mg in doses before meals | 2–4 | Activity depends on α-phase Useful in renal failure |

**Table 37**: Oral hypoglycaemic agents — B. biguanides

| Drug | Pharmacokinetics | Dose | Duration of action | Special features |
|---|---|---|---|---|
| Phenformin (Dibotin) | 50% absorbed from gut. 1/3 of absorbed drug metabolised. 2/3 excreted unchanged in urine. $T_\frac{1}{2}$ = 3–5 h. | 50–200 mg in single dose or divided doses | 6–8 h | Phenformin more often responsible for lactic acidosis than metformin. Now rarely used as lactic acidosis has high mortality. |
| Metformin (Glucophage) | All excreted unchanged in urine | 0.5–3 g in single dose or divided doses | 8–12 h | Drug of choice of this group |

3. Can produce hypoglycaemia in non-diabetics (and diabetics). Hypoglycaemic coma is chief danger.
4. Other toxicity: skin allergy; GI toxicity; cholestatic jaundice; haemopoietic changes, hypothyroidism.
5. Hypoglycaemia potentiated by clofibrate, phenylbutazone, monoamine oxidase inhibitors.
6. Hypoglycaemia reduced by steroids, thiazides, frusemide, the Pill, thyroxin, nicotinic acid.

## B. Biguanides
1. Reduce glucose absorption from gut and increase anaerobic glucose metabolism to reduce hyperglycaemia.
2. Reduce appetite and hence aid weight loss. Also metallic taste, vomiting, diarrhoea.
3. Lactic acidosis — uncommon but 60% mortality (contraindicated in renal, hepatic, cardiorespiratory disease and in alcoholism — because of increased risk of lactic acidosis). Main risk with phenformin and in renal, hepatic and cardiac failure.
4. Drug interactions less common than with sylphonylureas — but hypoglycaemia potentiated with salicylates.

## Special problems in diabetes

### a. Infections
 (i) Even minor viral infections may raise insulin needs 30%.
 (ii) Dose of insulin must be promptly reduced after infection.
(iii) Patients often stop insulin if vomiting and not eating.
(iv) Use sliding scale based on blood and/or urine tests with 4 hourly insulin: — see Table 35.

### b. Surgery
 (i) Admit to hospital 48 hours before operation.
 (ii) Change (if not treated normally in this way) to three times daily soluble insulin.
(iii) During surgery i.v. infusion of 3 U insulin/h plus 6 g glucose/h. Infusion rates may have to be modified to produce blood glucose levels of 6–8 mmol/l (monitor hourly).
(iv) Continue (iii) until oral feeding with intermittent insulin injections can be resumed — initially the sliding scale is used
 (v) Patients with such mild diabetes that insulin is not required during operations should have monitoring of glucose levels into the postoperative period.

## C. Pregnancy

(i) Increased risk to fetus and increased incidence of congenital malformations. Deterioration of established retinopathy and nephropathy in mother.

(ii) Supervision essential from the earliest stages of pregnancy to produce exemplary blood glucose control. Single dose insulin regimes changed to multiple doses.

(iii) Renal threshold for glucose falls during pregnancy and therefore urine testing is unsuitable. Change to blood testing with Dextrostix. Modify insulin and meals accordingly.

(iv) Renal glycosuria can cause starvation ketosis. Do not increase insulin dose but raise carbohydrate intake.

(v) Any problem with control is treated immediately in hospital. Check control with $HbA_{1c}$ and with preprandial blood glucose (should be < 7.2 mmol/l).

(vi) Obstetrician and physician together see patient: 4 weekly up to 28 weeks, 2 weekly up to 36 weeks and weekly up to delivery. Accurate assessment of fetal development needed to choose time of delivery.

## d. Labour

(i) Induce on morning of chosen day. No breakfast but set up drip of 10% glucose with 10 U soluble insulin/500 ml and infuse 100 ml/hr.
*Alternatively*: 10 g/h glucose by drip and 1–2 U insulin/hr by syringe pump.

(ii) Monitor blood glucose hourly and change rate of drip if necessary.

(iii) After rupture of membranes, apply electrodes to fetal scalp and monitor ECG. Measure fetal blood pH. Deliver rapidly if bradycardia, tachycardia or pH falls below 7.2.

(iv) Paediatrician present at delivery. Increased risk of hypoglycaemia, hypocalcaemia, hyperbilirubinaemia and congenital malformations.

## General care of diabetics

(i) Maintain blood glucose in ideal range, avoiding preprandial hyperglycaemia and post insulin hypoglycaemia.

(ii) Continuing education. British Diabetic Association very helpful particularly with diabetes in childhood.

(iii) Many problems in children: increases in physical activity and emotional crises can lead to hypoglycaemia; low renal threshold; failure to empty bladder.

(iv) Stop smoking; treat hypertension; treat hyperlipidaemia.

(v) Regular symptom enquiry and examination of eyes, feet and urine.

## THYROID GLAND

Excessive production of $T_3$ and $T_4$ produces thyrotoxicosis: deficiency produces myxoedema or cretinism.

Secretion of $T_3$ and $T_4$ increased by TSH (released in response to low plasma levels of $T_3$ and $T_4$) and by immunoglobulins with TSH activity (not affected by $T_3$ and $T_4$ levels).

### Actions of $T_3$ and $T_4$

| Hormone action | Clinical consequence in hyper- or hypothyroidism |
|---|---|
| 1. Stimulation of metabolism | Heat intolerance, increased appetite with weight loss, raised metabolic rate in hyperthyroidism; hypothermia and coma in myxoedema |
| 2. Promotion of growth and development | Dwarfism and mental deficiency in cretinism |
| 3. (Possible) sensitisation to sympathetic effects and to catecholamines | Eyelid retraction, tachycardia, tremor, hyperactive reflexes in hyperthyroidism |

| Pharmacokinetics | Thyroxine ($T_4$) | Liothyronine ($T_3$) |
|---|---|---|
| Gut absorption | Complete | Complete |
| Latency before action starts | 24 h | 6 h |
| Peak effect | 7–10 d | 24 h |
| $T_{\frac{1}{2}}$ | 6–7 d | 2 d or less |
| Metabolism | Conjugation and enterohepatic circulation 20% is converted to $T_3$ in tissues. | Conjugation and enterohepatic circulation |
| Normal levels | 50–10 µg/l (80% of circulating thyroid hormone) | 1–1.6 µg/l (20% of circulating thyroid hormone) |
| | 99.95% bound to thyroid binding globulin | 99.5% bound to plasma protein |

Therefore, ratio of free $T_4$ : $T_3$ is 4–5:1.

## Uses of $T_3$ and $T_4$

$T_4$ is standard treatment for hypothyroidism.
$T_3$ is sometimes used in the initial treatment of myxoedema coma.
$T_4$ may reduce the size of goitres which have not responded to iodine alone.

*Toxicity*
Cardiac — tachycardia, angina, myocardial infarction, congestive failure, arrhythmias, sudden death.
Diarrhoea
Tremor, restlessness, heat intolerance.

## Treatment of hyperthyroidism

*1. Medical*
Children and young adults
Preparation for surgery
Mild – moderate disease
Thyroid gland not greatly enlarged
Elderly patients rendered euthyroid on drugs, can then be left indefinitely on a small maintenance dose.

*2. Surgery*
Large gland
Compression of neighbouring structures
Nodular gland, toxic adenoma

*3. Radioactive iodine ($I^{131}$)*
Postoperative recurrence
Surgery contraindicated
Failed drug therapy in an adult

## Medical management

### a. Long-term treatment

| | Drug | Dose | Toxicity |
|---|---|---|---|
| Block iodination of tyrosyl residues | Methimazole | Can be administered but is the active metabolite of carbimazole | Common: maculopapular rashes. Less common: arthralgia, jaundice, lymphadenopathy, nausea, vomiting, pyrexia (these respond to antihistamine & change of drug). Uncommon: (1:1000 patients) agranulocytosis, often preceded by sore throat (stop drug, isolate patient. Neutrophils reappear in 1–2 weeks). Most toxicity occurs in first 2 months. |
| | Carbimazole (Neo-Mercazole) | 30–60 mg daily till euthyroid then 5–15 mg daily for 12–18 months | |
| | Propylthiouracil | 300–600 mg daily then 50–150 mg daily for 12–18 months | |

Potassium perchlorate blocks iodine uptake by thyroid, only used if toxic reactions occur with other drugs because it may cause aplastic anaemia.

Drugs usually given for 1–2 years then slowly withdrawn. 50% relapse when drugs stopped and require continued treatment.

### b. Short term management
Preparation for surgery
Treating severe disease until I[131] starts to become effective
1. Start antithyroid drug
2. Add propranolol (initially 40 mg 6- or 8-hourly) — reduces restlessness, tremor, sweating, anxiety, within 12–48 hours. Raise dose after 48 hours if inadequate response. β-blockers act by:
   (i) reducing peripheral sympathetic activity
(ii) blocking formation of $T_3$ from $T_4$
   Drug cover must continue during and after operation, and start 4–8 weeks beforehand.

3. 7–10 days before surgery, iodine (0.5 ml Lugol's aqueous iodine solution 8 hourly) is given. This is a powerful but short-lived inhibitor of hormone release.

c. *Pregnancy*
1. Operate if severe disease or large goitre in early or mid-pregnancy.
2. Antithyroid drugs can be given throughout pregnancy if surgery is not undertaken.
3. Radioactive iodine is contraindicated.

d. *Thyroid crisis*
1. Drugs by nasogastric tube if swallowing difficult.
2. Carbimazole 60–120 mg or propylthiouracil 600–1200 mg.
3. Lugol's iodine or potassium iodide given at least 1 hour after starting antithyroid drugs.
4. Propranolol, e.g. 1.5 mg i.v. or 20–80 mg orally 8 hourly.
5. Dexamethasone 2 mg 6-hourly inhibits formation of $T_3$ from $T_4$ in tissues.
6. Correct fluid balance.
7. Treat heart failure or arrhythmias.
8. Treat hyperthermia with ice packs.
9. Plasmapheresis and exchange transfusion if no response to above.

e. *Eye signs*
1. Usually resolve with treatment but 5% guanethidine eye drops may improve appearance.
2. Visual failure — prednisolone 60 mg daily with surgical decompression if unsuccessful.

**Treatment of hypothyroidism**
1. Oral L-thyroxine 100–200 μg daily. Response monitored clinically and biochemically. In elderly patients and those with heart disease, start with 25–50 μg daily and increase dose by 25–50 μg daily every 2–3 weeks until maintenance dose reached.
   *Toxicity*:  myocardial ischaemia, psychosis.
2. Myxoedema coma:
   L-thyroxine 400–500 μg i.v. or by nasogastric tube (alternatively tri-iodothyronine can be given)
   Cortisol
   Intravenous fluids containing electrolytes and glucose if respiratory acidosis: give $O_2$, tracheostomy and assisted ventilation if required.
   Rewarm in normal ambient temperature.
   On recovery initiate lifelong thyroxine.

## OSTEOPOROSIS

No known measure reverses osteoporosis.
Treatment aims to maintain current skeletal integrity and prevent
  further loss.
1. Patient education: stress
   a. benign nature and remitting course
   b. importance of exercise and avoidance of bed rest.
2. Diet should contain adequate protein, minerals and vitamins:
   Vitamin D (1000 U calciferol/day) or its metabolites should not
   be given in absence of deficiency or osteomalacia.
   Supplementary calcium (as lactate or carbonate 1 – 1.5 g
   elemental calcium/day) is almost as effective as oestrogens in
   postmenopausal osteomalacia. Soft tissue calcification is rare;
   renal stones avoided by giving adequate fluids.
3. Low dose conjugated oestrogens (Premarin 0.625 mg/day) of
   some benefit if started shortly after menopause but possible risk
   of endometrial cancer (thus add progestogen for last 5 days of 28
   day cyclical therapy and do regular pelvic exams, with vaginal
   smears) and thromboembolism.
4. Anabolic steroids, e.g. stanozolol — helpful in males with
   Kleinefelter's syndrome and hypogonadal states.
5. Experimental therapies: fluoride; calcitonin; growth hormone;
   phosphates and diphosphonate — not yet evaluated.

## OSTEOMALACIA

### A. Nutritional osteomalacia and rickets
1. Low dose vitamin $D_2$ (calciferol) as Calcium with vitamin D
   tablets (calcium lactate 300 mg; calcium phosphate 150 mg,
   ergocalciferol 12.5 mg = 500 units) — one or two daily.
2. If due to malabsorption use 50 000 units calciferol daily given as
   Calciferol tablets Strong (12.5 mg ergocalciferol = 50 000 units).
3. 1-α-hydroxycholecalciferol ie alfacalcidol (One-alpha) may
   be used in doses of 0.5–1 $\mu$g/day for nutritional rickets to
   give a more rapid response although the drug is more
   expensive.
Effects of treatment:
increased muscle strength; initial fall of serum $Ca^{++}$ with normality
in 3 months
initial rise then fall of alkaline phosphatase
healing of pseudofractures within 3 months.

### B. Familial hypophosphataemic rickets and adult onset
hypophosphataemic osteomalacia
1. Phosphate supplements (1 – 1.5 g/day)
2. Vitamin D 50 000 U orally/day as Calciferol tablets Strong.

### C. Osteomalacia with renal tubular acidosis
1. Correct acidosis with bicarbonate.
2. Calciferol supplements.

## RENAL BONE DISEASE

Defective renal parenchyma

↓

Failure to 1 – hydroxylate ⟶ Osteomalacia
25 (OH) cholecalciferol

↓

Low $Ca^{++}$ and raised $PO_4$

↓

Parathyroid stimulation ⟶ Secondary hyperparathyroidism

1. Osteomalacia or hyperparathyroidism: give 1,25
   dihydroxycholecalciferol (Rocaltrol) or
   1-α-hydroxycholecalciferol (one-alpha), but avoid
   hypercalcaemia (1,25 dihydroxcholecalciferol contraindicated in
   hypercalaemia or soft tissue calcification: parathyroidectomy
   may be required).
2. Hypocalcaemia also treated by oral calcium and phosphate
   binding agents (e.g. aluminium hydroxide). Reduction of
   phosphate may inhibit secretion of PTH.

## TREATMENT OF HYPERPARATHYROIDISM

1. Vitamin D preparations are treatment of choice:
   a. vitamin D 1 – 2 mg daily (49 000 – 80 000 U) oral but slow
      onset of action and can give prolonged phases of
      hypercalcaemia.
or
   b. Dihydrotachysterol (AT 10) 0.25 – 1 mg daily oral.
or
   c. 1-α-hydroxycholecalciferol (one-alpha) 1 – 2 μg daily oral.
or
   d. 1,25 dihydroxycholecalciferol (Rocaltrol) 0.5 – 10 μg daily oral.
   c. and d. produce a rapid response, and if hypercalcaemia recurs
   it will resolve in days (not weeks) on drug withdrawal.
2. Synthetic PTH (injected) is an alternative treatment.
3. Essential: regular follow-up every 3 – 6 months.

## PAGET'S DISEASE

Most patients are asymptomatic and require no treatment.
Indications for treatment are:
a. Bone pain unresponsive to simple analgesics.
b. Hypercalcaemia due to immobilisation.
c. Nerve root or cord compression — paraplegia may be reversed
   but deafness rarely improves.
d. Juvenile Paget's disease — only some types respond.
e. Reduction of high cardiac output failure (rare).

Progression of disease, especially in young patients, may be prevented (unproven). No improvement in rate of fracture healing with treatment.

Treatment monitored by symptomatic response, alkaline phosphatase, urinary hydroxyproline excretion. Additional methods — X-rays, bone scans, skin temperature, radio-calcium kinetics.

Two main treatments:

## 1. Calcitonins
32 amino-acid polypeptide hormone secreted by parafollicular cells of mammalian thyroid. Inhibits osteoclast activity so reducing bone resorption. Degree of hypocalcaemia produced related to prevailing bone resorption rate so produces greater fall in children, thyrotoxicosis and Paget's than in normals.

| Source | Potency | Therapeutic use in Paget's |
|---|---|---|
| Porcine calcitonin (Calcitare) from pig thyroid | 100 i.u./mg | 160 i.u. daily for 3–6 months reducing to 80 i.u. 3 times weekly by s.c. or i.m. injection. |
| Salcatonin-synthetic salmon calcitonin (Calsynar) | 4000 i.u./mg | 50–100 i.u. daily for 3–6 months reducing to 50 i.u. 3 times weekly by s.c. or i.m. injection. |

Human calcitonin (synthetic) not commercially available and supplies limited. Antibodies to porcine and salmon calcitonins develop but rarely cause treatment failure.

Response 50% patients: improvement in pain occurs within 1–2 weeks. Urinary hydroxyprolone excretion falls in a day or two, alkaline phosphatase falls more slowly: they reach a nadir which is not decreased by increasing dose although etidronate may further improve response. After withdrawal of calcitonin, symptoms can remain controlled despite deterioration of biochemical features.

*Adverse effects*
Nausea after injection.
Flushing of face, paraesthesiae, fever, metallic taste.

## 2. Disodium etidronate (Didronel)
Diphosphonate analogue of pyrophosphate in which unstable phosphorous oxygen (P–O–P) bonds replaced by stable phosphorus carbon (P–C–P) bonds.

*Pharmacology*
Inhibits growth and dissolution of hydroxyapalite crystals, reduces bone absorption and turnover.

10% absorbed after oral dosing; rapidly cleared from blood by bone and renal excretion (unchanged) so caution needed in renal impairment. Biological effects largely confined to bone. Within 24 hours half absorbed drug is excreted in urine but release from skeleton has $T_{\frac{1}{2}}$ of 2–4 weeks.

*Clinical use*
Dose 5 mg/kg/day as single oral dose at bedtime 2 hours after food — especially avoid foods high in calcium or antacids containing calcium, magnesium or iron. This dose given for not more than 6 months.

10 mg/kg/day may be used for not more than 3 months when rapid suppression of disease, e.g. to lower cardiac output, is necessary.

60% patients achieve pain relief, maximal after 6 months which may persist after drug stopped. Cycles of 6 months on and off treatment used for prolonged suppression. Can be used together with calcitonin.

*Adverse effects*
GI intolerance, especially with higher dose.

# Anti-infective chemotherapy

## ANTIBACTERIAL DRUGS

### Antibiotics
Compounds synthesized by microorganisms which kill or inhibit the growth of cells which produce disease (mainly microorganisms and neoplasms).

### Chemotherapeutic substances
All compounds (synthetic and produced by living cells) which kill or inhibit the growth of cells which produce disease in the body.

### Bactericidal
i.e. kills bacteria (e.g. penicillins, aminoglycosides).

### Bacteriostatic
i.e. stops bacterial division: bacteria eliminated by host defences (e.g. tetracyclines, erythromycin).

N.B. Bactericidal/static distinction of little importance under most conditions in practice. However, bactericidal drugs should be used when phagocytic cells cannot get to site of infection (e.g. endocarditis) or in leucopenia. Giving bacteriostatic and cidal drugs together may be synergistic, additive or antagonistic, but usually no measurable disadvantage occurs.

## SULPHONAMIDES

Use has declined in recent years but still have some clinical applications.

### Action
Block bacterial folic acid synthesis by combining with pteridine to form an inactive complex. This metabolic step is absent in man.

## Pharmacokinetics
Lipid soluble so most are well absorbed from small intestine.
Penetrate into CSF and nasopharynx. Variable degree of plasma
protein binding. Main metabolites are (inactive) sulphate,
glucuronide and acetyl derivatives. For some
genetically-determined acetylator status influences rate of
metabolism. Mainly excreted in urine by glomerular filtration and
tubular secretion and best avoided in renal failure.

## Toxicity
Rashes are common (include Stevens-Johnson syndrome)
Highly sensitising when applied topically.
Drug fever, dizziness, headache, malaise, crystalluria (especially
  with sulphadiazine). Can produce anuria.
Acute renal toxicity can also occur due to intrarenal damage.
Kernicterus (when given in last 2 weeks of pregnancy or to a
  neonate) because of displacement of unconjugated bilirubin from
  plasma protein binding.
Haemolytic anaemia in G6PD deficiency.
Agranulocytosis, aplastic anaemia
Bacterial resistance (especially *N. meningitidis*).

## Interactions
Potientate oral sulphonylurea hypoglycaemic agents and oral
anticoagulants.

## Sulphonamides

| Sulphonamide | Dose | Special features & use |
|---|---|---|
| Sulphacetamide (Albucid) | Eye drops 10%, 20%, 30% 2–4 drops 2–6-hourly (also eye ointment 2.5%, 6%, 10%) | Used topically for ocular infections including neonatal conjunctivitis and chlamydial eye infections |

**Short acting**

| | | |
|---|---|---|
| Sulphadimidine | 2 g initially then 0.5 – 1 g 6 – 8-hourly. | $T_{\frac{1}{2}} = 7$ h used in uncomplicated urinary infections |
| Sulphamethizole | 200 mg 5 times daily | $T_{\frac{1}{2}} = 2.5$ h used in uncomplicated urinary infections |
| Sulphafurazole | 2 g initially then 1 g 6 – 8-hourly | $T_{\frac{1}{2}} = 6$ h used in uncomplicated urinary infections |

**Medium acting**

| | | |
|---|---|---|
| Sulphadiazine | 1 – 1.5 g every 4 h | $T_{\frac{1}{2}} = 16$ h Given i.v. for meningococcal meningitis with i.m. penicillin — use for this is declining. Effective in treating nasopharyngeal carriers. |

**Long acting**

| | | |
|---|---|---|
| Sulphamethoxydiazine | 0.5 g every 24 h | $T_{\frac{1}{2}} = 37$ h Has been used to prevent urinary infections but particularly prone to produce Stephens-Johnson syndrome |
| Sulphadoxine | 2 g every week | $T_{\frac{1}{2}} = 150$ h Malaria prophylaxis (with pyrimethamine = Fansidar) |

**Uses of sulphonamides**

| Drug | Application |
|---|---|
| *Sulphacetamide* | Local use in eye infections esp. chlamydia |
| Silver sulphadiazine | Local use for burns (active against pseudomonas) |
| Sulphapyridine | Low dose over long periods for dermatitis herpetiformis |
| *Short acting sulphonamides* | Uncomplicated urinary infections |
| Sulphadiazine | Meningococcal meningitis |
| Succinylsulphathiazole Phthalylsulphathiazole | Sulphonamides not now used for gut infections, gut sterilisation |
| Short acting sulphonamides | Nocardiosis |
| Sulphonamide plus pyrimethamine | Toxoplasmosis |

## Sulphonamide mixtures

| Composition | Approved name | Trade name | Dose |
|---|---|---|---|
| Trimethoprim 80 mg Sulphamethoxazole 400 mg | Co-trimoxazole | Bactrim Fectrim Septrin | 2 tabs twice daily (injection also available) |
| Trimethoprim 80 mg Sulphamoxole 400 mg | Co-trifamole | Cofram | 2 tabs initially then 1 twice daily |
| Trimethoprim 90 mg Sulphadiazine 410 mg | Co-trimazine | Coptin | 1 tab twice daily |

### Uses

Acute exacerbations of bronchitis
Urinary tract infections and prostatitis    First time treatment
Pneumocystis carinii

Enteric fever
Otitis media
Bacillary dysentery                         Second line treatment
Brucellosis
Gonorrhoea

## TRIMETHOPRIM (Ipra; Monotrim; Syraprim; Trimopan)

### Action

Competitive inhibitor of dihydrofolate reductase with affinity for bacterial enzyme 50 000 times that for human. Thus inhibits formation of 'active' folate.

Potent broad-spectrum bacteriostatic agent. Resistance due to resistant dihydrofolate reductase is increasing.

### Pharmacokinetics

Well absorbed from gut.
$T_{\frac{1}{2}}$ 6–12 h; 70% renally excreted and $T_{\frac{1}{2}}$ is increased 2–3 times by renal failure.

### Toxicity

Nausea, vomiting, diarrhoea; rash; folate deficiency anaemia (only in those with initially low folate stores).

**Use**

For urinary tract infection — 200 mg 12-hourly — as effective as
co-trimoxazole.
For prophylaxis of urinary tract infection — 100 mg nightly.
Probably effective in respiratory tract infections.

**Trimethoprim-Sulphonamide mixtures**

Suggested advantages:
a. Delayed emergence of trimethoprim resistance — evidence
   equivocal.
b. Synergy due to action at two sites in folic acid metabolism —
   only demonstrable when both drugs present at sub-inhibitory
   concentrations so probably of dubious clinical relevance.
c. Wider spectrum — mixtures also effective for gonococcus and
   some anaerobes.
d. Although absorption and elimination of trimethoprim and
   admixed sulphonamides similar, tissue penetration and urinary
   excretion differ.
e. Except in gonorrhoea, no clinical trial has shown mixtures to be
   superior to trimethoprim alone.
f. Toxicity of sulphonamide mixtures =

         Toxicity of sulphonamide + Toxicity of trimethoprim
   Therefore trend is to use trimethoprim alone (it's cheaper) for
urinary infections.


THE PENICILLINS

Penicillanic nucleus + side chains = penicillins.
Penicillanic acid = β-lactam ring fused with thiazolidine ring.
Action on bacterial cell wall.
In general penicillins have $T_{\frac{1}{2}}$ 1–2 h and are mainly eliminated in
the urine (tubular secretion is blocked by probenecid).

**Organisms sensitive to benzyl penicillin**

G +ve cocci:
   *Staph aureus* — not β-lactamase (penicillinase) producing strains
   *Strep. pneumoniae* β-haemolytic streptococci (Lancefield group A
   *Strep. pyogenes*)
   *Strep. viridans*
G −ve cocci:
   *Neisseria gonorrhoeae*
   *Neisseria meningitidis*
G +ve bacilli:
   *Bacillus anthracis*
   *Corynebacterium diphtheriae*
   *Listeria monocytogenes*
   *Clostridium* sp. (and many other anaerobes except *Bacteroides
   fragilis*)

Spirochaetes:
  *Treponema pallidum*
  *Treponema pertenue*
  *Leptospira icterohaemorrhagiae*
Actinomyces

**Some resistant strains**
*Strep. faecalis*
*Neisseria gonorrhoeae*
*Haemophilus influenzae*
Penicillinase-producing staphylococci
*Escherichia coli*
Klebsiella
*Proteus mirabilis*
Serratia
*Pseudomonas aeruginosa*
*Bacteroides fragilis*

**Penicillin toxicity**

*1. Hypersensitivity*
Type 1 reactions (early)
a. rash (common) — urticaria, erythema
b. anaphylaxis (rare) — circulatory collapse, bronchospasm,
   laryngeal oedema
Serum sickness (type III reactions) — delayed by 2–12 days:
fever, malaise, arthralgia, angioedema, erythema nodosum,
   exfoliative dermatitis, erythema multiforme, Stevens-Johnson
   syndrome.

*2. Neurotoxicity*
a. Only high doses (those which may be used with carbenicillin)
b. Anuria
c. Intrathecal injection of over 50 000 U
Encephalopathy can present as:
  fits, coma
  permanent sequelae
  death

*3. Haemolytic anaemia*
Only high doses

4. *Ampicillin, talampicillin and pivampicillin* produce rash (usually
morbilliform) in about 8% of patients, more commonly in young
women. A very high incidence of this reaction occurs in infectious
mononucleosis and chronic lymphatic leukaemia.

*Note*: The penicillins are relatively non-toxic and safe drugs.

**Table 38** Penicillins I — Benzylpenicillin and related drugs

| Drug | Administration | Special features | Main uses |
|---|---|---|---|
| Benzylpenicillin (soluble penicillin; Penicillin G) | i.m. (or i.v.) 4–6-hourly 1–20 × 10⁶ U daily. High doses for infective endocarditis and meningitis. Intrathecal 10 000–40 000 (never more) (10⁶ units ≅ 600 mg) | Highly active against susceptible organisms but destroyed by penicillinase. Partly inactivated by gastric acid. Does not penetrate well into the CSF. | 1. Serious infections needing parenteral antibiotic, e.g. meningitis, endocarditis, septicaemia. 2. Infections due to susceptible organisms, e.g. pneumococcal pneumonia, streptococcal pharyngitis, gonorrhoea, syphilis, soft tissue infections due to streptococci pyogenes & microaerophilic streptococci. |
| Phenoxymethyl penicillin (Penicillin V) | Oral 250 mg 4–6-hourly | Resistant to acid hydrolysis, otherwise same properties as benzylpenicillin. Moderately well absorbed from gut. Destroyed by staphylococcal penicillinase. | Streptococcal pharyngitis (& its prophylaxis) |
| Procaine penicillin G | i.m. 300 mg 12–24-hourly | Prolonged action, but otherwise same properties as benzylpenicillin | As with benzylpenicillin apart from severest infections; prevention of endocarditis after dental procedures |
| Benzathine penicillin (Penidural LA) | i.m. 229–916 mg every 5–7 days. Rheumatic fever prophylaxis 916 mg every 3 weeks. | Prolonged action, effective blood levels persist for 1–2 weeks. Otherwise, same properties as benzylpenicillin. | When poor patient compliance suspected. Prophylaxis of streptococcal infections. |

**Table 39** Penicillins II — Broad-spectrum penicillins

1. Spectrum includes many strains of *E. coli, H. influenzae,* Proteus and Salmonellae
2. Inactivated by β-lactamases including those of *Staph. aureus* and some *E. coli* Almost all Staphs and one-third *E. coli* strains now resistant
3. Can be given p.o., i.m., i.v.

| Drug | Administration | Special features | Main uses |
|---|---|---|---|
| Ampicillin (Penbritin) | Oral 250 mg — 1 g 6-hourly. i.m. or i.v. 250–500 mg 6-hourly. | High concentrations in urine & bile. *Toxicity:* GI intolerance, rashes (including morbiliform rash esp. with young females and in glandular fever and chronic lymphatic leukaemia). | Urinary infections, acute exacerbations of chronic bronchitis, cholecystitis, Infections due to *H. influenzae* (e.g. meningitis, arthritis, otitis media). |
| Amoxycillin (Amoxil) | Oral 250 mg 8-hourly. i.m. or i.v. 500 mg 8-hourly or 1 g 6 hourly. | Better (× 2) intestinal absorption than ampicillin & higher tissue levels. Otherwise same as ampicillin but possibly more active against *Strep. faecalis* and Salmonella. | As with ampicillin. Also large single dose (3 g) before dental & other instrumental procedures, in particular with valvular heart disease as SABE prophylaxis. Also 2 × 3 g doses in acute urinary infections. May penetrate sputum better than ampicillin. Typhoid (as good as chloramphenicol). |

**Table 39** (continued)

| Drug | Administration | Special features | Main uses |
|------|----------------|------------------|-----------|
| *Prodrugs of ampicillin* | | | |
| Inactive compounds better absorbed than ampicillin which are split by gut and/or liver on absorption to give higher levels of ampicillin in blood and tissues. More expensive than ampicillin. | | | |
| Talampicillin (Talpen) | Oral 500 mg twice daily | Phthalidyl ester of ampicillin. Less diarrhoea than after ampicillin. | As with ampicillin |
| Pivampicillin (Pondocillin) | Oral 500 mg 12-hourly | As with talampicillin, better absorption than ampicillin & higher blood levels for the same mg dose | As ampicillin; 1.2 – 2 g as a single dose for gonorrhoea |
| Bacampicillin (Ambaxin) | Oral 400 mg 8 – 12-hourly | As pivampicillin | As ampicillin |

**Table 40** Penicillins III — Active against β-lactamase producing bacteria
Acid stable so can be given p.o.

| Drug | Administration | Special features | Main uses |
|---|---|---|---|
| *1. Inherent resistance to β-lactamase* | | | |
| Cloxacillin (Orbenin) | p.o.: 500 mg 6-hourly. i.v./i.m.: 500 mg 4–6-hourly. | | Infections due to β-lactamase producing Staph. is sole indication. |
| Flucloxacillin (Floxapen) | p.o.: 250 mg 6-hourly i.v.: 250–500 mg 6-hourly i.m.: 250 mg 6-hourly | Twice as well absorbed orally than cloxacillin which it has largely replaced | As cloxacillin |
| *2. β-lactamase inhibition* Clavulanic acid has little intrinsic antibacterial activity but inhibits β-lactamase | | | |
| Amoxycillin + Potassium Clavulanate (Augmentin) | 1–2 tablets 8-hourly | Activity against most amoxycillin-resistant *Staph. aureus*, *H. influenzae*, *Kl. aerogenes*, *E. coli* and *Bacteroides* sp. Not active against resistant *Strep. pneumoniae*. Significant number of amoxycillin-resistant G −ve bacilli are resistant and efficacy should not be assumed. Expensive relative to amoxycillin. | When sensitivity of amoxycillin-resistant organism demonstrated. Place in therapy not clear yet. |

**Table 41** Penicillins IV — Active against *Pseudomonas aeruginosa*
1. Despite broad spectra solely used for suspected or proven Pseudomonas (or occasionally ampicillin-resistant Proteus) infections
2. All hydrolysed by β-lactamases so 90% *Staph. aureus* and 40% *E. coli* resistant
3. Synergistic with aminoglycosides (but should be put in same container together)
4. All given i.v. (except carpecillin — not recommended)
5. Very expensive

| Drug | Administration | Special features | Main uses |
|---|---|---|---|
| *1. Carbenicillin and related drugs* | | | |
| Carbenicillin (Pyopen) | 25–30 g/day (1 g/h) | Neurotoxicity (like correspondingly large doses of other penicillins). N.B.: 30 g carbenicillin contains 163 mM $Na^+$ so danger of overload. Dose reduction needed in renal failure. | Severe infections due to Pseudomonas and Proteus |
| Carpecillin (Uticillin) | 0.5–1 g 8-hourly orally | Phenyl ester of carbenicillin acts as pro-drug but does not give high enough carbenicillin blood levels to be useful for severe infections. | Reserved for rare Pseudomonas urinary infections and G −ve infections resistant to other drugs |
| Ticarcillin (Ticar) | 15–20 g/day | Twice as active as carbenicillin but ineffective against carbenicillin resistant strains. 20 g has 107 mM $Na^+$. Reduce dose in renal failure. | As carbenicillin |
| *2. Ureidopenicillins* | | | |
| Mezlocillin (Baypen) | 15–20 g/day at 6–8-hourly intervals | Twice as active as carbenicillin. Effective on some carbenicillin resistant strains. 20 g has 37 mM $Na^+$. Usual doses appropriate in renal failure until GFR < 25 ml/min. | Spectrum wider than rest (= ampicillin + carbenicillin) so could be used for infections with other enterobacteria |

| | | | |
|---|---|---|---|
| Azlocillin (Securopen) | 15 g/day at 8-hourly intervals | 2–4 times more active than mezlocillin or ticarcillin on Pseudomonas but less potent than mezlocillin on other G −ve bacteria. 15 g = 33 mM $Na^+$. Usual doses in renal failure until GFR < 25 ml/min. when same dose given at 12-hourly intervals. | As carbenicillin but also penetrates CSF so can be used in Pseudomonas meningitis |
| Piperacillin (Pipril) | 16 g/day as 4 g 6-hourly | As active as azlocillin against Pseudomonas. Spectrum is wide (= azlocillin + mezlocillin) 80% renally excreted, 20% in bile so in renal failure only minor dose reduction needed (GFR 20–40 ml/min 4 g 8-hourly; GFR < 20 ml/min 4 g 12-hourly). 16 g has 32 mM $Na^+$. | As carbenicillin |

**Table 42** Agents closely related to the penicillins

| Drug | Administration | Special features | Main uses |
|---|---|---|---|
| Mecillinam (Selexidin) | Parenteral administration only 5–15 mg/kg every 6–8 hours | An imidinopenicillin chemically related to penicillins but with different action on bacterial cell wall. Destroyed by some but not all penicillinases. Not absorbed from gut. Excreted in urine. *Toxicity:* GI upsets. Possible cross allergy with penicillin. | Active against G –ve bacilli, including Salmonellae & Shigellae but excluding *Ps. aeruginosa, H. influenzae* and Neisseria. Used for infections resistant to ampicillin. |
| Pivmecillinam (Selexid) | Oral 200 mg 6–8-hourly for urinary infections and 1.2–2.4 g daily for salmonella infections | Pivaloyloxymethyl ester, a prodrug of mecillinam. Absorbed from gut and hydrolysed to free mecillinam. | As for mecillinam, particularly urinary and systemic infections |

## CEPHALOSPORINS AND CEPHAMYCINS

Inhibit bacterial cell wall synthesis by inhibiting transpeptidase formation of cross links in mucopeptide (as does penicillin).

Broad spectrum agents although individual agents have enhanced activity against some pathogens.

### Pharmacokinetics
Nearly all need to be injected.

Most eliminated unchanged renally (like penicillins) with some exceptions, e.g. cephalothin, cefotaxime. Therefore usually need to reduce dose in renal failure.

Half-lives usually 1–2 h.

In general, penetrate sputum poorly.

### Toxicity
Hypersensitivity (10% penicillin sensitive patients cross-reacted to first generation cephalosporins — may not be true for more recent agents).

Renal tubular necrosis occurred with older cephalosporins, e.g. cephaloridine, cephalothin, especially if given with gentamicin or frusemide. Later cephalosporins have not been implicated.

Direct Coombs test (interferes with blood cross-matching).

False positive urine test for reducing agents: cefotaxime, cefoxitin, cephalexin, cephradine, cephazolin.

### Indications for cephalosporins and cephamycins
They should not be used where a narrower spectrum drug is available.

1  Severe undiagnosed sepsis.
   Cefoxitin active against most important anaerobes, thus could be used in sepsis complicating intestinal or genital disease.
   Cefuroxime or cefamandole used if chest or kidney primary site (if *Pseudomonas aeruginosa* present then gentamicin, carbenicillin, piperacillin, azlocillin or ticarcillin must be used as well).
2. Can be used in staphylococcal sepsis but flucloxacillin preferable.
3. Cefuroxime, cefoxitin, cefotaxime or cephamandole active against penicillin-resistant gonococci (also spectinomycin could be used).
4. Urinary tract infections — ONLY if resistance to usual drugs. None are useful in prostatic infections.
5. Chest infections — ONLY if patient seriously ill and *H. influenzae* resistant to ampicillin (but these strains usually sensitive to cotrimoxazole). *Klebsiella pneumonia* is indication for cefotaxime. No cephalosporin is first or even second choice in treatment of acute exacerbations of chronic bronchitis.

**Table 43** Cephalosporins — First generation

1. Rarely agents of first choice: becoming obsolete
2. Some oral agents in this group
3. All hydrolysed by β-lactamases

| Drug | Administration | Special features | Main uses |
|---|---|---|---|
| Cephaloridine (Ceporin) | 500 mg i.m. 6–8-hourly (30 mg/kg/day for children) Intrathecal: 25–50 mg (0.5 mg/kg for children) | Large doses can produce renal failure (esp. in renal failure or if frusemide or gentamicin used simultaneously). Rashes Minor degrees of reversible leucopenia. | Rarely used now because of toxicity |
| Cephalexin (Ceporex; Keflex) | 500 mg p.o. 8-hourly | Probably not nephrotoxic but nevertheless not to be used with frusemide. | Less active than cephaloridine against G +ve cocci but more resistant to *E. coli* β-lactamase. Poor activity against haemophilus and staphylococci. |
| Cephazolin (Kefzol) | 0.25–0.5 mg i.m. or i.v. 6-hourly | Low renal toxicity. Significant biliary excretion. As active as cephaloridine. | Substitute for cephaloridine but more expensive |
| Cephradine (Velosef) | 1 g twice daily p.o. Parenterally: i.m. or i.v. 0.5–1 g 6-hourly. | Rashes, GI upsets, vulvovaginitis. Possible renal toxicity. | Low activity, but useful in urinary tract infections and gonorrhoea. Relatively resistant to β-lactamase from *E. coli* and staphylococci. |

**Table 44**: Cephalosporins — Second Generation

1. Greater activity against G –ve bacteria
2. Stability against β-lactamases widens spectrum
3. All require injection (may cause thrombophlebitis)
4. All relatively expensive

| Drug | Administration | Special features | Uses |
|---|---|---|---|
| Cefuroxime (Zinacef) | i.v. or i.m. 0.75–1.5 g 6–8-hourly | No evidence of nephrotoxicity — high urinary concentrations even in renal failure | Less active than cephaloridine against Staph. aureus but is effective in penicillinase producing strains and also for enterobacteria, pneumococci, gonococci and Haemophilus |
| Cefoxitin (Mefoxin) | i.v. 1–2 g 6–8-hourly | Cephamycin not a cephalosporin. Very stable against β-lactamases. Too painful to be given i.m. | High activity against B. fragilis and coliforms so useful in postoperative infection of bowel or pelvic origin (not drug of first choice) |
| Cefamandole | i.v. or i.m., 1–2 g 6–8-hourly | Least active of the group, e.g. not resistant to β-lactamases of penicillin-resistant gonococci. Antabuse-like reaction with alcohol. | No special advantage over others |

**Table 45** Cephalosporins — Third generation

1. Variable stability to β-lactamase
2. Variable activity against *Pseudomonas aeruginosa*, inactive against *Strep. faecalis*
3. All require injection
4. Expensive

| Drug | Administration | Special features | Uses |
|---|---|---|---|
| Cefotaxime (Claforan) | i.v. or i.m. 1–2 g 8-hourly | Metabolised (to metabolite more active than cefuroxime) so no need to reduce dose in renal failure. Active against all Enterobacteriaceae (including some resistant to gentamicin) but less active against G +ve organisms, e.g. *Staph. aureus*. | Specific G −ve infections rather blind therapy. Second line of therapy of meiningitis, gonorrhoea, salpingitis. First line for Klebsiella pneumonia. |
| Cefsulodin (Monaspor) | i.v. (over 20 mins) or i.m. 0.5–2 g. 6–8-hourly | No action on G −ve bacteria and relatively little on G +ve. High activity on *Pseudomonas aeruginosa*. Little resistance to β-lactamase. | Specifically for Pseudomonas infections |
| Latamoxef (Moxallactam) | i.v. or i.m. 0.25–4 g 8-hourly | Like cefotaxime but higher activity against *B. fragilis* and *Pseudomonas aeruginosa*. High biliary excretion results in reduced vitamin K synthesis by gut flora and consequent hypoprothrombinaemia and bleeding tendency. Disulfiram reaction with ethanol. | G −ve meningitis Intra-abdominal infections in place of gentamicin |

6. Intra-abdominal sepsis — cefoxitin, latamoxef and cefotaxime effective but clindamycin + gentamicin probably still drugs of first choice.
7. Bone and joint infections: cefazolin is second line (after flucloxacillin) for Staphylococcus; for *H. influenzae* cefotaxime is effective.
8. Pseudomonas infections: role of cefsulodin is presently uncertain: an aminoglycoside + ureidopenicillin is first choice.

ERYTHROMYCIN

A macrolide.
Spectrum similar but not identical to benzylpenicillin so useful for patients allergic to penicillin.

**Pharmacology**
Bacteriostatic.
Binds to bacterial but not human ribosome 50S subunit to inhibit protein synthesis.
Erythromycin base destroyed by acid so given as enteric coated tablets or as esters (succinate or estolate) which are less susceptible and better absorbed. The stearate salt is also given but is acid labile. Both estolate and succinate are inactive until hydrolysed to free base. Food does not alter estolate absorption (which gives higher erythromycin plasma levels than other preparations). Base and stearate are poorly absorbed if given with food, *but* estolate (Ilosone) not recommended because of possibility of jaundice.
Erythromycin is excreted partly in the urine and partly in the bile but is mainly metabolised. $T_{\frac{1}{2}} = 1-2$ h.
No need for dose adjustment in renal failure.

**Dosage**
Oral:  250–500 mg 6-hourly in adults
       20 mg/kg/day in 2 divided doses in children.
i.v. 500 mg 6-hourly as lactobionate — insolubility makes i.m. injection in reasonable volume impossible.

**Toxicity**
Serious toxicity unusual but mild GI upset common with oral drug.
Reversible hepatotoxicity uncommon, usually associated with estolate; presents as cholestatic jaundice with eosinophilia.

**Uses**

Drug of first choice for:

1. Penicillin sensitive patients, e.g. for strep., staph. and pneumococcal infections, prophylaxis bacterial endocarditis, syphilis.
2. Legionnaires' disease.
3. Diphtheria and diphtheria carriers.
4. Pertussis.
5. Campylobacter enteritis.
6. Chlamydial pneumonia in infants.
7. Chlamydial infection in pregnancy (tetracycline would harm fetus).
8. Mycoplasma pneumonia in infants (tetracycline used in adults).


## AMINOGLYCOSIDES

Common properties:

1. Inhibit bacterial ribosomal protein synthesis.
2. Spectrum includes aerobic and facultatively anaerobic Gram −ve bacilli and cocci and staphylococci but streptococci and other Gram +ves and strict anaerobes are resistant.
3. Three main types of acquired resistance:
    (i) ribosome level (streptomycin only)
    (ii) decreased transport of antibiotic into bacterium — may affect several aminoglycosides
    (iii) plasmid transmitted enzymes which adenylylate, phosphorylate or acetylate antibiotic.
4. Often synergistic with β-lactam antibiotics.
5. Poorly absorbed p.o. so given parenterally or topically.
6. Narrow therapeutic range — variably nephrotoxic and/or ototoxic. Also neuromuscular blockade and sensitisation.
7. Plasma $T_{\frac{1}{2}}$ about 2 h. Monitoring of levels important for safe parenteral use.
8. Renal excretion so caution in renal failure.
9. Avoid in pregnancy — cross placenta to cause 8th cranial nerve damage.

**Table 46** Aminoglycosides

| Drug | Dosage | Toxicity | Comments |
|------|--------|----------|----------|
| Streptomycin | 1 g/day in adults i.m. or i.v. 750 mg if age > 40 and 500 mg if small. | Ototoxicity Hypersensitivity, especially in nurses giving injections. | Less used now for TB but useful in hepatic failure. Acquired resistance now common in other infections. |
| Gentamicin (Cidomycin; Genticin) | i.m. or i.v. 2–5 mg/kg/day in divided doses every 8 h. Use blood levels to control therapy — aim for peak < 10 $\mu$g/ml and trough < 2 $\mu$g/ml. Also given intrathecally for Gram negative meningitis. | Vestibular damage Reversible nephrotoxicity | Broad spectrum with activity against Pseudomonas so used for 'blind' treatment of serious infections with $\beta$-lactam |
| Tobramycin (Nebcin) | i.m. or i.v. 3–5 mg/kg/day in divided doses every 8 h. Use blood levels to control therapy. | Vestibular damage Less nephrotoxic than gentamicin. | More active than gentamicin against Pseudomonas but less active for other bacteria |
| Amikacin (Amikin) | i.m. or i.v. 15 mg/kg/day in 2 divided doses. | Mainly high-tone deafness | Potentially widest spectrum as stable to 8 of the 9 bacterial aminoglycoside-inactivating enzymes. Used for gentamicin resistant organisms. Expensive. |
| Kanamycin (Kannasyn; Kantrex) | i.m. 500 mg 12-hourly. p.o. 250–500 mg 6-hourly. Not recommended i.v. | Deafness mainly but mild nephrotoxicity relatively common | Largely superseded by gentamicin. Gut sterilisation. Topical application. |
| Neomycin | Not now used systemically because of deafness. 4 g/day orally. | Sensitisation if used topically. Prolonged oral administration may produce malabsorption syndrome. | Topical for Staphylococcal and Gram-negative infections. Gut sterilisation in liver disease. |

**Table 47** Antibacterial agents with special uses

| Drug | Dose | Pharmacokinetics | Toxicity | Uses |
|------|------|------------------|----------|------|
| Sodium fusidate (Fucidin) | 500 mg 6-hourly oral or i.v. (also local application to skin) | Usual oral dose gives peak plasma levels of 25 $\mu$g/ml within 3 h. $T_{\frac{1}{2}}$ = 4–6 h. Good organ penetration (but not into CSF). Penetrates pus and bone. Mainly metabolised. No cumulation in renal failure. | Low toxicity: mild GI disturbances. Allergy. Reversible changes in liver function tests and occasionally jaundice. | MIC *Staph. pyogenes* = 0.07 $\mu$g/ml. Reserved for serious staphylococcal infections especially osteomyelitis. Effective against penicillinase-producing & methicillin-resistant strains. Useful in penicillin allergic patients. |
| Vancomycin (Vancocin) | 1 g i.m. or i.v. twice daily. For enteritis & colitis 500 mg in water orally 6-hourly. | Not absorbed from gut. Enters pleural & ascitic fluid and CSF is meninges inflamed after 1 g i.v. plasma level of 2.5 $\mu$g/ml. 90% excreted in urine. Cumulation in renal failure. | Irritant: thrombophlebitis, necrosis if injection extravasates. Ototoxicity, proteinuria, rash, fever. | MIC for *Staph. pyogenes* = 0.16–1.8 $\mu$g/ml. MIC for *Strep. viridans* = 0.3–2.5 $\mu$g/ml. Use restricted to serious, refractory Gram-positive infections, e.g. *Staph. enterocolitis* & pseudo membranous colitis. Prophylaxis of bacterial endocarditis. |
| Chloramphenicol | 1.5–3.0 g daily in 3 or 4 divided doses orally or parenterally. Eye ointment. | Well absorbed from gut. Penetrates well into bile, eye, fetus, saliva, sputum & CSF. Metabolised and conjugated in liver with glucuronic acid. $T_{\frac{1}{2}}$ = 1.5–3 h. Impairs metabolism of phenytoin, tolbutamide, phenobarbitone. | Reversible, dose-dependent inhibition of erythropoiesis; irreversible idiosyncratic marrow aplasia (1 : 30 000). Rarely encephalopathy and optic neuritis. In neonates: grey-baby syndrome (circulatory collapse) due to failure of immature liver to glucuronidate chloramphenicol. | Typhoid & other serious Salmonella infections. *Haemophilus influenzae* meningitis. Topically for eye infections. |

**Table 48** Drugs used solely for urinary infections

| Drug | Dose | Pharmacokinetics | Toxicity | Uses |
|---|---|---|---|---|
| Nitrofurantoin (Furadantin) | 200–400 mg daily oral | Absorbed well by mouth. 1/3 excreted unchanged in urine (100 $\mu$g/ml urine attained on usual oral dose — but low concentrations in plasma) $T_{\frac{1}{2}}$ = 1 h. | Nausea common. Peripheral neuropathy if blood levels high, thus contraindicated by renal failure. Hypersensitivity (5%), produces rashes, fever & hepatitis (with +ve ANF). Rarely: bone marrow depression; pulmonary infiltration. Haemolytic anaemia if G6PD deficient. | Gram-negative urinary pathogens: $E.\ coli$ }  MIC for $< 35\ \mu$g/ml Klebsiella spp. } (Proteus spp. usually resistant; Pseudomonas always resistant) |
| Nalidixic Acid (Negram) | 1 g 6-hourly | Absorbed well by mouth. Peak plasma levels 25 $\mu$g/ml on usual oral dose. $T_{\frac{1}{2}}$ = 1–1$\frac{1}{2}$ h. Metabolised to hydroxynalidixic acid (active) which is excreted as glucuronide (inactive). Urinary concentration of active substances = 25–250 $\mu$g/ml after usual dose. Dose does not cumulate in moderate renal failure but toxic cumulation in severe renal disease. | Toxicity uncommon; GI disturbances; rashes; visual disturbances; raised intracranial pressure & fits. Haemolytic anaemia if G6PD deficient. | Gram-negative organisms MIC 10 $\mu$g/ml (apart from Pseudomonas and Bacteroides spp.) |
| Cinoxacin (Cinobac) | 500 mg twice daily for 2 weeks | Rapidly absorbed by mouth. 60% excreted unchanged in urine. $T_{\frac{1}{2}}$ = 1–1$\frac{1}{2}$ h. | Toxicity increased in renal failure. GI disturbances. Hypersensitivity. (urticaria; rashes; oedema). Transient changes in liver function tests. Not known if safe in pregnancy. | Similar spectrum to nalidixic acid. Used in acute and chronic urinary tract infections. |

**Table 49** Drugs for anaerobic and other infections

| Drug | Dose | Pharmacokinetics | Toxicity | Clinical use |
|---|---|---|---|---|
| Metronidazole (Flagyl) | Oral.: Anaerobic infections — 400 mg 6-hourly; Trichomonas vaginalis & acute ulcerative gingivitis — 200 mg 8-hourly for up to 7 days; Acute amoebic dysentery — 800 mg 8-hourly for 5 days. Rectal: 500 mg & 1 g suppositories. i.v.: Anaerobic infections 500 mg 8-hourly. | Well absorbed from gut and across mucosae. $T_{\frac{1}{2}} =$ 6–10 h. Penetrates into abscesses, bone, CNS & milk. Excreted in saliva & urine. Undergoes extensive hepatic metabolism so reduce dose in hepatic failure. | CNS: Reversible peripheral neuropathy (1–3%), ataxia, vertigo, headaches, fits. GI: (5–10%) nausea, vomiting, metallic taste, diarrhoea. Others: fever, reversible neutropenia. Interactions: Disulfiram-like with ethanol; potentiates warfarin and coumarins. | Anaerobic infections. Trichomonas vaginalis. Acute ulcerative gingivitis. Giardia lamblia infections. Acute amoebic dysentery, hepatitis & abscess. Tropical ulcer, dracontiasis, Dracunculus medinensis infestations. ? Crohn's disease. |
| Clindamycin (Dalacin C) — Lincomycin similar. | Oral: 150–300 mg 6-hourly. i.v. or i.m.: 0.6–2.7 g/day in 2–4 divided doses. | Well absorbed from gut. $T_{\frac{1}{2}} =$ 2 h. 85% undergoes hepatic metabolism and $T_{\frac{1}{2}}$ increased by cirrhosis, hepatitis or old age. Concentrated in bile and macrophages and polymorphs (so enters abscesses) but poor penetration into CNS. Levels in bone about 40% plasma level. | GI: diarrhoea (10–20%) — dose-related due to toxic effect on mucosa. Also more serious pseudomembranous colitis (2%). Allergy: Rash (3–5%) eosinophilia. | Anaerobic infections. Effective also in staphylococcal and pneumococcal infections. |

## PROPHYLAXIS OF INFECTIVE ENDOCARDITIS

### Required by patients with
a. Rheumatic and 'degenerative' valvular disease — especially mild aortic and mitral incompetence and mitral valve prolapse.
b. Congenital heart disease — especially small VSDs, Patent ductus and biscuspid aortic valves.
c. Prosthetic heart valves.

### For the following procedures
a. Dental, e.g. extractions, scaling.
b. Genito-urinary, e.g. instrumentation, complicated vaginal delivery.
c. Gastro-intestinal endoscopy and surgery.
d. Cardiac surgery.

### Principles
a. Bactericidal antibiotics required.
b. Administration immediately prior to procedure — prevents bacterial antibiotic resistance.
c. Effective antibiotic levels maintained for at least 10 hours after procedure.

### Methods

A. *Outside hospital*
(i) Oral amoxycillin  — 3 g 1 hour before procedure
                      — 3 g 8 hours after — optional
(ii) If allergic to penicillin
     Oral erythromycin  — 1 g 30 mins before procedure
                         — 500 mg 6-hourly × 4 after procedure

B. *In hospital*
(i) i.m. injection of mixture of benzylpenicillin, procaine penicillin and benzathine penicillin (e.g. Penidural, Triplopen) 20 minutes before procedure
(ii) If allergic to penicillin slow i.v. injection 1 g vancomycin 20 mins before procedure
(iii) If prosthetic valve present, give i.m. gentamicin 80 mg in addition to (i) or (ii).

## ANAEROBIC BACTERIAL INFECTIONS

Likely pathogens in:
  intra-abdominal sepsis
  non-venereal infections of genital tract
  aspiration pneumonia and lung abscess
Less common in:
  cutaneous and breast abscess
  brain abscess
  pelvic inflammatory disease
  chronic sinusitis and otitis media
  decubitus ulcers
  diabetic foot ulcers
  dental abscess

## Treatment

A.  *First line drugs*
1.  Metronidazole — 400 mg 6-hourly orally or by suppository
    500 mg 6-hourly (well absorbed rectally).
    i.v. — 15 mg/kg over 1 h then 7.5 mg/kg every 6 h.
N.B.  parenteral metronidazole is relatively expensive.
2.  Clindamycin — oral 300 mg 6-hourly p.o. or as i.v. infusion of
    clindamycin phosphate 200–300 mg every 6 h given over
    10–60 mins.

B.  *Second line drugs*
1.  Chloramphenicol — active against most anaerobic bacteria and
    enters CNS, but use reserved because of bone marrow toxicity.
2.  Penicillins — *B. fragilis* and several others are resistant.
    Benzylpenicillin agent of choice for gas gangrene and other
    clostridial infections; orodental and pulmonary infections by
    anaerobes. β-lactamase resistant penicillins are inferior but
    broad spectrum penicillins and carbenicillin-piperacillin group
    are alternatives to benzylpenicillin.
3.  Cephalosporins — first generation drugs similar to
    benzylpenicillin; cefoxitin useful for intra-abdominal sepsis;
    latamoxef most active against *B. fragilis*.

## Note on Pseudomembranous colitis (antibiotic associated colitis)

*Colitis*
— diarrhoea (rarely bloody)
— colicky abdominal pain
— tenesmus
— fever
Develops 4–10 days after beginning antibiotic. May be fatal.

*Associated with*

| *Common* | *Uncommon* |
|----------|------------|
| Clindamycin | Tetracycline |
| Lincomycin | Co-trimoxazole |
| Ampicillin | Cephalosporins |
| | Benzylpenicillin |
| | Chloramphenicol |
| | Metronidazole |

*Cause*
Enterotoxin from antibiotic-resistant overgrowth of *Clostridium difficile* in colon.

*Treatment*
1. Oral vancomycin 500 mg — 2 g/day for 2 weeks — kills *Cl. difficile*.
2. Cholestyramine 4 g 8-hourly for 2 weeks — binds toxin.

TREATMENT OF UNKNOWN SEVERE INFECTION IN THE IMMUNOSUPPRESSED OR DEBILITATED

Pending specific information from swabs, blood cultures etc, use:
1. Bactericidal antibiotics
2. Intravenous route
3. High doses of drugs
4. Antibiotics in combination to
   (i) achieve synergistic effect
   (ii) prevent emergence of resistance
   (iii) cover wide spectrum including anaerobes
   (iv) treat infection due to two or more organisms not equally susceptible to single agent.
Common combinations are:
Ampicillin + Gentamicin + Metronidazole
Piperacillin + Gentamicin
Cephotaxime
or Latamoxef  + Clindamycin + Metronidazole

PROPHYLACTIC ANTIBIOTICS IN SURGERY

1. Antibiotic should be present at high concentration when bacteria are inoculated — give drugs just prior to operation, e.g. with premedication, preferably i.v. or i.m.
2. Bactericidal drugs preferable.
3. Oral agents, e.g. for bowel preparation, require longer preoperative use so encouraging bacterial resistance; allow overgrowth of staphylococci, fungi; may result in pseudomembranous colitis.

**Table 50** First line anti-tuberculous drugs

| Drug | Pharmacology | Pharmacokinetics | Adverse effects |
|---|---|---|---|
| Isoniazid | Bactericidal. Interferes with mycolic acid synthesis in bacterial cell wall. Active against intracellular organisms. | Well absorbed with high CSF levels. Mainly hepatic elimination by genetically determined acetylation (see page 33) $T_{\frac{1}{2}} < 80$ min fast, $> 140$ min slow. Inhibits phenytoin and warfarin metabolism. | Peripheral neuropathy (mainly slow acetylators) — prevented by pyridoxine 10 mg/day. Disturbance of hepatic function — rarely hepatocellular failure, usually in old or alcoholics (? mainly fast acetylators). Occasionally fever, rash, lymphadenopathy, convulsions, psychosis. |
| Rifampicin (Rifadin) | Bactericidal. Inhibits bacterial DNA dependent RNA polymerase. | Well absorbed with high CSF levels. Deacetylated by liver and excreted in bile. $T_{\frac{1}{2}} = 1\frac{1}{2}$–5 h. Enzyme induction causes interactions with pill, anticoagulants, etc. | Transient elevation of hepatic enzymes — serious hepatotoxicity uncommon (mainly in alcoholics or in pre-existing liver disease). 'Flu' syndrome after high doses. Colours urine, tears, sweat, sputum red. |
| Ethambutol (Myambutol) | Bacteriostatic | Well absorbed but CSF poorly penetrated. Mainly eliminated unchanged in urine. $T_{\frac{1}{2}} = 5$–6 h. | Retrobulbar neuritis, 1% on high doses (usually reversible) — important to test vision. Polyneuritis. Pruritis. |
| Pyrazinamide (Zinamide) | Bactericidal | Well absorbed with high CSF levels — used for TB meningitis | Hepatotoxicity with occasional acute necrosis. Nausea and vomiting. Arthralgia, hyperuricaemia and gout. |

**Table 51** Second line anti-tuberculous drugs

| Drug | Dose | Special features & usefulness | Toxicity |
|---|---|---|---|
| Prothionamide* (Trevintix) | Up to 0.5 g twice daily or as a single evening dose with sedation | Rarely used because of GI toxicity | Gastric irritation Liver damage Neuropathy Mental disturbance |
| Thiacetazone | 2 mg/kg oral | Cheap, but use limited because of toxicity | High incidence of rashes |
| Cycloserine | 1 g/day oral | Main use in resistance to more conventional drugs. The most toxic of the second line drugs. | Mental disturbance Fits |
| Capreomycin (Capastat) | 15 mg/kg i.m. daily | Similar to streptomycin in actions and toxicity — but may be useful in patients with hypersensitivity or for resistant organisms | Ototoxicity } with high Nephrotoxicity } plasma levels Hypokalaemia Hypocalcaemia Hypomagnesaemia |
| PAS (Paramisan) | 10–12 g/day oral | Largely abandoned because of low efficacy and high toxicity. $T_{\frac{1}{2}} = 1$ h. | Gastric irritation Hepatitis Rashes (5–10% of patients) |

*Ethionamide (Trescatyl) is similar

4. Choice of agent:
   Biliary surgery — co-trimoxazole, cephazolin
   Vascular surgery — flucloxacillin
   Orthopaedic implantation — flucloxacillin
   Gastroesophageal surgery — cefuroxime
   Small/large bowel surgery — metronidazole + co-trimoxazole
   Gynaecological surgery — metronidazole + co-trimoxazole
   Amputation of gangrenous limbs — benzylpenicillin

## TREATMENT OF TUBERCULOSIS

**General principles**
1. At least 2 drugs given together prevent emergence of resistance.
2. Combination includes one first line bactericidal drug.
3. Poor compliance is commonest cause of failure, so drugs often given in combined formulations.
4. Tubercle bacillus grows slowly so treatment lasts months.

*First line drugs*
Isoniazid
Rifampicin
Streptomycin
Ethambutol
Pyrazinamide

*Reserve drugs*
Para aminosalicylic acid
Ethionamide
Prothionamide
Cycloserine
Thiocarlide
Capreomycin

**Standard regimen**
(British Thoracic and Tuberculosis Association 1976)
For 9 months:
Isoniazid    — 300 mg/day (+ 10–20 mg pyridoxine/day)
Rifampicin   — 450 mg/day if weight < 50 kg
             600 mg/day if weight > 50 kg
   Plus any of the following for first 2 months only:
Ethambutol   — 25 mg/kg/day or
Pyrazinamide — 20–30 mg/kg/day or
Streptomycin — 750 mg i.m. for 6 days a week.

Oral therapy given together once daily where possible (improves compliance; prevents acquired resistance due to failure to take one drug), e.g.:

Mynah  = isoniazid + ethambutol
Rifinah = isoniazid + rifampicin

Produces 100% sputum conversion and 1% relapse rate within 2 years of stopping treatment.

*Extrapulmonary TB* is treated similarly but for at least 12 months.

### Resistance to antituberculosis drugs

1. Mainly due to erratic drug taking (if patient unreliable — twice weekly streptomycin + high dose INH supervised)
2. Primary resistance: 4% with INH, rare with rifampicin and ethambutol.
3. Atypical mycobacteria: resistant to most standard anti-TB drugs, but may require no treatment or other drugs such as erythromycin.
4. Parenteral treatment is possible only with streptomycin, capreomycin, isoniazid and rifampicin.

### Use of steroids in TB

1. Suppression of drug allergy.
2. Large pleural effusions which have persisted despite drug therapy and repeated aspiration.
3. Resolution of large lymph nodes.
4. Reduction of toxaemia in severe disease.

LEPROSY

Mainstay still dapsone (because cheap) but resistance increasing and rifampicin (expensive) and clofazimine also used, often with dapsone.

### Dapsone

*Pharmacokinetics*
Well absorbed from gut.
$T_{\frac{1}{2}}$ 20 h. Metabolised in liver partly by polymorphic acetylation.

*Dose*
25–50 mg increasing to 400 mg twice weekly or 100 mg daily.
Given for 3–10 years in patients with few bacilli and for life in those with many.

*Adverse effects*
Neuropathy
Allergic dermatitis
GI effects (nausea, vomiting)
Anaemia
Lepra reactions (fever, erythema nodosum, iritis, polyneuritis)
  during treatment of leprosy.

*Uses apart from leprosy*
Dermatitis herpetiformis
Prophylaxis of chloroquine-resistant malaria (with pyrimethamine
as Maloprim).

## ANTIMALARIALS

### 1. Prophylaxis
Drugs used to prevent malaria:

*a. 4-amino quinolines*

 (i)  Chloroquine 300 mg weekly. Not usually toxic at this dose.
(ii)  Amodiaquine 400 mg weekly. Bone marrow suppression (rare).

*b. Folate reductase inhibitors*
 (i)  Pyrimethamine 25–50 mg weekly
(ii)  Proguanil 200 mg daily — effective if pyrimethamine resistance
      present.

*c. Chloroquine-resistant falciparum malaria*
  (i)  Dapsone 25 mg with proguanil 200 mg daily
 (ii)  Maloprim (pyrimethamine 12.5 mg with dapsone 100 mg)
       weekly
(iii)  Fansidar (pyrimethamine 25 mg with sulphadoxine 0.5 g)
       weekly

### 2. Treatment of acute attack

*a. Chloroquine*
In vivax terminates acute attack but not radically curative.
In falciparum usually curative.
Total oral dose 1.5 g (or 30 mg/kg):
   600 mg initially
   300 mg after 6 h
   300 mg daily for 2 days.

In severe falciparum m.:
  5–10 mg/kg i.v. every 12–24 h (each dose given over 4 h).
Toxicity in these doses:
  headache, visual disturbances
  pruritus
  GI disturbances.

|  | *Chloroquine* | *Quinine* |
|---|---|---|
| Absorption | Almost completely absorbed from intestine. Can be given i.v. and i.m. Excretion accelerated by acidifying urine. High concentration in all tissues. | Complete absorption from intestine. Peak levels at 1.3 h. Irritant and poor absorption i.m. and s.c. |
| $T_{\frac{1}{2}}$ | 120 h | 10 h (but prolonged in falciparum m.) |
| Elimination | 50–70% renal excretion unchanged, some hepatic metabolism. | 95% metabolised in liver |
| Non-malarial uses | Rheumatoid arthritis; Discoid lupus; Possible benefit in SLE; Photoallergic reactions; Clonorchis sinensis, Fasciola hepatica, & Paragonimus infestations. | Myotonia congenita 0.3–0.6 g 8-hourly Dystrophia myotonica 0.3–0.6 g 8-hourly Nocturnal leg cramps 0.2–3 g at night. |
| Toxicity | Prolonged treatment with large doses: retinopathy with loss of central acuity, macular pigmentation, retinal artery constriction. Lichenoid skin eruptions, bleaching of hair. Reduced T waves on ECG. Weight loss. Ototoxicity. | Large doses: cinchonism — tinnitus, deafness, headache, nausea, visual disturbances. GI disturbances. Rashes, Fever, Delirium, Tremor, Fits, Coma, Renal failure Haemolytic anaemia, Purpura. |

### b. Quinine
Mainly used to treat an acute attack of chloroquine-resistant falciparum.

Usual oral treatment: 10 mg/kg every 12 h for 4 doses, followed by 3 tablets of Fansidar (pyrimethamine 75 mg with sulphadoxine 1.5 g) to ensure eradication of disease. For recrudescence of treated malaria or for severe falciparum by i.v. infusion (10 mg/kg over 4 h, then repeat after an interval of 12 h).

### c. Mefloquine
Used with quinine in the treatment of chloroquine-resistant falciparum. 50% of patients develop GI disturbances, dizziness, nausea, weakness.

### 3. Treatment of relapse
Not usually required with *P. falciparum* and *P. malariae*. Following treatment of acute attack of *P. vivax*, prevent or treat febrile episodes with primaquine 15 mg of base (26.3 mg of phosphate) daily for 2 weeks. If G6PD deficient, may have to give proguanil HCl continuously (100 mg daily) for 3 years.

**Table 52** Antifungal agents — 1. Polyenes (Bind to fungal cell membrane sterols to increase permeability, leakage of cell constituents and cell death)

| Drug | General properties | Dose | Clinical use |
|---|---|---|---|
| Nystatin (Nystan) | Mainly for *Candida albicans*, but effective against other yeasts and fungi. Too toxic for systemic use so limited to superficial infections — topically not toxic or allergenic. Not absorbed from gut. Can be inhaled as aerosol for pulmonary infections and injected into cavities around a mycetoma without systemic absorption. Very safe — nausea if oral dose > 5 millin U/day. | One pessary per night for 14 nights. Sexual partner applies nystatin cream to glans for 14 days. Both take oral nystatin 500 000 U 8-hourly for 10 days. Nystatin suspension (100 000 U/ml) | Drug of choice for vaginal candidosis<br><br>Effective in oropharyngeal candidosis but nasty taste |
| Candicidin (Candeptin) | Similar properties to nystatin | Nystatin ointment, cream gel and dusting powder (100 000 U/g)<br><br>Candicidin vaginal tablets (3 mg) and ointment (0.6 mg/g) Natamycin vaginal tablets (25 mg) and cream (2%) | Cutaneous candidosis<br><br>Candicidin and natamycin effective in vaginal candidosis |
| Natamycin (Pimafucin) | | Natamycin 1% suspension for oral infections and 2% suspension for inhalation | Natamycin effective in oral and pulmonary candidosis |

| Drug | General properties | Dose | Clinical use |
|---|---|---|---|
| Amphotericin B (Fungilin; Fungizone) | More powerful action than nystatin against yeasts and fungi. Tolerated well topically and orally. Not absorbed from gut. Can be given systemically but toxic. High protein binding; poor penetration into body fluids.<br>*Toxicity:*<br>Renal damage common (reversible if drug stopped early and i.v. mannitol given). | Amphotericin lozenge 10 mg 3–4-hourly. | Drug of choice in oral candidosis |
| | | 1 mg i.v. test dose then 5 mg/day in 500 ml dextrose over 4–6 h. Increase daily by 5 mg increments to max 0.5 mg/kg for 5–6 weeks. With flucytosine give 0.3 mg/kg/day amphotericin. | Drug of choice in systemic mycoses — amphotericin must be started early |
| | | 0.025–1 mg intrathecal diluted in CSF. | Fungal meningitis |
| | Headache, chills, hypotension. Drug fever (give 50 mg cortisol i.v.). Anaemia. | 5–16 mg intra-articular injections. | Mycotic joint infections |
| | Vomiting (give chlorpromazine 50 mg). | 1 ml amphotericin B suspension (100 mg/ml) | Oesophageal candidosis |
| | Hypokalaemia. | Amphotericin B tablets 100 mg. | Reduction of carriage of yeasts in gut |

**Table 53** Antifungal agents — 2 Non-polyenes

| Drug | General properties | Dose | Clinical use |
|---|---|---|---|
| Flucytosine (Alcobon) | Interferes with fungal RNA and DNA synthesis. Narrow spectrum synthetic antifungal — but effective against candida, cryptococcus and torulopsis. Ineffective against filamentous fungi (e.g. aspergillosis). Well absorbed from gut and widely distributed in body fluids including CSF. Low protein binding. Can be used with amphotericin B and imidazoles. Resistance can develop during treatment: little toxicity at levels below 100 $\mu$g/ml serum; above this can cause depression of marrow and liver function. Cumulation in renal failure. | Normal renal function: 50 mg/kg i.v. or oral 6-hourly. (Monitor levels in renal failure 25–100 $\mu$g/ml). | Drug of choice in systemic yeast infections (if strain is sensitive): particularly candida infections in immuno-suppressed patients and cryptococcal meningitis. Given with amphotericin B to prevent emergence of resistant organisms which occurs rapidly when flucytosine given alone. |
| *Imidazoles:* | Inhibit ergosterol synthesis in cell membrane and block peroxidase | Main use in topical infections due to candida and dermatophytes. | |
| Miconazole (Daktarin) | Can also be given i.v. (for systemic candida and coccidioides immitis). Parenterally has mild toxic effects similar to amphotericin. ?Potentiates warfarin. | Miconazole: gel 25 mg/ml 2% cream; 2% dusting powder. 250 mg miconazole tablets. | Oral candidosis skin infections by candida and dermatophytes. Fungal infections of oropharynx and GI. |
| | | Miconazole injection (10 mg/ml): 600 mg 8-hourly i.v. in 500 ml saline. | Systemic candidosis and coccidioides in patients who cannot tolerate amphotericin B. |

**Table 53** (continued)

| Drug | General properties | Dose | Clinical use |
|---|---|---|---|
| Ketoconazole (Nizoral) | Well absorbed from stomach if pH < 3. Does not enter CSF. Relatively non-toxic: rashes, gynaecomastia. | 200 mg p.o. once daily with food (important not to take fasting or with antacids, $H_2$-blockers or anticholinergics). | Systemic aspergillosis (given as oral capsules or i.v.). Tinea — all forms. Chronic mucocutaneous candidosis. |
| Other imidazoles include Econozole and Clotrimazole. | | | |
| Griseofulvin (Fulcin; Grisovin) | Inhibits polymerisation of tubular protein into microtubules in fungi at mitosis. Well absorbed from gut (especially with fatty food). Low plasma levels but concentrated in keratin. Effective in dermatophyte infections. Not effective against yeasts or topically. *Toxicity:* headache, nausea and vomiting, potentiates action of alcohol. Contraindicated in porphyria and in serious lung disease. Decreases efficacy of coumarin anticoagulants. | 500–1000 mg daily orally with meals as single or divided dose. For children 10 mg/kg/day. 4 week treatment for skin and hair. 1 year treatment for nails. | Indicated for dermatophyte infections which have not responded to topical treatment. |
| Iodides | Oral toxicity: GI discomfort, lymphadenopathy, lacrimation, rashes, exacerbates dermatitis herpetiformis. | Saturated KI (1 g/ml) orally: 1 ml 8-hourly increasing to 4 ml 8-hourly. Treatment continues for 6 weeks after lesions have healed. | Indicated for lymphocutaneous spororotrichosis and for subcutaneous phycomycosis due to *Basidiobolus haptosporus*. |
| | Local irritation | Povidone-iodine (Betadine) 200 mg pessary twice daily for 10 days. | Effective in vaginal candidosis. |

**Table 54** Antiviral drugs

| Drug | Mechanism of action | Clinical use | Dose | Adverse effects |
|---|---|---|---|---|
| Vidarabine | Phosphorylated then competitively inhibits herpes virus DNA-polymerase. ? incorporated into viral and cellular DNA, i.e. not selective for viral DNA. | Herpes simplex eye infections (as effective as IDU for herpes keratitis and essential for IDU resistant viruses). Herpes simplex encephalitis varicella or herpes zoster in immuno-compromised patients (possible benefit in chronic hepatitis B carriers). | 3% eye ointment. 200 mg/ml of monohydrate for i.v. injections (Vira-A) 15 mg/kg/day 10 mg/kg/day | GI — nausea, anorexia, diarrhoea CNS — confusion, ataxia, dizziness Marrow — suppression |
| Idoxuridine | Antimetabolite like vidarabine | Herpes zoster and herpes labialis Genital herpes Herpes simplex eye infections | 5% IDU in DMSO solution (Herpid) 20% IDU in DMSO topically 0.5% IDU ointment or 0.1% IDU drops topically | Avoid contact of conc. solutions with mucous membranes |
| Acyclovir (Zovirax) | Phosphorylated by specific enzyme in herpes infected cells then inhibits herpes DNA-polymerase 10–30 × more than host DNA-polymerase, i.e.: *selective toxicity.* | Herpes simplex corneal ulcers Herpes simplex and zoster in immuno-compromised patients. Possibly effective in herpes encephalitis. Genital herpes | 3% ointment as effective as IDU. i.v.: 5 mg/kg in 1 hr every 8 hours. p.o. 200 mg 4-hourly | Raised urea and creatinine. Inflammation if extravasates. Reduce dose in renal failure. |
| Amantadine (Symmetrel) | Interferes with uncoating of Influenza A virus prior to cell penetration. | Prophylaxis and reduction of severity of influenza A in vulnerable patients. | 100 mg 12-hourly p.o. | CNS: Confusion, excitement, hallucinations (N.B. has an amphetamine-like action — see page 116). |

# Cancer chemotherapy

**Definitions**
*Doubling time* — time for tumour to double cell number.
*Cell cycle time* — time for cell to go through cell cycle.
*Growth fraction* ($G_F$) — proportion of tumour in cell cycle. This fraction may be very large (75–80%) in small tumours which are thus sensitive to treatments which kill dividing cells.

Many tumour cells grow rapidly but cycle times overlap with normal, e.g.
Polychromatophil normoblast — 15–18 h
Leukaemic blast — 50–80 h
Large intestinal epithelium — 25–53 h
Myeloma cell — 2–6 days.

Slow growth implies long period of tumour growth before clinical presentation — as tumour grows doubling time increases and $G_F$ decreases.

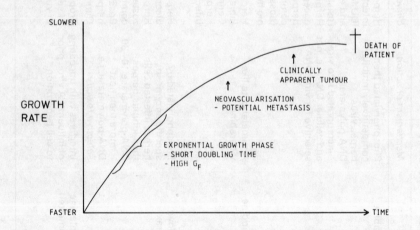

| No. of doublings | 0 | 10 | 20 | 30 | 40 |
|---|---|---|---|---|---|
| No. of cells $10^0$ | | $10^3$ | $10^6$ | $10^9$ | $10^{12}$ |
| Tumour weight | | $1\,\mu g$ | $1\,mg$ | $1\,g$ | $1\,kg$ |

Note:
1. Clinical presentation of tumours is late — after about 30 doublings — death occurs after only another 10 doublings.
2. Metastasis occurs early — 1 mg tumour burden.

## Cell cycle and phase specificity of cytotoxic drugs

$G_0$ — quiescent, resting non-replicative phase
$G_1$ — pre-replicative
S — DNA replication ⎫ Cellular
$G_2$ — post-replicative ⎬ Proliferation
M — mitosis (prophase, metaphase, anaphase, ⎭
 telophase)

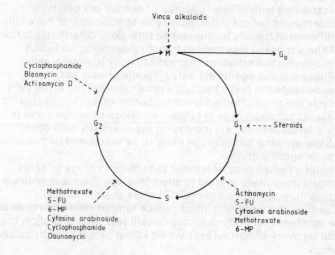

| Group | Specificity | Part of cycle affected | Dosage limitation |
|---|---|---|---|
| Alkylating agents | Non-cycle dependent | $G_0$ M $G_1$ | Total dose |
| Antimetabolites | Phase | S or $G_1$/S | Time of dose |
| Antibotics | Cycle | $G_2$ M some $G_1$ | Time and to lesser extent dose |
| Plant alkaloids | Phase | M or /$G_1$ | Time of dose |
| Corticosteroids | Probably non-cycle dependent | ? $G_1$ | ? |

Cell kills of neoplastic cells (‗ ‗) vs normal bone marrow (‗‗‗)

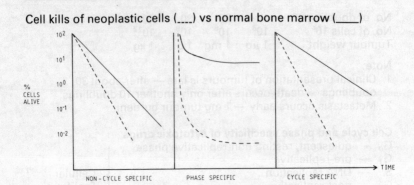

N.B.
1. For each agent same degree of killing of neoplastic cells associated with different degree of normal cell death, i.e. therapeutic indices differ. Non-cycle specific agents have little differential toxicity for tumour so total dose determines toxicity. Others more or less toxic to tumour depending on $G_F$ but increasing dose does not increase toxicity to normal cells.
2. Phase specific agents act only on some phases so dose-response curve reaches a maximum but the faster cells cycle the more effective the drug becomes; cycle non-specific agents act on all cells in tumour and dose-response curve is log-linear with cell kill increasing exponentially with dose.
3. Slow growing tumours not likely to be eradicated by phase or cycle specific drugs.

High $G_F$ means greater tumour sensitivity to drugs so small tumours most likely to yield to chemotherapy (hence sometimes 'debulk' tumour with surgery/DXT before chemotherapy).

Curative chemotherapy must reduce tumour cells to nil or to such low numbers that body defences can kill rest. Aim is to allow more rapid recovery of normal cells whilst killing cancer cells by pulsed therapy.

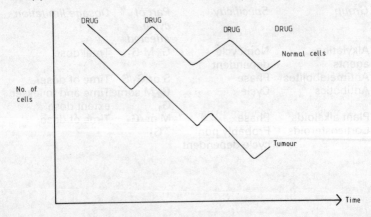

Drug combinations given as intermittent pulses:
 (i)  each drug of mixture has different toxicity so each used in optimal dose
 (ii)  each acts at different biochemical site
(iii)  combination is additive or synergistic
(iv)  some agents chosen to penetrate certain site, e.g. CNS
Clinical remission does not indicate cure: treatment for inapparent disease and micrometastases is needed — adjuvent or maintenance therapy. Cycle or phase-specific drugs useful here because micrometastases have high $G_F$ — if non-cycle dependent drugs used dose must be low to avoid toxicity.
May be necessary to prevent recurrence from tumour nest in *sanctuary site* (immune from drug penetration), e.g. CNS, testis by specific drug therapy e.g. inject methotrexate into CSF.
*Adjuvent chemotherapy* — to destroy disseminated microfoci of malignancy when no clinical evidence of residual disease present. Eradication should be easier because:
 (i)  tumour small so greater blood supply; $G_F$ higher
 (ii)  less immunosuppression when tumour small
(iii)  less bone marrow suppression/infiltration allow greater tolerance to chemotherapy.
But because disease clinically inapparent some cured patients will be exposed to hazards of treatment. Evidence of improved survival in Wilms' tumour, Ewing's tumour, acute lymphoblastic leukaemia; osteogenic sarcoma but in breast cancer it is controversial.

## Toxic effects of cancer chemotherapy
Major problems dur to inability of drug action to differentiate normal from neoplastic cells:
1. Bone marrow
   — leucopenia; thrombocytopenia; rarely anaemia or total aplasia.
   — immunosuppression and infections.
2. GI tract
   — ulceration of mouth and intestine.
   — diarrhoea.
3. Testis
   — azoospermia.
4. Ovary
   — infertility; premature menopause.
5. Hair follicles
   — alopecia.
6. Induction of second malignancies — e.g. acute myeloid leukaemia, non-Hodgkin's lymphoma.
7. Hyperuricaemia due to rapid tumour lysis.
   Many drugs also locally irritant or have special toxicity.

## DRUGS USED IN CANCER CHEMOTHERAPY

Various groups:
1. Alkylating agents
2. Anti-metabolites
3. Plant alkaloids
4. Anti-tumour antibiotics
5. Random synthetics and enzymes
6. Hormones

## 1. ALKYLATING AGENTS

Act via reactive alkyl ($R\text{-}CH_2\text{-}CH_2^+$) groups which react with nucleic acids (also proteins, enzymes) and inhibit function. Most important sites of attack are: guanine (7 position), cytosine (3 position) and adenine (1 and 3 positions). Most powerful agents are bifunctional with 2 reactive alkyl groups and can form strong inter- and intrastrand bridges within and between DNA and RNA strands preventing DNA replication and RNA translation.

### Cyclophosphamide (Endoxana)

*Mode of action*
Not itself cytotoxic — activated in vitro by mainly hepatic microsomal enzymes to several reactive metabolites which when taken up by cells may liberate other alkylators: phosphoramide mustard most likely to be main active metabolite.

*Pharmacokinetics*
Given orally or i.v. $T_{\frac{1}{2}}$ 6–12 h — inactivation by hepatic (? kidney) enzymes. Little excreted unchanged by kidneys but renal excretion of more polar active metabolites results in 'chemical' cystitis. Activation and elimination enhanced by enzyme inducers: effect on therapeutic efficacy unknown.

*Adverse effects*
Nausea and vomiting (50%) — frequently occurs following day, may last 72 h.

Alopecia — often marked in young (? because hair grows rapidly). Regrowth sometimes during treatment usual — takes 6–9 months.

Cystitis — drink 2 l/water/day for at least 48 h after drug and empty bladder frequently. Bladder irrigation with cysteine may help.

Myelosuppression at 7–10 days — platelets relatively spared.

Visual effects; hyponatraemia (? due to inappropriate ADH secretion or ADH potentiation by drug); hyperpigmentation; myocarditis.

*Uses*
Hodgkin's and non-Hodgkin's lymphoma
Leukaemias and Myeloma
Breast, lung, ovarian carcinomas
Soft tissue and bone sarcomas
Powerful immunosuppressant

**Ifosfamide (Mitoxana)**
Isomer of cyclophosphamide activated to some of the same active metabolites but also some different ones. Has less myelosuppressant but greater renal toxic effects. Only used i.v. for lung, pancreatic, testicular cancer.

**Nitrosoureas**
Carmustine or BCNU
Lomustine or CCNU
Methyl-CCNU
Streptozotocin

Alkylate nucleic acids and proteins via chloroethyl ($CH_2CH_2Cl$) groups.
Carbamylate proteins via isocyanate (R-NCO) group.
Highly lipid soluble so enter CNS.

*Pharmacokinetics*
Methyl-CCNU, CCNU rapidly and completely absorbed orally.
BCNU given i.v. Rapid hepatic metabolism to active metabolites — also spontaneous degradation.

*Adverse effects*
Myelosuppression occurs late (30–40 days after treatment)
   Nausea and vomiting 2–6 hrs after drug, often severe but rarely lasts > 24 hrs.
   Nephrotoxicity and hyperglycaemia only with streptozotocin.
   BCNU injection is painful.

*Uses*
CCNU and BCNU useful in Hodgkins lymphoma
BCNU — malignant gliomas
Streptozotocin — islet cell tumours of pancreas

**Dacarbazine (DTIC)**
Probably alkylating agent.
   Poorly absorbed given orally and irritant if injected so given slowly into fast i.v. drip.
   Short $T_{\frac{1}{2}}$ (30 mins) with hepatic metabolism and renal excretion (50% as active metabolite).
   Nausea and vomiting common; myelosuppression at about 3 weeks. Other effects: 'flu-like illness; fever; paraesthesiae.
   Used in Hodgkin's lymphoma; melanomas.

**Table 55** Commonly used alkylating agents

| Drug | Pharmacokinetics | Adverse effects | Comments | Uses |
|---|---|---|---|---|
| Mustine or Nitrogen mustard | Short plasma $T_{\frac{1}{2}}$ 10 mins so only given i.v. or into pleural cavity for malignant effusions | *Venous thrombosis* (give non-steroidal anti-inflammatory agent orally 12 h before to 36 h after mustine). *Myelosuppression* — nadir at 7 days. *Nausea and vomiting* — common within 1 h of dosing, often severe. | Solution unstable (given into fast-flowing drip) and irritant (avoid contact with skin, eyes; extravasation) | Hodgkin's lymphoma |
| Chlorambucil (Leukeran) | Rapid and extensive absorption from gut. Plasma $T_{\frac{1}{2}}$ 1–2 h. Hepatic metabolism to phenylacetic mustard. Minimal (< 1%) renal excretion. | Myelosuppression seen at 3–4 weeks — may be prolonged possibly because it is especially toxic to stem cells. Other effects (nausea, stomatitis, alopecia, diarrhoea) rare. | Effective orally and usually given over long periods (month or more) | Lymphomas. Chronic lymphatic leukaemia. Ovarian and breast carcinoma. |
| Melphalan (Alkeran) | L-phenylalanine mustard. Incomplete and erratic absorption from gut. Plasma $T_{\frac{1}{2}}$ 1–2 h. Mainly spontaneous hydrolysis to inactive mono and dihydroxymelphalan but 10–20% excreted via kidneys. | Myelosuppression occurs later (21–24 days) than after most other alkylating agents. Other effects (nausea, stomatitis, alopecia, diarrhoea) rare. | Used mainly orally but i.v. preparation available and better GI absorption of chlorambucil makes latter likely to replace oral melphalan. | Multiple myeloma; Ovarian and breast carcinoma; Melanoma. |

| Busulphan (Myleran) | Hepatic metabolism to inactive compounds. Pharmacokinetics little known. Given orally. | *Myelosuppression* can occur unexpectedly days or weeks after starting treatment. Toxic to stem cells and irreversible marrow failure can occur. *Skin pigmentation; Addisonian-like wasting syndrome* rare and not associated with adrenal failure. *Irreversible interstitial pneumonitis and pulmonary fibrosis after several months treatment. Depression ovarian function and amenorrhoea* | Unlike other drugs active groups are methone sulphoxy radicles | Chronic myeloid leukaemia |

## 2. ANTIMETABOLITES

**Methotrexate**

*Mode of action*
Inhibits dihydrofolate reductase.

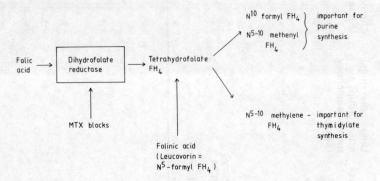

Methotrexate (MTX) blocks formation of active folates required for 1 carbon transfers, e.g. in DNA synthesis. Block bypassed by administration of folinic acid. Cell cycle dependent — acts on S-phase.

*Pharmacokinetics*
Low doses ($< 30$ mg/m$^2$) completely absorbed from gut. Higher doses absorbed slowly and incompletely — ? saturable absorption process — therefore better given i.v.

Three half-lives (i.e. 3-compartment pharmacokinetic model):
$T_{\frac{1}{2}}\alpha$: 15–40 mins (distribution).
$T_{\frac{1}{2}}\beta$: 3–6 h (renal elimination + metabolism) — chief determinant of toxicity with low doses.
$T_{\frac{1}{2}}\gamma$: 6–70 h (enterohepatic recirculation + redistribution) — chief determinant of toxicity after high doses.

MTX after high doses distributes into CSF but more usual to give intrathecally. Redistribution from CSF and deep compartments (especially if effusions present) causes toxicity.

Renal elimination most important (caution in renal failure) — tubular secretion (reduced by probenecid) also biliary secretion but MTX is recycled and little is lost in faeces although some metabolised by gut bacteria. Variable hepatic and gut flora metabolism (20–60% dose) — important metabolite is 7-hydroxy MTX since low solubility at acid pH causes crystalluria and renal damage.

*Dose*
Conventional low dose — 15 mg/m$^2$ twice weekly.
   High dose infusion therapy (30–250 mg/kg) with folinate rescue. MTX toxicity depends upon duration plasma concentration remains above the toxic threshold beyond 24 hours. Monitoring of plasma MTX and administration of folinate (100–1000 mg/m$^2$ calcium leucovorin i.v.) until plasma level < 20 nM gives maximum anti-tumour effect with marrow protection.
   Intrathecal — given via Ommeyer reservoir into cranial CSF for treatment of intracranial deposits (lumbar injection inadequate).

*Adverse effects*
Myelosuppression.
Gastro-intestinal mucositis; nausea and vomiting.
Hepatitis and cirrhosis with chronic oral therapy (e.g. for psoriasis).
Nephrotoxicity.
Neurotoxicity mainly after intrathecal injection:
— arachnoiditis (mimics meningitis)
— motor dysfunction
— necrotising, demyelinating leukoencephalopathy.
   Before initiation of high dose therapy creatinine clearance and IVP required.

*Interactions*
Increased toxicity:
salicylates, sulphonamides (decreased renal clearance + altered protein binding).
phenytoin (displaced binding).
probenecid (decreased renal excretion).
Decreased efficacy:
steroids, 1-asparaginase, bleomycin, penicillin, kanamycin (decreased cellular MTX uptake).
? allopurinol (increased intracellular purines).
neomycin, sulphathiazole (decreased GI absorption).

*Uses*
Chorioncarcinoma
Acute lymphatic leukaemia
Osteogenic sarcoma
Many malignancies including head and neck, epidermal carcinomas, breast, teratoma, non-Hodgkin's lymphoma.

**Table 56** Commonly used antimetabolites

| Drug | Mode of action | Pharmacokinetics | Adverse effects | Uses |
|---|---|---|---|---|
| 5-fluorouracil (Fluoro-uracil) | Inactive until converted in cell to nucleosides (Fluorouridine + Fluorodeoxyuridine) then phosphorylated. These block thymidylate synthetase and also incorporate into RNA. | Incomplete GI absorption + extensive hepatic metabolism so usually given i.v. $T_{\frac{1}{2}}$ = 10–40 mins. Some renal excretion (20%). Sometimes given via hepatic artery infusion for hepatic metastases. | *Oral ulcers, diarrhoea, nausea* but rarely vomiting. *Bone marrow depression Cerebellar ataxia* (2%) after intrathecal injection (? forms toxic fluorocitrate) | Cancer of GI tract Breast, Ovary, Skin |
| 6-mercaptopurine-6MP- (Puri-Nethol) | Inhibit enzymes of purine synthesis so block DNA & RNA synthesis. Incorporated into DNA and RNA causing strand breaks and misinformation. | Complete GI absorption. Hepatic metabolism by xanthine oxidase (so ↑ toxicity if allopurinol given — reduce 6MP dose by 2/3). + renal elimination (20%). | *Myelosuppression* (leucopenia > thrombocytopenia) *Hepatotoxic* (jaundice 30% adults) *Nausea, vomiting, diarrhoea* only with high doses | Childhood acute lymphatic adult myeloid leukaemia. Immunosuppression. |
| Cytosine arabinoside (Cytosar) | Converted to triphosphate in cell which inhibits DNA polymerase | Poor GI absorption and hepatic metabolism (activation by kinases + inactivation by deaminases) so given i.v. $T_{\frac{1}{2}}$ 1–3 h. Renal metabolism (deamination) and elimination also occurs. Penetrates CSF. | *Myelosuppression; Nausea and vomiting; Fever* during treatment | Acute leukaemia Intrathecal use for meningeal carcinoma; leukaemia or lymphoma |

## 3. PLANT ALKALOIDS

**Vinca alkaloids**
Derived from periwinkle plant (Vinca rosea): Vincristine (Oncovin); Vinblastine (Velbe); Vindesine (Eldisine).

*Mode of action*
Bind to microtubules and disrupt spindle thus blocking mitosis. Other microtubular functions (maintenance cell shape, membrane mobility and integrity) also affected.

*Pharmacokinetics*
Erratic oral absorption so given i.v. but both are very irritant if extravasated.
$T_\frac{1}{2}$ approx 3 h. Undergo extensive binding to formed blood elements. Hepatic metabolism + biliary excretion — some metabolites cytotoxic. Increased toxicity with hepatic impairment so dose modification indicated.

*Adverse effects*
*Vincristine*:
Neurotoxicity — motor, sensory and autonomic (usually constipation) neuropathy — usually dose-limiting effect.
Jaw pain.
Inappropriate ADH secretion.
Leucopenia and nausea and vomiting relatively uncommon.
*Vinblastine*:
Myelosuppression nadir at 7–10 days (leucopenia > thrombocylopenia) — usually dose-limiting effect.
Nausea and vomiting.
Neurotoxicity does occur but is uncommon.
*Both drugs*:
Alopecia (5–10%) usually patchy.

*Uses*
*Vincristine*:
Acute lymphatic leukaemia.
Hodgkin's and non-Hodgkin's lymphoma.
Breast, testicular carcinoma.
Sarcomas.
Wilms tumour.
Neuroblastoma.
*Vinblastine*:
Non-Hodgkin's lymphoma.
Breast, testicular carcinoma.
Chorionepithelioma.

## Podophyllotoxin VP 16-213 (Etoposide)

Alkaloid from May Apple.

Spindle poison preventing cells entering mitosis but unlike vinca alkaloids no interference with microtubules. May also block DNA synthesis.

Can be given orally or i.v. $T_{\frac{1}{2}} = 11.5$ h.

Dose limiting adverse effect is myelosuppression with nausea, vomiting and reversible alopecia also common.

New agent but very active in small cell lung cancer; also active for acute lymphatic leukaemia and lymphoma.


## 4. ANTITUMOUR ANTIBIOTICS

### Doxorubicin (Adriamycin)

Anthracycline antibiotic produced by *Streptomyces peucetius*.

*Mode of action*

Intercalates DNA helix thus uncoiling and preventing DNA and RNA synthesis.

*Pharmacokinetics*

Poor (< 5%) absorption from gut.

$T_{\frac{1}{2}} = 16-20$ h. Extensive hepatic metabolism and biliary secretion (before use determine liver function and reduce dose if plasma bilirubin increased) only 10% excreted in urine. Some metabolites may be active. Active drug uptake by cells.

*Adverse effects*

Irritant — avoid contact with skin or eyes and extravasation. Must be given slowly i.v. to avoid venous irritation and cardiac arrhythmias.

Myelosuppression — 12-14 days after dose (later than many cytotoxics).

Cardiotoxicity — dose-related cardiomyopathy with cardiomegaly and cardiac failure. Total doses > 550 mg/m$^2$ associated with 20-30% risk cardiotoxicity. If mediastinal radiotherapy or cyclophosphamide used dose should not exceed 450 mg/m$^2$.

Nausea and vomiting common, may be moderate to severe.

Alopecia — common and often total if used with cyclophosphamide. Head cooling may prevent but is cumbersome.

Radiation-recall phenomenon — erythema and skin oedema in skin previously irradiated.

Red urine passed after drug (not haematuria!).

*Uses*

Hodgkin's and non-Hodgkin's lymphomas.

Breast, lung, ovarian, gastric, bladder (sometimes injected into lesions), endometrial and testicular carcinomas.

Bone and soft-tissue sarcomas.

**Table 57** Some antitumour antibiotics

| Drug | Mode of action | Pharmacokinetics | Adverse effects | Uses |
|---|---|---|---|---|
| Bleomycin | Fragments DNA strand. Inhibits incorporation of thymidine into DNA. | Mixture of polypeptides. Renal excretion (60% unchanged in urine), rest undergoes hepatic metabolism. Plasma $T_{\frac{1}{2}}$ 9 h. Elimination prolonged by renal failure (caution when used with nephrotoxic drugs, e.g. aminoglycosides, high dose methotrexate). Highly bound to skin, lungs. | *Oral ulcers* — unusual if dose not greater than 30 mg/week. *Skin* — hyperpigmentation, erythema, oedema, pain. All reversible. Also radiation-recall skin damage. *Lungs* — fibrosis and pneumonitis — irreversible and sometimes fatal. Minimise risk by keeping total dose < 200 mg and doing regular X-rays. *Flu-like illness* — fever, chills within 4–8 h dose in 10% patients. N.B. Bleomycin not associated with clinically important marrow toxicity. | Lymphomas. Testicular and squamous cell carcinoma of head and neck. |

| Drug | Mode of action | Pharmacokinetics | Adverse effects | Uses |
|---|---|---|---|---|
| Mithramycin (Mithracin) | Binds to DNA and inhibits DNA-directed RNA synthesis | Unknown. Renal impairment enhances toxicity. | *Hepatotoxicity*—raises transaminases. *Myelosuppression and Haemorrhage* (↓ platelets + vascular toxic effect + ↓ clotting factors) Nausea and vomiting | In dose of 25 μg/kg every 2–4 days inhibits osteoclasts and reduces Ca$^{++}$ in hypercalcaemia from any cause |
| Actinomycin (Cosmegen Lyovac) | Binds to DNA and inhibits RNA polymerase and thus RNA synthesis | Poorly absorbed from gut. Very short plasma $T_{\frac{1}{2}}$ but long tissue $T_{\frac{1}{2}}$ (50–90%) and renal (5–20%) excretion of unchanged drug. | Ulceration of mouth Myelosuppression Alopecia | Wilms' tumour Chorioncarcinoma Some sarcomas |

## 5. RANDOM SYNTHETICS AND ENZYMES

### Procarbazine (Natulan)
Hydralazine monoamine oxidase inhibitor.

*Mode of action*
Depolymerises DNA without affecting double helix structure.
Mechanism unknown? acts as alkylating agent — methylates
adenine and guanine residues.

*Pharmacokinetics*
Requires activation to azo-derivative.
  Rapid and almost complete GI absorption. Plasma $T_{\frac{1}{2}}$ of
procarbazine $\sim$ 10 mins. Undergoes hepatic metabolism to
compounds (? cytotoxic) which are renally excreted. Procarbazine
and metabolites can penetrate CNS.

*Adverse effects*
Dose-related myelosuppression (nadir 7 – 10 days).
  Nausea and vomiting initially but less prominent after several
doses.
  Procarbazine is weak, MAOI-food interactions rare but alcohol
sometimes causes blotchy, purplish facial flush. Care with tricyclic
antidepressants, sympathomimetics and CNS depressants.

*Uses*
Hodgkins and non-Hodgkins lymphomas.

### Cisplatin (Neoplatin)
Platinum diamminodichloride — heavy metal coordination
compound (expensive), only inorganic compound used in cancer
chemotherapy.

*Mode of action*
Cycle non-specific agent.
Relatively selective DNA synthesis inhibitor (? acts like bifunctional
  alkylator).
? enhances tumour immunogenicity.

*Pharmacokinetics*
Only given by i.v. injection or infusion.
Elimination $T_{\frac{1}{2}}$ 58 – 73 h but low urinary excretion up to 1 month
  after treatment.
High protein and tissue binding.
Urinary elimination.

*Dose*
Schedules vary from bolus to 5 day infusions.
   Before treatment creatinine clearance and audiogram necessary.
Do not give if serum creatinine > 130 $\mu$mol/l. Important to
maintain high urine flow as cisplatin is nephrotoxic by fluid
infusion, sufficient to maintain output > 200 ml/h.
   Renal toxicity cumulative so measure serum creatinine before
each course.

*Adverse effects*
Vomiting and diarrhoea 2–4 h after starting drug and severe for
several hours — may last mildly for up to a week.
   Nephrotoxicity: dose-related, cumulative, irreversible tubular
necrosis.
   Ototoxicity: high tone deafness (up to 30% patients) ± tinnitus.
May be irreversible.
   Myelosuppression: dose-related and cumulative especially with
radiotherapy or other chemotherapy.
   Others: neuropathy, rashes, hypomagnesaemia.

*Uses*
Testicular and ovarian cancer.
Possibly bladder and head and neck cancers.

**Colaspase (Crasnitin)**
L-asparaginase produced by *E. coli*.

*Mode of action*
Some tumour cells (unlike normal cells) cannot synthesise
asparagine. Colaspase hydrolyses free plasma and tissue
asparagine so depriving tumour of exogenous amino acid.

*Pharmacokinetics*
Hydrolysed in gut so given i.v. — does not penetrate CNS so given
intrathecally if required.
   $T_{\frac{1}{2}}$ 8–30 h — probably taken up by reticulo-endothelial cells.

*Adverse effects*
Nausea, anorexia and vomiting.
Allergic reactions to foreign protein (fever, chills, anaphylaxis).
N.B. No effect on bone marrow.

*Clinical use*
Acute leukaemias and some lymphomas.

## 6. HORMONES

May produce remission in some cancers but do not eradicate disease.

### 1. Oestrogen used for 2 cancers which are partially hormone-dependent

a. *Prostatic carcinoma*
Oestrogens block androgen production with remission in 60% patients with advanced disease.

Diethylstilboestrol 1 mg 8-hourly as effective as high dose stilboestrol. Fosfestrol (Honvan) 100–200 mg 8-hourly reducing to once daily is activated by acid phosphatase to stilboestrol but is no more effective and can produce pain in metastases.

Main adverse effects are nausea, fluid retention (hypertension, oedema, heart failure), thromboembolism, feminisation and loss of libido.

b. *Breast cancer*
Oestrogens give remission in 30% women with advanced disease who are 5 years post-menopausal but may exacerbate disease in younger women. Tumours with oestrogen receptors 6 times more likely to respond (60%) than receptor negative tumours (10%). Hormone responsiveness inversely proportional to tumour aggressiveness; tumours metastates only to skin or bone have 30% response but lung or liver metastases show 10% response.

Diethylstilboestrol 1–15 mg/day in divided doses.

*Adverse effects*
Nausea
Fluid retention
Hypercalcaemia — serum $Ca^{++}$ may rise rapidly especially with bony metastases.

### 2. Anti-oestrogens for breast cancer

a. *Tamoxifen (Nolvadex)*
Competes with oestradiol for cytoplasmic receptor. Few side effects and as effective as diethylstilboestrol. Dose 10 mg 12-hourly. Main toxicity: nausea; secondary to anti-oestrogen effect (hot flushes; occasional vaginal bleeding and pruritus).

b. *Aminoglutethimide (Orimeten)*
Produces medical adrenalectomy making surgery unnecessary and inhibits peripheral tissue aromatisation of androgens to oestrogens.

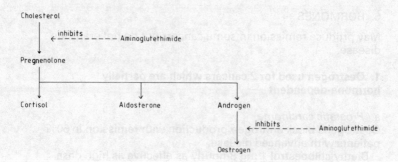

Reduction in cortisol produces rise in ACTH so 250 mg 6-hourly given with cortisone acetate 25 mg 12-hourly + fludrocortisone 0.1 mg alternate days (replaces aldosterone deficit). Side effects: lethargy, ataxia, dizziness (dose dependent and reduces with chronic therapy — self-induction of metabolising enzymes).

Rash sometimes with fever — usually self-limiting.

### 3. Progestogens
May produce remission in up to 30% breast cancer resistant to other hormones. Also used endometrial carcinoma. Nil side-effects.

Medroxyprogesterone acetate (Depo-Provera) — 200–800 mg i.m. weekly.

Megestrol acetate (Megace) — 40 mg p.o. daily.

### 4. Androgens
For breast cancer in post-menopausal women (pre-menopausal ovary converts androgen into oestrogen so should not be used). Response rate ~ 20%.

Fluoxymesterone (Ultandren) 10–30 mg daily.

Nandrolone phenylpropionate — 50–100 mg IM/week.

Adverse effects — Cholestatic jaundice; virilisation; fluid retention; hypercalcaemia.

### 5. Prednisolone
Inhibits lymphoid proliferation. Dose 10–100 mg p.o. daily. Adverse effects numerous (see page 265). Used in acute and chronic lymphocytic leukaemia; multiple myeloma; Hodgkin's and non-Hodgkin's lymphomas; breast carcinoma.

## ACQUIRED TUMOUR RESISTANCE TO CYTOTOXIC AGENTS

| Mechanism | Examples |
|---|---|
| 1. Reduced uptake of drug | Methotrexate; Daunorubicin |
| 2. Deletion of enzyme to activate drug | Cytosine arabinoside; 5-fluorouracil |
| 3. Increased detoxication of drug | 6-mercaptopurine |
| 4. Increased concentration of target enzyme | Methotrexate |
| 5. Decreased requirement for specific metabolic product | Asparaginase |
| 6. Increased utilisation of alternative metabolic pathways | Antimetabolites |
| 7. Rapid repair of drug-induced lesion | Alkylating agents |
| 8. Decreased number of receptors for drug | Hormones |
| 9. Alteration in proliferation rate (? underlying mechanism) | Myeloma, chronic myeloid leukaemia commonly terminate in a more aggressive phase |

### Longer term hazards of cancer chemotherapy
1. Gonadal damage — alkylating agents, vinca alkaloids, cytosine arabinoside. Azoospermia usual during treatment. Recovery often occurs but may take several years (N.B. many patients have low sperm count before treatment). Many women develop amenorrhoea after cytotoxic drugs but periods restart when treatment stopped. Women in late 30s – 40s may have premature menopause.
2. Second malignancy, e.g. after treatment of Hodgkins lymphoma with radio- and chemotherapy incidence of acute leukaemia increased 29-fold.
3. Teratogenesis: avoid pregnancy for at least 4 months after end of chemotherapy (in male and female).

## Treatment of side effects and complications common to cytotoxic drugs

1. *Vomiting* — practical problem — treatment only about 70% effective. Injection usually given $\frac{1}{2}$–1 hour before chemotherapy then continued or changed to oral therapy if no vomiting.

   (i) Phenothiazines
   Prochlorperazine (Stemetil)

   12.5 mg i.m.
   5– 10 mg p.o.
   8-hourly.

   Thiethylperazine (Torecan)

   6.5 mg i.m.
   10 mg p.o.
   8-hourly.

   (ii) Butyrophenones
   Haloperidol (Haldol; Serenace)

   2 mg i.m.
   1– 2 mg p.o.
   8-hourly.

   Droperidol (Droleptan))

   10– 15 mg i.v.
   5– 20 mg p.o.
   4– 8-hourly.

   (iii) Metoclopamide
   (Maxolon, Primperan)

   10 mg i.v.
   20 mg p.o.
   3-hourly.

   (iv) Steroids
   Dexamethasone

   10 mg i.m.

   Methylprednisolone

   250 mg i.v.
   6-hourly (up to 4 doses) starting 2 h before chemotherapy.

   (v) Experimental drugs
   Domperidone — dopamine antagonist acting mainly peripherally.
   Tetrahydrocannabinol and derivatives e.g. nabilone — main action probably on cerebral cortex.

   Combinations of drugs used, e.g. prochlorperazine 12.5 i.m. 1 hour before cisplatinum followed by promethazine 25 mg i.v. every hour to total 100 mg.

2. *Bone marrow depression* — Blood count required not more than 24 h before treatment.
   If  WBC 2500– 3500/mm$^3$  }  halve dosage.
       Platelets 50 000– 100 000/mm$^3$ }
   If  WBC < 2500/mm$^3$        without
       Platelets < 50 000/mm$^3$    treatment.

Patients with 600 neutrophils/mm$^3$ and platelet counts > 40 000/mm$^3$ require only observation — below this admission and screening for *infection*. If infected, regimes such as:
Gentamicin 120 mg 8-hourly i.v. (with monitoring)
Flucloxacillin 500 mg 6-hourly
Metronidazole 400 mg 6-hourly orally
Amphotericin lozenges 3-hourly
are used until bacteriological diagnosis made. Platelet transfusions often needed if count < 20 000/mm$^3$.
3. *Hyperuricaemia* — rare with solid tumours but common in leukaemia, myeloma etc. Give allopurinol 300 mg/day 24 h before therapy + high fluid intake.

# Drugs and the eye

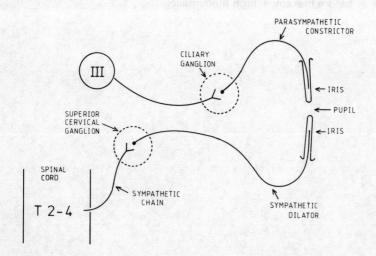

## Autonomic innervation of iris
*Dilator pupillae muscle*
— sympathetic dilator fibres activate α (mainly) and β-adrenergic receptors.
*Constrictor pupillae muscle*
— parasympathetic constrictor fibres activate muscarinic cholinergic receptors.
*Ciliary body*
— mainly innervated by parasympathetic nerves
— stimulation relaxes suspensory ligament of lens which becomes convex and accommodates for near vision.

MYDRIATICS (dilate pupil)

## A.  Parasympatheticolytics
*Eye drops*
Atropine sulphate 1% and 2% — long (days) action useful.

Homatropine hydrobromide, 0.1%, 0.2%, 1% — shorter action than atropine (onset 5 mins, lasts 24 h).

Hyoscine hydrobromide, 0.2% — shorter action and more rapid onset than atropine.

Tropicamide, 0.5% and 1% — action only 20 mins. 0.5% has no cycloplegic action.

Cyclopentolate hydrochloride, 0.1%, 0.5% and 1% — short action (4 hours) — reversed by physostigmine drops.

## B.  Sympatheticomimetics
Phenylephrine (10%)
Cocaine (2%)

## C.  Combined preparations
e.g. Homatropine and cocaine eye drops.
*Uses*
Ophthalmoscopic examination.
Cycloplegic action used in sight-testing infants.
Atropine used in iritis and cyclitis.
Phenylephrine also temporarily lowers intraocular pressure in glaucoma.
*Toxicity*
Precipitation of some forms of glaucoma.
Contact dermatitis, especially atropine.


MIOTICS (constrict pupil)

Parasympatheticomimetics — largely used in treatment of glaucoma (see below).

## Physostigmine (Eserine)
Cholinesterase inhibitor used as 0.25–0.5% drops. Effects last 12 hours.

## Pilocarpine
Cholinomimetic drug resistant to action of cholinesterase. Used as 1–4% drops. Effects last 6 hours and less powerful than physostigmine.

**Ecothiopate**
Irreversible anticholinesterase.
*Toxicity*
Systemic effects (diarrhoea, bronchospasm, bradycardia) unusual but nasolachrymal duct should be compressed for 2 minutes after application to block drainage into nose.
Eye pain due to ciliary muscle spasm — passes off in chronic use.
Glaucoma due to blockage of angle by cysts of the iris epithelium.

## GLAUCOMA

Increased intra-ocular tension with impaired vision.
Two types of primary glaucoma — entirely different diseases:

### 1. OPEN ANGLE GLAUCOMA (CHRONIC SIMPLE GLAUCOMA)

Generally painless chronic condition with slow progressive visual loss. Due to imbalance of *secretion* of aqueous (from ciliary epithelium) into posterior chamber, and *outflow* from anterior chamber (usually resistance to outflow lies in trabecular meshwork of angle or in cells of canal of Schlemm). Drugs used chronically to normalise intra-ocular pressure.

**Treatment**
a. Lowering of intra-ocular pressure in established disease: aim to lower pressure below 21 mmHg throughout 24 h.

*1. Topical preparations*
(i) Parasympatheticomimetics: constrict pupil and reduce resistance to outflow of aqueous by increasing tension in scleral spur, thereby opening up the trabeculae around Schlemm's canal.

*Pilocarpine* — 0.5–6% eye drops. 1 drop 4–6 times daily or sustained release units (Ocusert) 1 placed under eyelid every 7 days — release 20–40 $\mu$g of pilocarpine/h.
If pilocarpine inadequate, stronger miotics used:
*Physostigmine (eserine)* — see above.
*Neostigmine*, e.g. as neostigmine methylsulphate 3% (Prostigmin) — usually for initial lowering of ocular pressure.
*Carbachol* — 3% eye drops: 2 drops 8-hourly.
*Ecothiopate iodide* — 0.03, 0.06, 0.125 and 0.25% eye drops (Phospholine). Usually given as 0.03% 1 drop twice daily.
*Demecarium bromide* — 0.25 and 0.5% eye drops (Tosmilen).
Usually an initial treatment of 1 drop of 0.25% solution.

*Toxicity*: Irreversible anticholinesterases (especially demecarium) can aggravate asthma and bronchitis. Stronger miotics often cause pain due to spasm of the iris. Accommodation is stimulated. Demecarium can produce cataract.

(ii) Drugs acting on the sympathetic system:

*Adrenaline* 1 and 2% eye drops (Eppy) — useful addition to pilocarpine especially in early cataract by allowing a larger pupil. Adrenaline reduces resistance to outflow ($\alpha$-effect) and reduces secretion of aqueous ($\beta$-effect). Drops used twice daily: they are unstable and must be stored at 4°C (discard if discoloured). The benefit of adrenaline is further increased by the addition of *guanethidine* drops (3 or 5%). A combination of the two (Ganda — 3% guanethidine + 0.5% adrenaline) allows use of lower adrenaline concentration thus avoiding adrenaline side-effects (other concentrations available).

Problems with adrenaline:
— red eye as effect wears off
— conjunctival pigmentation
— irritation

*Timolol maleate* (non-selective $\beta$-adrenergic blocker without partial agonist or local anaesthetic activity). $\beta$-blockers reduce aqueous secretion without change in pupil size or accommodation. Unsuitable for closed angle glaucoma unless used with miotic.

As 0.25 and 0.5% drops (Timoptol), effect begins at around 3 hours and lasts about 24 hours so used twice daily.

No local irritation.

Adverse effects due to systemic absorption via nasal mucosa:
— bradycardia
— bronchospasm (avoid in asthma)
— depression, anxiety, confusion
— avoid in heart failure.

## 2. Oral drugs

*Acetazolamide* (Diamox): inhibits carbonic anhydrase responsible for aqueous secretion.

Given as 125 mg 8-hourly or 500 mg (Diamox Sustets) 12-hourly in open angle glaucoma with local treatment.

Adverse effects:
— diuresis — short-lived (few days) as acid-base status changes but effect on aqueous formation continues.
— paraesthesiae
— indigestion and nausea
— depression

*Dichlorphenamide* — carbonic anhydrase inhibitor used if acetazolamide side effects troublesome. Initial dose 100–200 mg then 100 mg 12-hourly.

### 3. Supervision
Essential part of treatment is regular observation of:
ocular pressure
retinal appearances
visual acuity
visual fields

### 4. Surgery
For failed medical management.
b. Prophylaxis
Intra-ocular pressure raised, but less than 35 mmHg with no glaucomatous cupping or field loss: such patients are not treated but are carefully observed with *serial* checks on ocular pressure.
  Hypotensive drugs in patients with glaucoma:
Clonidine can precipitate optic nerve ischaemia.
Methyldopa can dangerously lower perfusion pressure in optic nerve head.
Systemic β-blockers can help to relieve glaucoma.

## 2. ANGLE-CLOSURE GLAUCOMA

Due to occlusion of the filtration angle by the iris root coming into contact with the peripheral cornea.

a. Acute angle-closure glaucoma is an ophthalmic emergency which presents as a red and painful eye associated with photophobia and visual loss.
  Drugs used to control pressure prior to surgery.
**Treatment**
1. *Dehydrating agents*: intravenous infusions of hypertonic solutions of urea, mannitol, glycerol. Glycerol also given orally. Produce diuresis and dehydration of tissues.
2. *Oral acetazolamide* in high doses, e.g. 250 mg 6-hourly.
3. *Topical miotics*: pilocarpine used to prevent mydriasis *after* lowering of intraocular pressure has been attained in patients with a fixed pupil. Pilocarpine is given early when the pupil is not fixed.
4. *Analgesics*, e.g. pethidine, morphine, may be required to control pain.
5. *Iridectomy* is performed after the coincidental inflammation has settled.

b. Primary chronic (creeping) angle-closure glaucoma.
Avoid precipitating factors:
Pupil dilating drugs — local and systemic atropine-like agents contraindicated in closed angle glaucoma but have no harmful effect in chronic simple glaucoma.
  Steroid applied to the eye can raised ocular pressure in some individuals and worsen glaucoma (see page 38).
  Acute angle-closure glaucoma can arise in chronic angle-closure glaucoma and require urgent treatment.

## UVEITIS

The uveal tract is derived from the mesoderm surrounding the optic cup. It comprises the iris, ciliary body and choroid. Uveitis may be secondary to external trauma or arise due to systemic diseases.

Blindness results from obliteration of pupil aperture, secondary glaucoma, cataract and macular involvement.

1. Specific treatment of cause when possible.
2. Local and systemic steroids (except in infective uveitis due to Herpes simplex or zoster).

   Steroids increase intra-ocular pressure which is determined by penetration (greater the penetration, greater the increase) and heredity (see page 38). Increase also occurs with systemic steroids.

   Local steroid eye preparations include:
   betamethasone disodium phosphate 0.1% drops and ointment
   — application may be as frequent as hourly
   clobetasone butyrate 0.1% drops ⎫ have least effect on
   fluoromethalone 0.1% suspension ⎬ intra-ocular pressure
   prednisolone sodium phosphate 0.5% drops

   In severe inflammation a sub-conjunctival injection of methylprednisolone acetate (Depo-Medrone) gives a high anterior chamber steroid concentration over several days. Oral prednisolone (60–100 mg) is used systemically.

   N.B. Steroids should *never* be used indiscriminately in the eye as use in infection (bacterial or viral) encourages infective spread within the eye.
3. Occasionally increased intra-ocular tension + thinning of the cornea due to steroids ruptures the globe.
4. Azathioprine or oxyphenbutazone (10% ointment) can be applied locally to reduce steroid dose.
5. The pupil is maintained dilated.

## EYE INFECTIONS

Treatment often started before pathogen identified using clinical picture as a guide.

May need to change antibacterial within first 48 h.

Antibacterials given in 4 ways:
a. Drops
   — for superficial infections, e.g. conjunctivitis
   — need to give 2-hourly because tears dilute drug
b. Ointments
   — release drug more slowly especially if eye covered with pad.
c. Subconjunctival injection (0.5–1 ml) gives therapeutic levels for 8–12 hours.

d. Systemic administration
  — used for deep or posterior segment infections.
  — drug penetration variable, e.g. ampicillin, chloramphenicol, have good penetration especially in inflammation.
(i)  *Broad spectrum agents*
Chloramphenicol (0.5% eye drops or 1% ointment)
Neomycin sulphate (eye drops BNF or 0.25% ointment)
Framycetin sulphate (0.5% ointment) — effective against pseudomonas.
(ii)  *Other agents*
Sulphacetamide (eye drops 30%) used for trachoma and TRIC infection (the latter requires systemic tetracycline therapy as well)
  Tetracyclines (e.g. oxytetracycline 0.5% ointment) — used also in trachoma.
  Penicillin is used in gonococcal ophthalmia neonatorium
  (Chloramphenicol is used for most other forms of conjunctivitis in the newborn and tetracycline or sulphacetamide for TRIC agent conjunctivitis)
  Bacterial infections often produce damage by inflammatory response rather than bacterial toxicity. Steroids often used with antibiotics (but rarely in conjunctivitis unless there is specific indication because of danger of exacerbating infection). Various steroid/anti-infective drugs available e.g. betamethasone 0.1% + neomycin sulphate 0.5% (Betnesol-N) are available.

  *Herpes simplex* infections treated with:
Idoxuridine (0.1%) drops applied hourly in day and 2-hourly at night or ointment (0.5%) — Ophthalmidine — 4 times daily.
  Experts use steroids with antiviral agents to limit damage.
*Toxicity*
Allergic reaction
Corneal irritation
Avoid in pregnancy — effects unknown.
N.B.  Herpid (5% idoxuridine) is for use on skin not eyes which it may damage.
Vidarabine 3% (Vira-A) ointment applied 5 times daily.
or Acyclovir 3% ointment (Zovirax) applied 4-hourly also useful in herpes.

**Anti-inflammatory preparations**
Topical anti-histamines as drops are used in allergic conjunctivitis, e.g. antazoline sulphate 0.5% + xylometazoline hydrochloride 0.05% (Otrivine-Antistin). Sodium cromoglycate 2% drops (Opticrom) used as prophylactic 4 times daily.

**Local anaesthetics**
Eye is particularly suitable for effective local anaesthesia.

*Cocaine*
2 or 4% drops — acts in 10 mins, lasts about 4 hours.
   Prevents noradrenaline reuptake so is sympathomimetic, giving dilated pupil and vasoconstriction — useful at surgery, e.g. cataract extraction.
Adverse effects:
— clouding of corneal epithelium
— systemic absorption (very rare)

*Oxybuprocaine* (*Benoxinate*)
0.4% drops — best for local procedures.
Rapid onset last 20 minutes.
Minimal initial stinging so useful in children.

*Amethocaine*
0.5 and 1% drops — used for local procedures but may initially sting and can cloud corneal epithelium.

## DRUGS WHICH HARM THE EYE

1. Tricyclic antidepressants and anticholinergic anti-Parkinsonian drugs:
   Failure of accommodation
   Aggravation of angle-closure glaucoma
2. Phenothiazine neuroleptics:
   Pigmentary retinopathy (especially thioridazine)
   Anterior polar cataract (especially chlorpromazine)
   Anticholinergic effects
3. Glucocorticoids:
   Systemic steroids:  Posterior subcapsular cataracts (rare if dose
      < 10 mg prednisolone/day)
   Papilloedema (rare) due to raised intracranial pressure when
      steroid dose reduced — treat by raising steroid dose again
   Raised intra-ocular pressure (see above)
   Infections encouraged
   Local steroids:  Can also raise intra-ocular pressure, cause
      cataract and can aggravate Herpes simplex corneal ulcers.
4. Chloroquine (high doses)
   Subepithelial linear corneal deposits (reversible)
   Retinal pigmentation, arteriolar damage and macular damage
   cause field defects and loss of central vision (irreversible)
5. Amiodarone
   Corneal deposits — produce no visual impairment
6. Ethambutol (more than 15 mg/kg/day)
   Optic neuritis (produces blindness) — more likely in alcoholics
   or diabetics
7. Fetal damage to eye from taking the following during
   pregnancy:
   Thalidomide
   Phenytoin
   Busulphan

# Drug overdose

Approximately 10% of acute adult medical admissions are because of overdoses. Some evidence for increase over the past 20 years. Causes in order of frequency:

1. Parasuicide (manipulative self-poisoning)
2. Suicidal intent (often associated with depression and schizophrenia)
3. Accidental (commonest in children)
4. Homicidal (very rare)

Long-term management requires the distinction between these groups to be made.

N.B. also rare group of children who have been deliberately overdosed by parents as manifestation of parent's mental illness.

Overdosage is commonly with more than one drug (alcohol is the commonest component) and thus the clinical features are variable.

Overdose mortality overall in hospital < 1%.

Approximately 10% cases require treatment other than careful nursing.

## MANAGEMENT

1. Diagnosis
2. Supportive therapy
3. Specific measures
4. Psychiatric

1. Diagnosis

(i) History from patient or companion:
drug taken, alcohol taken in addition, treatment for other diseases, obvious signs in present illness, e.g. fits.
(ii) Past history of psychiatric illness
suicide attempts
drug abuse and alcoholism

(iii)  Physical signs, for example:
      *Fits*
      tricyclic antidepressants
      amphetamine, cocaine and other stimulants
      antihistamines
      narcotic analgesics
      neuroleptics
      solvents
      *Pulmonary oedema*
      narcotic analgesics
      glutethimide
      *Skin bullae*
      any cause of coma
      *Papilloedema*
      glutethimide
      *Involuntary movements or restlessness*
      salicylates
      antihistamines
      anticholinergics
      neuroleptics
      lithium
      tricyclic antidepressants
      *Coma*
      hypnosedatives
      alcohol
      narcotic analgesics
      tricyclic antidepressants
      *Also* look for jaundice, injection marks, scars, necrosis and
      gangrene.
 (iv)  Special diagnostic procedures: drug screen in blood, urine and
      gastric contents. Look for mixtures (including alcohol). Retain
      sample for forensic purposes.
  (v)  Grade level of consciousness:
        I.  drowsy, responds to verbal commands
       II.  unconscious but responds to minimally painful stimuli
      III.  unconscious, responds only to very painful stimuli
       IV.  unconscious, does not respond to stimuli
 (vi)  Monitor:
      respiratory function: respiratory minute volume (if <4l, then do
      arterial $PO_2$, $PCO_2$, pH and standard bicarbonate).
      circulatory: pulse rate and blood pressure.
      temperature: rectal temperature measurement.
      blood: urea, electrolytes, haematocrit.
      renal function: urine output (bladder catheterisation required in
      severely poisoned patients).

## 2. SUPPORTIVE THERAPY

 (i) Maintain airway and ventilation: most important initial procedure as respiratory failure is commonest immediate cause of death.
 (ii) Shock: treat with intravenous fluids (plasma, dextran) with monitoring of central venous pressure and clinical observation.
(iii) Hypothermia: contributes to shock, acidaemia and hypoxia and measurement of core temperature imperative.
Avoid active reheating.
Wrap patient in foil or 'space' blanket to conserve heat and nurse in warm atmosphere. Use warmed humidified air if on ventilator.
(iv) Monitor and control fluid and electrolyte balance.
 (v) Nursing care of unconscious patient: regular turning, eye and mouth care, attention to pressure areas etc. very important.

## 3. SPECIFIC MEASURES

### A. Prevention of further absorption

a. In a conscious child or adult, induce vomiting by irritation of pharynx with spatula. Alternatively give 15 ml syrup of ipecac which causes vomiting in 15–20 mins. Avoid apomorphine (causes protracted vomiting) and saline (causes electrolyte imbalance).
b. Gastric aspiration and lavage should be undertaken if known that drug ingested within previous 4 hours (exception salicylate, tricyclics and anticholinergics when it may be worthwhile at later times). Wide bore stomach tube is passed and 500 mg warm water repeatedly ($\times$ 5–8) introduced and emptied from stomach. As variants of this for:
   (i) opiates: use dilute potassium permanganate
   (ii) iron: use desferrioxamine
  (iii) glutethimide: use water and castor oil
       All lavage fluid should be removed at end of washout except in iron poisoning when 10 g desferrioxamine and in glutethimide poisoning when 50 ml castor oil is left in stomach.
       Danger of aspiration pneumonia so protective gag reflex must be present before starting washout. If reduced or absent, washout is performed with a cuffed endotracheal tube in place.
       Lavage can be traumatic and must be done cautiously if corrosive poisons taken. It is contraindicated in overdose with petroleum and related solvents.
       It is impracticable in children.
c. Activated effervescent charcoal (Medicoal) is an adjunctive treatment but 10 g charcoal absorbs about 1 g drug so that efficacy limited. Used in paracetamol, tricyclic overdoses.

## B. Enhancement of drug elimination

Applicable in few cases.

Reduces duration of coma and therefore of secondary complications like pneumonia, hypotension, thromboembolism. Little trial evidence that overall outcome altered.

*a. Forced diuresis*
1. Alkaline diuresis
— salicylates
— phenobarbitone, barbitone (only barbiturates that have sufficiently high renal excretion to make its enhancement worthwhile: others undergo hepatic metabolism).

*Principle*: To increase proportion of ionised drug in renal tubules thus reducing tubular reabsorption since only lipophilic unionised molecules cross cell membranes readily. Ionisation of acids is increased in alkaline urine and vice versa.

*Method:*
a. Ascertain that
  (i) BP adequate (i.e. patient not shocked)
  (ii) pulmonary oedema absent
  (iii) CVP line and peripheral venous line in place
  (iv) current electrolyte status is known
  (v) as far as possible that renal function normal.
b. Follow scheme below:

Catheterise bladder and set up input / output chart.
Measure BP and pulse every 30 mins or more frequently.
Initiate diuresis with 20 mg frusemide IV.

Forced alkaline diuresis
In first hour give:
1. 500 ml 5% dextrose
2. 500 ml 1.2% sodium bicarbonate
3. 500 ml 5% dextrose

Forced acid diuresis
In first hour give:
1. 1000 ml 5% dextrose
2. 10g arginine HCl or lysine HCl over 30 mins
3. 500 ml 0.9% saline

At end of first hour:
Check i. lung bases, JVP
Check ii. Input / output chart

If urine flow <3 ml/min

Stop procedure — patient unsuitable.

If urine flow >3 ml/min

1. Give IV fluid + frusemide to maintain urine flow 500 ml/h.
2. Add 20 mmol $K^+$/l to infusion. Check electrolytes and modify input accordingly.
3. Maintain urine pH at 7.5 – 8.5 (alkaline diuresis) or 5.5 – 6.5 (acid diuresis) by appropriate infusion of alkali or acid infusions.

N.B. This is a dangerous procedure — monitor JVP, lung bases, CVP (chest X-ray) and electrolytes frequently. Discontinue as soon as drug level has fallen adequately and patient's clinical condition improved.
2. Acid diuresis.
Rarely used for amphetamine and other bases. Urinary acidification difficult to achieve because respiratory stimulation produces consequent respiratory alkalosis.

### b. Haemoperfusion
Passage of blood over column of activated charcoal or ion-exchange resin via extracorporeal circuit.
  Used for barbiturates, glutethimide, chloral hydrate, meprobamate, methaqualone, paracetamol, theophylline.
  Available only in specialist centres and danger of haemorrhage, infection, platelet and leucocyte consumption on column, air embolism.

### c. Haemodialysis
Used rarely for severe lithium intoxication. No advantage over forced alkaline diuresis for other drugs when renal function normal.
N.B. Measurement of plasma drug concentration is only rarely important in management but it is in these cases in which active elimination measures are used where it is most useful.

## Special features of particular drug overdoses
Only rarely is there a specific antidote for a given drug. Most patients recover with simple nursing measures.
*Benzodiazepines*, one of the commonest overdoses, exemplify this approach.

## Paracetamol

### Effects
Patient is conscious, but may be nauseated and vomit. Main hazard is delayed hepatocellular necrosis after 2–3 days. As little as 10–15 g may produce dangerous toxicity.

### Mechanism of toxicity
In overdose, the usual metabolic pathway ($\rightarrow$ sulphate + glucuronide) is overloaded and more drug is metabolised via mixed function oxidase. Usually products of this minor pathway are detoxified by glutathione, but in overdose this protective mechanism is overwhelmed and reactive intermediates covalently combine with hepatic intracellular enzymes and other proteins. Toxicity more likely if patient's liver enzymes induced by other drugs.

*Management*
1. Assess severity of overdose from plasma paracetamol concentration (> 1 mmol/l at 4 hours or more after ingestion suggests hepatic necrosis likely).
2. If seen within 12 hours of overdose attempt to increase hepatic glutathione levels with either (a) oral methionine 2g 2-hourly for 5 doses, or (b) N-acetylcysteine 150 mg/kg in 200 ml, 5% dextrose over 15 mins then 50 mg/kg in 500 ml, 5% dextrose over 4 hours then 100 mg/kg in 1000 ml, 5% dextrose over next 16 hours.

   Methionine is cheaper and easier to give than N-acetylcysteine but latter useful in unconscious patients after mixed overdoses.

## Salicylates

*Effects*
Excitement, talkative and aggressive behaviour.
Nausea and vomiting (sometimes haematemesis) commonly.
Tinnitus, vertigo, headache, deafness.
Sweating and fever.
Hyperventilation causes respiratory alkalosis with occasional tetany but salicylate also causes metabolic acidosis due to itself and accumulation of tricarboxylic acids from an inhibited Krebs' cycle acting as fixed acids.
Haemorrhage from hypoprothrombinaemia, interference with platelet function and gastric irritation.
Unconsciousness rare except with very severe overdose.
Easy to underestimate severity of poisoning clinically.

*Management*
1. Never too late to start gastric lavage.
2. Take blood for salicylate level. If > 3.5 mmol/l consider forced alkaline diuresis (see above).
3. If abdominal pain give magnesium antacids.
4. In severe poisoning give 10 mg vitamin K i.m.

## Opiates

*Effects*
Stupor and coma.
Respiratory depression with cyanosis.
Pinpoint pupils.
Possibly pulmonary oedema and/or cardiac arrhythmias.

*Management*
1. Ventilate with oxygen, preferably via endotracheal tube to prevent aspiration.
2. Give naloxone 0.4 mg i.v., wait 3 mins, if no effect give 1.2 mg i.v., wait 3 mins, if no effect give 3.6 mg i.v. Repeat doses as required. Remember (a) naloxone $T_{\frac{1}{2}}$ effect shorter than opiates; (b) naloxone precipitates acute withdrawal reactions in opiate addicts.
3. Give i.v. glucose and thiamine in addicts.

**Mixed opiate preparations**
a. Distalgesic (dextropropoxyphene + paracetamol) requires treatment with naloxone + methionine or N-acetylcysteine. Common overdose. Potentially very toxic (especially with alcohol).
b. Lomotil (diphenoxylate + atropine) Usually taken by children in overdose. Slowed gastric emptying delays narcotic effects for several hours so gastric lavage can often be useful several hours after ingestion. Treat with naloxone and symptomatic measures for anticholinergic effects.

**Digitalis**

*Effects*
See page 150

*Management*
1. Maintain normal plasma $K^+$ by infusion (N.B. vomiting produces hypokalaemia.)
2. Treat:
   bradycardia with atropine
   ventricular tachycardia with phenytoin
3. Consider insertion of prophylactic pacemaker
4. EDTA to lower plasma $Ca^{++}$ rarely used.
5. Recently administration of digoxin antibodies has been found effective.

**Barbiturates and glutethimide**

*Effects*
Coma, sometimes with fluctuation of consciousness
Dilated, unresponsive pupils, sometimes with flat EEG may be confused with brain death
Respiratory depression and sudden apnoea (especially glutethimide)
Papilloedema (with glutethimide)
Hypotension with shock and renal failure
10% develop bullous eruption: no diagnostic value as occurs in other overdoses.

*Management*
1. Supportive
2. Phenobarbitone and barbitone only can be removed by forced alkaline diuresis
3. Haemoperfusion effective in severe overdose.

## β-adrenergic blockers

*Effects*
Bradycardia, hypotension, low cardiac output, conduction defects in heart
Bronchospasm in asthmatics
Convulsions
Coma

*Management*
1. Gastric lavage (even several hours after overdose)
2. Insert i.v. line, estimate blood gases and pH
3. 500 mg cortisol i.v. initially
4. If hypotensive give isoprenaline 10–20 μg/min i.v. If bradycardia give atropine 2 mg i.v. as a single dose, but a pacemaker may have to be inserted.
   If low cardiac output does not respond to isoprenaline, give glucagon (in dextrose) 5–15 mg/h i.v.
   If persistent hypotension give dopamine, dobutamine or noradrenaline.
   Persistent refractory low cardiac output may require and aortic balloon pump.
5. For bronchospasm i.v. or aerosol salbutamol
6. Correct acidosis
7. Correct fluid retention with frusemide

### Labetalol overdose
As with β-blockers but α-blockade can cause peripheral vasodilation with lowered cardiac output and require i.v. infusion of isoprenaline with noradrenaline.

### Tricyclic antidepressants

*Effects*
Hyperreflexia; tremor; excitement; fits.
Supraventricular and ventricular tachycardias; intracardiac blocks; cardiac arrest can occur 4–6 days after overdose
Anticholinergic effects: dilated pupils, paralytic ileus, retention of urine.
Coma, hypotension or hypertension, respiratory depression

*Management*
1. Insert intravenous line
2. Gastric lavage (even 1 day after overdose)
3. Put activated charcoal in stomach after lavage (25 g/g of drug ingested)
4. Repeated blood gas estimations (treat acidosis with i.v. bicarbonate but ventilate when required)
5. i.v. diazepam if repeated fits
6. i.v. infusion of a plasma expander if hypotension due to peripheral circulatory failure
7. Continuous cardiac monitoring (correction of hypoxia and acidosis may correct arrhythmias but treat persistent supraventricular tachycardia with propranolol); ventricular tachycardias with lignocaine or disopyramide; bradycardia with conduction defects requires insertion of a pacemaker.

**Iron**
Commonly in children who take their pregnant mother's iron tablets which resemble sweets.

*Effects*
Gastritis, vomiting, diarrhoea, haematemesis. This settles in 12–24 hours and patient becomes well but will develop hepatocellular necrosis, renal failure, cardiac damage, haemorrhagic enterocolitis, convulsions and coma after a further 12–24 hours.

*Management*
1. Gastric lavage using chelating agent desferrioxamine (see above)
2. Desferrioxamine 2 g i.m. then i.v. at not greater rate than 15 mg/kg/h (max 80 mg/kg/day).
3. Continue treatment until serum iron concentration < 200 mmol/l or transferrin no longer 100% saturated.

### 4. PSYCHIATRIC ASSESSMENT

Patients should usually be seen by a psychiatrist prior to discharge from the medical unit. Approximately equal number of patients fall into the categories:
1. Depressive illness
2. Personality disorder (often 'repeat overdoses')
3. Drug addicts and alcoholics
4. No psychiatric disorder (intolerable socio-economic pressures; unhappy love affairs; adolescent tantrums, etc.)
   Not all of these will benefit from further psychiatric follow-up or social help.

## Some specific antidotes for overdose

| Drug | Antidote |
|---|---|
| Lithium | NaCl infusion |
| Monoamine oxidase inhibitors | Hypertensive reactions: $\alpha$-blocker (e.g. chlorpromazine) Tachycardia: $\beta$-blocker |
| Coumarin anticoagulants | Water soluble analogues of vitamin K (e.g. menaphthone) |
| Cyanide | Cobalt edetate (Kelocyanor) 20 ml of 1.5% solution given over 1 minute. *Stat.* and 50 ml of 50% glucose i.v., *or* sodium nitrite 10 ml of 3% solution given i.v. over 3 minutes, then sodium thiosulphate 25 ml of 50% solution i.v. |
| Methanol | i.v. ethanol (e.g. 5% solution) slows down conversion to formaldehyde. |
| Organophosphorus anticholinesterases | Pralidoxime (30 mg/kg) in 5 ml water, slow i.v. injection, repeat after 1 min, *plus* atropine 2 mg i.v. followed by 1 mg i.v. every 10 mins until bradycardia and meiosis reversed. |
| Mercury and arsenic | D penicillamine up to 1.5 g/day oral *or* injection of BAL 2.5 mg every 4–6 hours for first day; 2 injections/day for next 3 days; then 1 injection daily until recovery. |
| Lead and copper | Calcium disodium edetate 15–25 mg/kg slow i.v. injection twice daily (as a 0.5–3% solution in 5% glucose) *or* BAL *or* penicillamine. |

# Drug dependence

**Definition**
State of chronic intoxication produced by repeated drug administration which is detrimental to individual and society. There is compulsion to continue taking the drug and individual may exhibit one or more of:
1. Tolerance — increasing amounts of drug required to produce same effect.
2. Physical dependence — body adapts to drug and abnormal reactions (withdrawal reactions) occur if drug administration stopped abruptly.
3. Psychic dependence — drug produces satisfaction and pleasure such as to require further administration to maintain the sense of pleasure or to avoid discomfort.

Characteristic features of drug dependence vary with drug. Caffeine (in tea, coffee, chocolate, cocoa, coca-cola) produces dependence with a physical withdrawal syndrome (headache, yawning, tiredness) but this is generally regarded as harmless.

**WHO classification:**

| Type | Compounds |
|---|---|
| Alcohol-barbiturate | Ethanol, barbiturates and other hypnotics and sedatives, e.g. benzodiazepines |
| Amphetamine | Amphetamine, dexamphetamine, methylamphetamine, methylphenidate and phenmetrazine |
| Cocaine | Cocaine and coca leaves |
| Cannabis | Preparations of *Cannabis sativa*, e.g. marihuana and hashish |
| Opiates | Opium, morphine, heroin, methadone, pethidine, etc. |
| Hallucinogens | Lysergic acid diethylamide (LSD), mescaline and psilocybin |
| Volatile compounds | Acetone, carbon tetrachloride and other solvents, e.g. 'glue-sniffing' |
| Nicotine | Tobacco, snuffs |

## Alcohol

1 unit = a single of spirits = 1 glass of wine = 1 pint of beer.
1 unit of alcohol raises blood alcohol by 10 mg/100 ml.
Urinary concentration is 1.3 × blood concentration.

*Acute intoxication*
N.B. Rate limiting enzyme is alcohol dehydrogenase which can
metabolise about 10 mg pure ethanol/hour (spirits about 50%
ethanol). Thus pharmacokinetics show saturation and rapid
accumulation once metabolic capacity exceeded.

*1. Main CNS effects*
reduced judgment and discrimination
reduced learning and attention span
impaired body-mind-eye coordination
social disinhibition

| *Blood level* (mg/100 ml) | *Usual result* (but much individual variation) |
|---|---|
| 20 | Feeling of warmth and relaxation |
| 30 | Mild relief from anxiety; facilitation of conversation |
| 50 | Incoordination; slowed reactions; speech mistakes |
| 100 | Ataxia; slurred speech |
| 100–200 | Vertigo; difficulty walking; vomiting |
| 300 | Stupor |
| 400 | Deep anaesthesia; respiratory depression |

*2. Other actions*
cutaneous and conjunctival vasodilatation
sweating
tachycardia
suppression of ADH production
increased gastric acid secretion; gastritis
metabolic and respiratory acidosis
hyperuricaemia
hypoglycaemia

*Chronic effects of alcohol*
1. *Nervous system*
   (i) Dependence:
   withdrawal states:
       tremor
       fits
       delirium tremens
       anxiety, insomnia, panic attacks

  (ii) Chronic neuronal degeneration:
      cerebral atrophy — dementia
      cerebellar syndromes
      psychiatric syndromes, e.g. depression, paranoia
  (iii) Consequences of vitamin deficiency:
      Wernicke's encephalopathy (features of
      acute and/or chronic organic psychosis +
      ophthalmoplegia + nystagmus)
      Korsakoff's psychosis (amnesic syndrome)
      Pellagra dementia — nicotinic acid lack
2. *Alimentary*
  chronic gastritis; peptic ulcer
  haematemesis (ulcer, varices, gastritis, Mallory-Weiss syndrome)
  acute, sub-acute and chronic pancreatitis
  hepatitis; cirrhosis
3. Myopathy
4. Bone marrow suppression
5. In some patients: hypertriglyceridaemia, hyperglycaemia, harm
  to fetus
6. Gout and accelerated atherogenesis


*Fetal alcohol syndrome*
*CNS*
mild to moderate mental retardation
poor coordination, hypotonia
irritability and hyperactivity
*Facial features*
microcephaly
short, upturned nose
hypoplastic maxilla
micrognathia
thinned upper vermilion of lips
retarded pre-natal and post-natal
*Growth*
Small baby


*Drug interactions*
May have medico-legal implications:
1. Potentiation of central depressants:
  anticholinergics, e.g. atropine, benztropine
  antihistamines ($H_1$-receptor blockers)
  barbiturates and glutethimide
  benzodiazepines
  chloral
  codeine

dextropropoxyphene
mianserin
phenothiazines
propranolol (? other β-blockers)
tricyclic andidepressants
2. Disulfiram reaction (flushing, palpitations, tachycardia,
hypotension, giddiness, nausea and vomiting)
Disulfiram (use as Antabuse in aversion therapy)
Metronidazole
Sulphonylureas especially chloropropamide
Procarbazine
Moxalactam
Cefamandole
Cefoperazone
Griseofulvin (?)
Trichlorethylene (industrial exposure)
3. Potentiates hypoglycaemia due to other agents.
4. Enzyme induction reduces action of some drugs, e.g.
tolbutamide, warfarin, phenytoin, but liver metabolism reduced
following a binge so action of drugs can be potentiated, e.g
phenylbutazone.
5. Enhanced gastric irritation by non-steroidal anti-inflammatory
agents.
6. Brain sensitivity to benzodiazepines reduced in chronic
alcoholics (cross tolerance).

*Treatment of alcohol abstinence syndromes*
Develops within hours of last drink, peaks 24–48 hours, gone
at 3–4 days. Less than 10% progress to delirium tremens.
Characterised by tremor, tachycardia, gut upsets. In all but mild
cases treat in hospital. Use benzodiazepines with long $T_{\frac{1}{2}}$ in large
doses (cross-tolerance with alcohol).
Diazepam — 40 mg daily for 4 days
           30 mg daily for 3 days
           20 mg daily for 2 days
           10 mg daily for 1 day
Chlormethiazole is also an excellent sedative, anxiolytic and
anticonvulsant but has an addiction risk. Lorazepam is useful if
there is serious hepatic dysfunction.
Chlorpromazine reduces panic but can precipitate fits and is thus
not recommended.
Also give Parenterovite ± folic acid.

*Delirium tremens (DTs)*
A serious physical illness accompanied by physical illusions and hallucinations which are typically unpleasant and often visual (e.g. small animals or insects crawling over body). There is profound confusion and disorientation and terrifying nightmares ('the horrors').

Diazepam used as above or given intravenously (10 mg stat then 5 mg every 5 minutes until calm) supplemented with haloperidol 2–4 mg i.m. every 4–6 hours. Haloperidol can be discontinued without tapering dose.

Fluid and electrolyte balance may required adjustment.

Give vitamins.

Treat any concurrent illness, especially infections, which can precipitate DTs.

Physical restrains occasionally required to protect patient and staff.

*Rum fits*
Grand mal seizures 7–48 hours after drinking stopped (~5% develop status).

I.V. diazepam treatment of choice.

Check $Mg^{++}$ level — give 1 g $MgSO_4$ i.m. four times daily for 2 days prophylactically.

*Overall treatment*
Also requires:
a. counselling and attention to behavioural and social factors.
b. treatment of any underlying psychiatric disorder, e.g. depression
c. group therapy (as with Alcoholics Anonymous).
d. follow-up.

A few patients are helped to aversion therapy using disulfiram or other alcohol sensitising drugs.

## Barbiturates and other hypnosedatives

Taken orally, i.v. or subcutaneously.
**Chronic abuse**
drowsiness
ataxia, nystagmus
reduced quality and quantity of work
increased appetite

**Withdrawal**
anxiety
insomnia
panic attacks
anorexia
fits (sometimes status epilepticus)

**Benzodiazepines**
Less prone to produce dependence but can cause the same picture
3– 13 days after stopping drug.
   Patients at risk usually on large doses (5– 10 times therapeutic)
for several months but few cases described after therapeutic
dose.
*Treatment*
Stop benzodiazepine gradually.
Replace with 40 mg propranolol 8-hourly for 2 weeks.

**Amphetamine and cocaine**
Taken orally i.v. or sniffed (cocaine).
These have similar effects — both have central catecholamine
effects.
Psychic dependence only.

*Acute administration*
excitement, euphoria, little need for sleep
anorexia
psychotic schizophrenia-like reactions, sometimes violent tremor,
tachycardia, dangerous arrhythmias
hypertension
fits

*Withdrawal*
depression
hyperphagia
hypersomnia
   Cocaine when sniffed can lead to ischaemic perforation of the
nasal septum (vasoconstriction due to inhibition of catecholamine
uptake).

**Cannabis**
Taken orally or smoked.
Cannabis = products of *Cannabis sativa*. Two forms:
1.  Hashish = resin from flowering tops.
2.  Marihuana = chopped leaves and stalk.
   Psychic dependence only.

*Acute effects*
distorted perception of time, colour, music
social relaxation
short term memory is impaired
hallucinations
incoordination
tachycardia
panic and delirium (bad trip) which may recur after intoxication has
     worn off (flashbacks)

*Chronic effects*
Mild dementia and personality changes — effects disputed.

## Opiates
Taken orally, i.v., subcutaneously, smoked.
     Several opiates abused — morphine, diamorphine, methadone,
pethidine, dipipanone, dextropropoxyphene are commonest. May
be taken with other drugs of addiction.
     Produce marked physical and psychic dependence with
tolerance.

*Acute overdose reactions*
Pulmonary oedema
Hypoxic reaction — acute respiratory depression (due to irregular
                                   potency of street supply or loss of tolerance).
                              — reaction to adulterants or particles in street
                                   drug.

## Complications of opiate abuse

*Infections*
Common:
1. Hepatitis
2. Endocarditis (50% on tricuspid valve; *Staph. aureus*
    commonest, but also fungal)
3. Septicaemia
Rare:
Malaria, syphilis, tetanus, osteomyelitis.

*Immunological*
1. Nephropathy and nephrotic syndrome.
2. Acquired immune deficiency syndrome with *Pneumocystis
    carinii* pneumonia and Kaposi's sarcoma.
3. False positive serology for syphilis and rheumatoid factor.

*Cardiovascular*
1. Arrhythmias
2. Emboli

*Pulmonary*
1. Ventilation/perfusion defects
2. Embolism by foreign particles
3. Aspiration pneumonia

*Gastro-intestinal*
1. Constipation
2. Biliary hypertension with raised transaminases, alkaline phosphatase and amylase.

*Skin*
1. Needle tracks, cellulitis and thrombophlebitis
2. Urticaria

*Nervous system*
1. Post-anoxic encephalopathy
2. Transverse myelopathy and paraplegia

*Obstetric*
1. Low birth weight or prematurity
2. Neonatal withdrawal syndrome (mortality 50%)

**Withdrawal syndrome**
At ~ 8 h — Yawning; sweating; rhinorrhoea; tearing; anxiety.
   ~ 20 h — Gooseflesh ('cold turkey'); chills; sweating; panic.
   ~ 24–48 h — Nausea and vomiting; diarrhoea; hypertension; fever.
   Up to 1 week — Muscle cramps.
   Up to several months — Insomnia.
Syndrome accompanied by craving for drug.
Syndrome suppressed with methadone (20 mg in divided doses first 3 days then 10 mg for 3 days) or clonidine (experimental).
Syndrome precipitated by opiate antagonists.

**Nicotine**
Tobacco smoke is a complex mixture which includes nicotine.
Nicotine is an alkaloid in the leaves of *Nicotiana tabacum*.

*Actions*
1. Stimulates then blocks nicotinic cholinergic receptors (raised blood pressure, tachycardia, cutaneous and splanchnic vasoconstriction).
2. Stimulates: vomiting centre, ADH secretion.
3. Stimulation of respiration (carotid body reflex).

4.  Cocaine-like stimulatory action on brain due to blockade of
    amine reuptake by neurones.
    Powerfully addicting with psychic and physical elements.
Tolerance occurs. Withdrawal state (constipation, increased
appetite, nicotine craving).
Smokers have *accelerated metabolism* of:
Nicotine
Imipramine
Phenacetin
Caffeine
Propoxyphene
Pentazocine
Theophylline
but *normal metabolism* of:
Diazepam
Desipramine
Pethidine
Warfarin
Ethanol

*Adverse effects*
Strong correlation with ischaemic heart disease
Cancers of lung, trachea, oesophagus, lip and tongue
Chronic bronchitis and emphysema, tuberculosis, cor pulmonale
Aortic aneurysm
Hernia
Peripheral vascular disease
Premature delivery, small babies, raised perinatal mortality

*Possible beneficial effects*
Associated with decreased incidence of ulcerative colitis.

*Treatment*
High degree of motivation important
Some can abruptly stop
Others can undertake gradual withdrawal or use graded filters
    (allow decreasing amount of smoke inhalation).
Nicotine chewing gum (Nicorette) in 2 mg and 4 mg/piece can be
    prescribed. Nicotine in gum is resin bound so absorption is
    slower than during smoking (and so less satisfying) and depends
    on speed of chewing. Most of the nicotine is absorbed in first 30
    minutes: chewing one 4 mg piece of gum every hour produces
    plasma nicotine levels similar to those of heavy smokers.
    Nicorette is used to control withdrawal symptoms while
    behavioural components are overcome.
Success rate 15–30% at 1 year.

**Solvents**
Volatile hydrocarbons — petrol, lighter fuel
                          — glue solvents (toluene, acetone)
                          — paint thinners, hair lacquer
Inhaled from a bag or rag — often a group activity.

*Produces*
Euphoria and exhilaration (like alcohol) followed by
Auditory or visual hallucinations
Then cerebral depression: ataxia, blurred vision, disorientation,
   drowsiness.

*Adverse effects*
Rarely serious in most cases BUT:
Occasionally renal damage
Toluene encephalopathy sometimes with abdominal pain, nausea
and vomiting.
Asphyxial death.
May produce tolerance and occasional withdrawal symptoms.

# Legal and practical aspects of prescribing

## 1. Medicines Act (1968)
Classifies medicines into three categories:
1. *General sales list preparations*: may be purchased from any shop or even a vending machine.
2. *Pharmacy only medicines*: supplied to a patient by a registered pharmacist without prescription.
3. *Prescription only medicines* (*POM*): only supplied by pharmacist on the prescription of registered medical (or dental) practitioner.
   a. provisionally registered doctors cannot write prescriptions for POM for dispensing outside hospital.
   b. provision for supply of small quantities of POM in emergency to patient provided that it has been prescribed previously by a doctor and it is not a controlled drug (see below) or one of a number of other substances such as barbiturates (except for epilepsy).

## 2. Misuse of Drugs Regulations (1973)
Categories the *controlled drugs* as:

### Schedule 1
Preparations of certain controlled drugs in which drugs are in such small amounts or combined in such a way that there is no risk of abuse, e.g. dihydrocodeine tablets (but not injection), all common preparations of codeine, preparations with less than 0.2% morphine e.g. kaolin and morphine mixture.

### Schedules 2 and 3
Includes opiates and other narcotics, cocaine and amphetamines. A prescription for a drug in these schedules must conform to the following rules:
a. In the doctor's own handwriting in ink or other indelible medium it must state:
   (i) name and address of patient
   (ii) dose to be taken

      (iii)  form (e.g. tablets, mixture) and, where appropriate, concentration of the drug
      (iv)  total quantity of preparation to be supplied
      (v)  quantities and concentrations written in figures and words
      (vi)  doctor's signature and date
  b.  The doctor's address need not be written but must appear on the prescription.
    In addition:
  a.  The prescriber's address must be within the UK
  b.  The prescription must be presented within 13 weeks of the date on the prescription
  c.  The pharmacist must be assured of the genuineness of the signature before dispensing.
    Doctors have a general right to possess these drugs and to administer and prescribe them subject to:
  a.  The keeping of a register of prescriptions and stocks of these drugs (usually done for the doctor by the nurses or pharmacist in hospital or retail practice). Entries must be indelible and chronological. Alterations must be accompanied by an explanation.
  b.  The keeping of such drugs in a locked receptacle (not a locked car or case).
    Patients may possess such drugs only if prescribed. It is an offence to fail to disclose to a prescribing doctor that another doctor has already prescribed a controlled drug.

*Schedule 4*
Drugs liable to abuse which are not used in medicine, e.g. LSD, coca leaf, cannabis.

**Notification and Supply to Addicts Regulations (1973)**
1. Doctors are *obliged* to notify (within 7 days) to the Chief Medical Officer at the Home Office the name, sex, date of birth, address, date of attendance, and NHS number of any patient suspected of addiction to: cocaine, dextromoramide, diamorphine, dipipanone, hydrocodone, hydramorphone, levorphanol, methadone, morphine, opium, oxycodone, pethidine, phenazocine and piritramide.
2. Failure to notify is an offence and can result in withdrawl of the right to prescribe controlled drugs.
3. Except for treatment of organic disease and injury, doctors are not allowed to prescribe controlled drugs to addicts unless they have a licence from the Secretary of State to do so. Thus prescription to addicts is limited to doctors specialised in their management.

**Practical aspects of prescribing.**
1. Write legibly with particular care to specification of dose (watch the decimal points, avoid confusing mg and $\mu$g, etc).
2. Clearly indicate the drug.
3. Specify full name, address and age of patient.
4. Specify precisely the strength of mixtures, creams, tablets.
5. Give clear instructions as to dose frequency, duration of treatment, and/or total amount to be supplied.
   Give dosage > 1 gram as fractions of gram, e.g. 1.5 g.
                 < 1 gram as milligrams, e.g. 500 mg, not 0.5 g.
                 < 1 mg as micrograms, e.g. 100 micrograms not 0.1 mg.
   Where decimals are unavoidable, a zero should be written before the decimal point.
   Liquid medicines are usually prescribed in multiples of 10 doses of 10 ml, the adult dose, i.e. 50, 100, 150, 200, 300 or 500 ml.
   Topical liquid preparations:  — 500 ml suitable for whole body
                                          — 200 ml for limbs
                                          — 100 ml for small areas, e.g. face.
   Eye and ear drops usually ordered in volumes of 10 ml; inhalations and sprays as 25 ml; eye lotions, gargles and mouth washes as 200 ml.
   Creams and ointments usually determined by the size of manufacturer's pack. As guide, whole body requires 100–200 g; medium areas 25–50 g; and small areas 5–25 g.
6. Do not leave large spaces which allow alteration or addition to your prescription.
7. Sign and date the prescription. Add your name and address. A telephone number is also helpful.
8. If in doubt, look it up or ask.
9. Unless otherwise specified, the name of the drug will automatically be written on the label by the pharmacist.
   Best to use simple English words and arabic numerals in writing prescriptions. Some Latin abbreviations are commonly used (not advised) by some prescribers:

| | |
|---|---|
| a.c., ante cibum | before food |
| b.d., bis in die | twice a day (b.i.d. is also used) |
| o.d., omni die | every day |
| o.m., omni mane | every morning |
| o.n., omni nocte | every night |
| p.c., post cibum | after food |
| p.o., per os | by mouth |

| p.r.n., pro re nata | as required |
| q.d.s., quater in die | four times a day (q.i.d. also used) |
| q.s., quantum sufficiat | a sufficiency, enough |
| rep., repetatur | let it be repeated |
| s.o.s., si opus sit | if necessary. Confine s.o.s. to prescriptions to be repeated once only and to use p.r.n. where many repetitions are intended. |
| stat., statim | immediately |
| t.d.s., ter in die | three times a day (t.i.d. also used) |

## Compliance with therapy

If after accurate diagnosis and appropriate prescribing the patient fails to take the drug the whole exercise is futile. Patients who fail to take therapy are called *non-compliers.*

*Incidence*
Much greater than expected or realised.
Always suspect non-compliance if treatment fails.
20% patients in general practice may not take their prescription for dispensing.
33% patients are non-compliers.
33% patients are poor compliers.
  Many determinants of compliance described but impossible to identify such individuals accurately.
  Patients may comply with one regimen but not another.
  Non-compliance more likely when:
a. Patients are very young or very old or psychiatrically ill.
b. Treatment is chronic.
c. No obvious connection between treatment and subjectively perceived benefit.
d. Failure to understand nature or importance of illness, side effects, and/or treatment.
e. Complex treatment — too many drugs or too frequent administration.
  Non-compliance may reflect failure of doctor to identify main reason for patient's visit: many patients do not always expect a prescription.

*Diagnosis*
Difficult in clinical practice. Can be done by:
a. Relaxed and friendly doctor-patient relationship may allow patient to discuss compliance.
b. Comparison of amount of drug left with expected consumption.
c. Assessment of clinical effect.
d. Plasma, urine or salivary drug level monitoring.

*Treatment*
Few trials to investigate effects of these measures. Probably important are:
a. Clear instructions about treatment, disease, etc. Write it down for patient if necessary.
b. Simple drug regime: twice daily regime known to be better than three or four times a day; reduce number of separate drug prescriptions (use combination tablets if appropriate).
c. In certain cases, e.g. schizophrenia, intramuscular depot injections can be used.
d. Regular follow-up and evaluation of patient response.
   If a drug is necessary, then so is compliance, and it is worth spending to time to obtain it.